# MOSQUITO WARRIOR

# MOSQUITO WARRIOR

## Yellow Fever, Public Health, *and the* Forgotten Career of General William C. Gorgas

Carol R. Byerly

THE UNIVERSITY OF ALABAMA PRESS
*Tuscaloosa*

The University of Alabama Press
Tuscaloosa, Alabama 35487-0380
uapress.ua.edu



Typeface: Garamond Premier Pro

Cover image: A deadly *Aedes aegypti* mosquito at feast (iStock.com);
General William C. Gorgas, c. 1901 (National Library of Medicine)
Cover design: Lori Lynch

Cataloging-in-Publication data is available from the Library of Congress.
ISBN: 978-0-8173-2193-2 (cloth)
ISBN: 978-0-8173-6142-6 (paper)
E-ISBN: 978-0-8173-9496-7

To my mother, Mary Ries

# Contents

*List of Illustrations* ix
*Acknowledgments* xi
*Abbreviations* xv
*Introduction* 1

PART I: TO MATURITY, 1854–1898

**1.** A Young Witness to War and Defeat 15
**2.** The Making of an Army Medical Officer 33
**3.** Love in the Time of Yellow Fever 48

PART II: NEW PURPOSE, 1898–1904

**4.** Trial by War and Disease, 1898 65
**5.** The Terror of Yellow Jack in Havana 81
**6.** War against Mosquitoes Begins 94
**7.** Will Panama Be Safe Enough to Build a Canal? 112

PART III: NATIONAL TO INTERNATIONAL RENOWN, 1904–1914

**8.** Dark Days at Home and in Panama 129
**9.** Halcyon Days for Panama Public Health 147
**10.** Fighting Mosquitoes and George Goethals 164
**11.** Making the Tropics "Safe for the White Man" 182
**12.** Fighting Mosquitoes Abroad 195

PART IV: TO FIGHT WAR AND DISEASE, 1914–1918

**13.** Public Health and the Bully Pulpit of the Army Surgeon General 211
**14.** Duty to Country vs. Mission for Humanity 225
**15.** Mobilizing the Nation for War 240

**16.** Doctors vs. Officers: Challenging the Army Hierarchy in the Name of Medicine 256

PART V: THE FINAL CAMPAIGNS, 1918–1920

**17.** General Gorgas Is "Retired for Age" 275

**18.** Fighting Disease to the Last 290

**Epilogue:** Remembering William C. Gorgas, 1920–2020 305

*Notes* 317

*Select Bibliography* 383

*Index* 389

# Illustrations

FIGURES

FIGURE I.1. *Conquerors of Yellow Fever*, 1939, painting by Dean Cornwell 6

FIGURE I.2. Female *Aedes aegypti* mosquito after a blood meal 8

FIGURE I.3. Life cycle of the *Aedes aegypti* mosquito 9

FIGURE 1.1. General Josiah Gorgas, c. 1863 17

FIGURE 1.2. Young William Crawford Gorgas, c. 1856 18

FIGURE 1.3. Willie Gorgas at Sewanee 31

FIGURE 2.1 "Shall We Let Him In?" *Frank Leslie's Illustrated Newspaper*, September 21, 1878 40

FIGURE 3.1. Marie and Aileen, c. 1891 58

FIGURE 3.2 Captain William C. Gorgas, 1893 59

FIGURE 4.1. USS *Relief* (hospital ship) 70

FIGURE 4.2. Yellow fever patient in hospital at Siboney, Cuba, July 1898 73

FIGURE 5.1. "Yellow Fever Cases, 1900," from William C. Gorgas's journal 82

FIGURE 6.1. Members of the US Army's yellow fever commission 97

FIGURE 6.2. R. Lillo sketch of Carlos J. Finlay and the Reed Commission 100

FIGURE 6.3. Yellow fever patient screened to prevent transmission of disease by mosquitoes 105

FIGURE 7.1. William C. Gorgas, n.d. 115

FIGURE 8.1. Plates from Halsted's "The Results of Operations for the Cure of Cancer of the Breast" 135

FIGURE 8.2. "The First Mountain to Be Removed," cartoon, *Harper's Weekly*, July 22, 1905 145

FIGURE 8.3. "A Deadlock Canal," *Piqua Daily Call*, Piqua, Ohio, July 5, 1905 146

FIGURE 9.1. Covering water sources to prevent mosquito propagation 149

FIGURE 9.2. Plates of water to prevent ant infestations 149

FIGURE 9.3. Fumigation brigades against yellow fever mosquitoes in Panama, 1905 150

FIGURE 9.4. Street in Colón before and after American sanitation efforts 152

FIGURE 9.5. Ancón Hospital medical staff, 1906 156

FIGURE 10.1. Section view of the American scheme for a lock canal 166

FIGURE 10.2. The life cycle of the malaria parasite 169

FIGURE 10.3. Female *Anopheles*, the malaria mosquito 170

FIGURE 10.4. Mowed lawns and screened housing were preventive measures against malaria 172

FIGURE 10.5. Department of Sanitation worker sprays larvicide to control mosquitoes 173

FIGURE 10.6. Chart showing the reduction of malaria cases in Panama from 1905 to 1913 175

FIGURE 10.7. Cartoon by William Gorgas 176

FIGURE 11.1. The Isthmian Canal Commission, 1909–1914 183

FIGURE 12.1. Portrait of Amelia Gorgas, 1890 200

FIGURE 13.1. Major General William C. Gorgas, Surgeon General of the Army 214

FIGURE 13.2. Marie Gorgas featured in *Ladies' Home Journal* 223

FIGURE 14.1. Rockefeller Foundation Yellow Fever Commission 233

FIGURE 15.1. General Medical Board of the Council of National Defense 251

FIGURE 16.1. Major General W. C. Gorgas, Surgeon General of the Army 269

FIGURE 18.1. Marie and William Gorgas in May 1920 298

FIGURE E.1. Stained-glass window in All Saint's Chapel at the University of the South 307

FIGURE E.2. Gorgas the Medical Hero in a Squibb Pharmaceuticals advertisement 308

FIGURE E.3. Marie D. Gorgas 311

FIGURE E.4. William C. Gorgas, portrait in oil by Alexander R. James 312

## MAPS

MAP 2.1. William Gorgas's United States 43

MAP 12.1. William Gorgas's overseas travels 196

# Acknowledgments

THIS BOOK IS THE PRODUCT of more than twenty years of work in the history of disease, military medicine, and American political history. I first encountered William Gorgas in the 1990s during my research on the influenza pandemic of 1918. My subsequent investigations into the US Army's management of tuberculosis, and the medical problems encountered in the construction of the Panama Canal, took me deeper into his life's work. The more I learned about this extraordinary medical officer and the more sources I found, including his journals and extensive correspondence with family and friends, the more surprised I was that no one had written a scholarly biography of him since the 1950s. So I determined to write one.

I have many people to thank for their help in negotiating such a rich and varied historical record. My early research was supported financially by John T. Greenwood and Col. William T. (Tom) Gray, ret., of the Office of Medical History of the Office of the Army Surgeon General, which enabled me to develop a broad outline of Gorgas's life. I have also relied on the expertise of many archivists and librarians. Mitchell Yockelson and other archivists at the National Archives I and II in the Washington, DC, area helped me explore the thousands of cubic feet of government records; archivists at the Library of Congress, the National Library of Medicine in Bethesda, Maryland, and the Rockefeller Archive Center in New York guided me to materials on Gorgas and on yellow fever. I would especially like to express my gratitude to the staff of the libraries of the University of Alabama and the University of Virginia for digitizing their extensive collections on the Gorgas family and the US Army's yellow fever work in Cuba respectively. This enabled me to conduct detailed research from my home office and to continue my work during the COVID-19 pandemic lockdown.

When I first visited the Gorgas Papers at the University of Alabama Library in Tuscaloosa in the late 1990s, I had no idea that I would be writing William

Gorgas's life story or that the University of Alabama Press would bring it to light. I heartily thank my editor there, Claire Lewis Evans, for her wisdom and enthusiastic support of this biography, as well as project director Jon Berry and copy editor Lisa Williams. Alex Boucher of the University of Alabama Library Special Collections, and Melissa Meyer, cartographer at the University of Alabama have also been most helpful.

Over the years, I've been able to visit important places in Gorgas's life with friends and family, and this has greatly enriched this project for me. Alma Moore accompanied me to Charleston, South Carolina, where as a boy Gorgas heard the first shots of the Civil War. Lee Panetta traveled with me to Brownsville, Texas, to see where Gorgas nearly died of yellow fever and met the love of his life, Marie. My sister Kathy Brandenburg accompanied me to Cuba, where we visited several sites of Gorgas's trials and triumphs. My late husband, Radford Byerly, and son Charles Byerly sailed with me through the Panama Canal and walked with me through the streets of old Panama City. Alice Goodman flew with me to London to see where Marie and William spent the final days of his life and to follow the path of his funeral procession to St. Paul's Cathedral.

Other friends and colleagues took time out of their own busy lives to read all or part of my work and have made it immeasurably better. My appreciation goes to Tina Gianquitto, Mary Griffin, Anne Meyering, Hannah Nordhaus, Nancy Vavra, and Peter Wood for their thoughtful comments and suggestions. I am also indebted to Dale Smith and Deanne Stephens Nuwer for their close reading of the manuscript and suggestions that have greatly improved it. Anne Davidson, Elizabeth Fenn, Julie Greene, Deb Grojean, Susan Kent, Christine Loromer, Jean Nordhaus, Peter Smith, and the members of my book group in Boulder have all listened to my Gorgas stories and supported my work in myriad ways. Thanks as well to Enrique Chaves-Carballo for providing me with Gorgas's Yellow Fever Log from Cuba. My able research assistants Megan Pielke, Mary Griffin, and Kate Foster helped me negotiate Gorgas's voluminous papers and records, and I give special thanks to Dr. Elene Mooney, OB-GYN, who deepened my understanding of the nature and significance of Marie's breast cancer treatment as well as Gorgas's approach to his work as a military officer and physician. I am also grateful to the members of the Boulder County Mosquito Control District board for their assistance, especially entomologist Melissa Kyer who helped me with the mosquito figures.

My extended family of Byerlys, Rieses, Brandenburgs, and Neuhausers offered me their continued support over the years, especially my mother, Mary Ries, who listened to my first full-length presentation on Gorgas's life, and who, along with my late father, Stanley Ries, has followed my love of history since I was sixteen years old. And finally, my love and appreciation to Lee Panetta for entering my life when this project was well under way and sharing the long months of COVID isolation. Thank you for listening to my multitude of Gorgas stories and writing problems, encouraging my work, and embracing the tradition of celebrating every incremental step toward publication.

# Abbreviations

| | |
|---|---|
| AEF | American Expeditionary Forces |
| AGG | Amelia Gayle Gorgas |
| AMA | American Medical Association |
| GPO | Government Printing Office |
| ICC | Isthmian Canal Commission |
| IHB | International Health Board, Rockefeller Foundation |
| *JAMA* | *Journal of the American Medical Association* |
| JGFP | Josiah Gorgas Family Papers, University of Alabama Libraries Special Collections |
| JJG | Josiah Gorgas |
| LoC | Library of Congress |
| *MDWW* | *Medical Department in the World War* |
| MG | Marie Doughty Gorgas |
| NARA | National Archives and Records Administration |
| NLM | National Library of Medicine |
| *NYT* | *New York Times* |
| OTSG | Office of the Surgeon General |
| *PHR* | *Public Health Reports* |
| PHS | Public Health Service |
| RHG | Richard Haynsworth Gorgas |
| RG | Record Group of the National Archives and Records Administration |
| WCG | William Crawford Gorgas |
| WCGP | William C. Gorgas Papers, University of Alabama Libraries Special Collections |
| *WDAR* | *War Department Annual Report* |

# MOSQUITO WARRIOR

# Introduction

William and Marie Gorgas arrived in style in London on May 29, 1920, on their way to yet another yellow fever expedition. They stayed in the posh Savoy Hotel on the Strand near Covent Gardens, where Gorgas had been feted in 1914 by the British Royal Medical Society. As chairman of the Rockefeller Foundation Yellow Fever Commission, he was traveling to West Africa to advise public health officials on the dreaded disease, stopping in London to consult with colleagues and friends on the way. The visit was to be a celebration. Among other events, Gorgas was scheduled to be decorated by King George V for his tropical disease work and his leadership of the US Army Medical Department during World War I. On May 30, however, in the middle of the night, he woke his wife to say that he had experienced a "slight paralytic stroke," and was rushed to the Queen Alexandra Military Hospital as a guest of the government.[1] When it was clear he was too disabled to go to Buckingham Palace for the knighting ceremony, George V visited Gorgas's hospital room on June 8 to bestow on him the Most Distinguished Order of St Michael and St George. While Marie was hopeful that William would recover, he suffered additional strokes and died on July 3, 1920. King George again honored Gorgas with a funeral ceremony at St. Paul's Cathedral usually reserved for general officers of the British Army.

An Englishwoman, May Thomas, sat by herself in the cathedral during the service and wrote a poem of sorrow. She sent it to Marie, explaining that the moment brought back "my own dark days of crushing grief and my heart flew out in sympathy to you and your irreparable loss."[2] The year before, Thomas had met William Gorgas in Panama just days after losing her young son to yellow fever. He had been so comforting to her that she now offered a poem of sorrow to his widow. Hers was one of dozens of condolences and tributes Marie received before she sailed back to the United States with her husband's coffin. Upon their return to Washington, Gorgas's casket lay in repose at the Church of the Epiphany before his funeral and burial with high military honors in Arlington Cemetery.

William Crawford Gorgas had lived a rich and exciting life of love and loss, adventure and achievement. At the time of his death in 1920, Gorgas was one of the most well-known physicians in the English-speaking world, but a century later few Americans recognize his name. Born in 1854, his life was shaped by three wars—the Civil War, the Spanish-American-Cuban War, and World War I. As an army medical officer, he participated in the transformation of medicine from a practice based on centuries-old humoral theory to one grounded in scientific germ theory and carried the messages of modern sanitation and public health to regions around the world. Gorgas witnessed the modernization of the nation's military from a network of dusty frontier outposts to a centralized, professional organization serving one of the most powerful armed forces in the world. He practiced medicine and science with some of the giants of the "golden age" of medicine, including his army colleague Dr. Walter Reed, and Johns Hopkins greats Dr. William Henry Welch and Dr. William Osler, and he worked alongside some of the most influential leaders of the century—Theodore Roosevelt, William Howard Taft, and Secretary of War Elihu Root—who helped elevate the United States to a position of international power and influence in the early twentieth century.

Gorgas is best known for his yellow fever work. In fact, it was a continuous thread in his life. His parents met during a yellow fever epidemic in Alabama, and a close medical school friend died in the epidemic of 1878. He met his wife, Marie, during another outbreak epidemic in Texas and soon became one of the army's experts on yellow fever in the 1880s and 1890s. Two crumbling leather notebooks in which he recorded the hundreds of yellow fever cases he treated in Havana during 1899 and 1900 after the Spanish-American-Cuban War testify to the suffering and death he witnessed from the disease. In 1901, however, he helped prove the US Army yellow fever commission's discovery that the *Aedes aegypti* mosquito transmitted yellow fever by clearing Havana of mosquitoes, and to the surprise of most, banishing the deadly disease from that city. Gorgas then took that knowledge and expertise to Panama to make it safe enough for American and West Indian workers to construct the most ambitious engineering project the world had ever seen. In recognition of Gorgas's accomplishments, President Woodrow Wilson appointed him army surgeon general in 1914, just months before the outbreak of World War I (1914–1918), and over the next four years Gorgas presided over the greatest expansion of the army medical service in US history. He continued to fight yellow fever throughout his career and, after retiring from the Army Medical Corps, died on his way to investigate the disease in West Africa.

Gorgas was not a saint or a man to emulate in all things. He was a white supremacist, born into a patriarchal family that held people in slavery, and he mourned the Lost Cause of the Confederacy. A leader in controlling tropical diseases, Gorgas did his work to a large degree in the interest of advancing white American imperialism and dominance overseas; his most famous speech was entitled, "The Conquest of the Tropics for the White Race."[3] Yet as a physician he cared for all kinds of people. His patients included white soldiers and Lakota Indians in the Dakotas; American engineers and West Indian canal workers in Panama; residents of the pestilent cities of Guayaquil, Ecuador and Lima, Peru; and Black miners in South Africa and Rhodesia. Gorgas's views on race, class, and nation were more nuanced than those of many of his contemporaries. He was a son of Alabama but married a northerner and chose New York City as his home. He wore the blue uniform of the US Army but pinned on his chest the Confederate Cross given to him by his mother. A lifelong Democrat, he nevertheless admired Republican Theodore Roosevelt, supported populist William Jennings Bryan, and espoused the views of Henry George, the popular reformer who advocated taxing the rich to improve living and working conditions for laborers. As the army surgeon general, Gorgas maintained the white, male character of the Medical Corps and helped to perpetuate a profoundly segregated society, yet he was also responsible for the health of the four million soldiers of all backgrounds during World War I and understood that good public health, like disease, does not follow the color line. Clean water and air, vaccines, safe food, and good hospitals can, if properly deployed, benefit everyone. And finally, while Gorgas prided himself on being a responsible physician and officer, devoted to his duty and his country, at times his zeal for fighting disease and mosquitoes caused him to neglect these obligations.

William Gorgas thus forged his own path across the landscape of region and race, war and disease, and lived purposefully, seizing every opportunity to carry new public health measures and education to populations in the United States and abroad. In this work he faced skeptical government officials and hostile business leaders as well as naive and beleaguered publics who did not always understand why they should do what he said to do. His immunity to yellow fever and his unshakable commitment to preventive medicine and sanitation enabled him, however, to calmly take on adversity and controversy and to make himself, as he liked to say, "useful." Gorgas knew that we take public health for granted at our peril.

I first encountered Gorgas doing research for a book on the influenza epidemic during World War I when as the US Army surgeon general he led the effort to control infectious diseases in the army's ranks. I was amazed by the amount of material available on this man: Gorgas's personal papers in the Library of Congress number twelve thousand documents; the University of Alabama Libraries Special Collections houses eight thousand documents; the National Archives contain thousands of records from his career as an army medical officer, 1880–1913, and as army surgeon general, 1914–1918; and the University of Virginia holds an extensive archive on the army yellow fever commission experiments of 1900–1902. Those records have informed this project. As a girl I had learned about William Gorgas and Walter Reed as "medical heroes" by reading Landmark Biographies, but despite the wealth of material, there are only two "standard" biographies: one by his wife, Marie, and journalist Burton J. Hendrick, *William Crawford Gorgas, His Life and Works* (1924), and the other, *Physician to the World: The Life of General William C. Gorgas* (1950), by John M. Gibson, which draws heavily on Marie's work.[4] In the absence of other biographies, the latter was republished in 1989 and again in 2012 without updating, so that one reviewer cautioned that readers might be put off by "racial and ethnic stereotypes found in this book, which seem to come as much from Gibson as from Gorgas."[5]

Public health policy is most successful, ironically, when it remains in the background of society, when we do not need to live in fear of deadly pathogens or worry about clean water and air or the safety of our food and medicines. As we struggle anew with infectious disease in the twenty-first century, Gorgas's life illustrates the challenges and rewards of building robust public health systems. It also shows that science alone cannot conquer disease. Harnessing scientific knowledge to benefit society requires political and diplomatic skill, because successful public health programs require public support for strong, well-funded sanitation systems, municipal codes, hospitals, medical personnel, vaccines, and disease surveillance. Gorgas became a leader in educating the public and government officials about the importance and usefulness of good sanitation so they could appreciate the benefits to themselves and their communities. A pioneer in the field, William Gorgas helped to marry emerging knowledge about the causes of infectious disease to institutions and instruments of control.

## SHAPING MEMORY AND HISTORY

Why, then, is there so little scholarship on William Gorgas? The answer involves the way individuals can shape memory and history, and, in this case, one man, Jefferson Randolph Kean, did much to efface Gorgas's memory. The story begins in 1902 after the army yellow fever commission headed by Walter Reed proved the long-held theory of Cuban physician Carlos Juan Finlay that the *Aedes aegypti* mosquito transmitted yellow fever. Reed and his colleagues bacteriologists James Carroll and Jesse Lazear, and Cuban pathologist Aristides Agramonte, conducted a series of experiments that confirmed the theory. Gorgas then proved it on a grand scale by eliminating mosquitoes from the city and freeing Havana of yellow fever in just ninety days; June 1901, was the first month in 150 years during which Havana had no recorded cases of yellow fever.

In the flush of this success, the secretary of war recommended to Congress that it recognize Reed and Gorgas, both army majors, by promoting Reed to full colonel and Gorgas to lieutenant colonel ahead of the regular order of advancement in the Medical Corps. But before the promotions could be formalized, Walter Reed died of appendicitis and peritonitis in an army hospital, in November 1902 at the age of fifty-one. With Reed's unexpected death, the surgeon general decided to promote Gorgas to the full colonelcy intended for his colleague. Congress agreed and jumped him ahead of some thirty other medical officers. The ensuing resentment and jealousy toward Gorgas persisted for decades and helps to explain why his legacy became eclipsed.

This is where Kean comes in. He made what he believed to be a deathbed promise to Walter Reed to watch over his widow and children and devoted himself to memorializing and advancing Reed's name. Kean's first and most appropriate accomplishment was to encourage Congress in 1909 to name the army's new hospital in Washington, DC, after his colleague, making the name Walter Reed synonymous with military medicine throughout the twentieth century. But Kean, the great-grandson of Thomas Jefferson, was a troubled man, and despite his career in the Army Medical Department in various administrative capacities, never held the top post himself. He felt that he never received proper recognition or reward for his work and detailed such grievances in his unpublished autobiography.[6] Kean did prevail in one way, however—by outliving almost everyone else involved in the Reed Commission experiments—and was thus able to shape the memory of those events and accomplishments until his death in 1950.

For example, Kean used his position in the Office of the Surgeon General to assist Congress in publishing detailed reports on the Reed Commission work in Cuba, and the resulting documents emphasized the role of American scientists and volunteers in the yellow fever experiments, diminishing that of Cuban scientists and Spanish volunteers. In 1928 Congress approved legislation to recognize the Reed Commission's work with a "Roll of Honor" awarding twenty-two men or their survivors a Congressional Gold Medal and a monthly pension of $150 for the rest of their lives.[7] Although Walter Reed recognized three Spanish volunteers in his seminal paper "The Etiology of Yellow Fever," Kean and the Congress omitted them from the honors.[8] The Roll of Honor also excluded the participants in the subsequent vaccine experiments—Gorgas, Cuban scientist Juan Guiteras, and the volunteer participants—because the experiments failed.[9] Such framing of the events in Cuba of 1900–1901 had consequences. This "Roll of Honor," with detailed reports, extensive documentation, and the imprimatur of Congress, became a primary historical document on the Reed Commission and effectively erased these participants.[10] By shepherding a comprehensive and "official" body of documentation of work in Cuba in 1900–1901, Kean gained control of the yellow fever story.[11]

One of Kean's most powerful accomplishments was to keep Gorgas out of a painting. In 1939 the pharmaceutical company Wyeth-Ayerst commissioned artist Dean Cornwell to do a series of paintings on "Pioneers of American Medicine." One of the first was *Conquerors of Yellow Fever*, portraying the work of the Reed Commission. It was an allegorical depiction of biologist Jesse Lazear inoculating

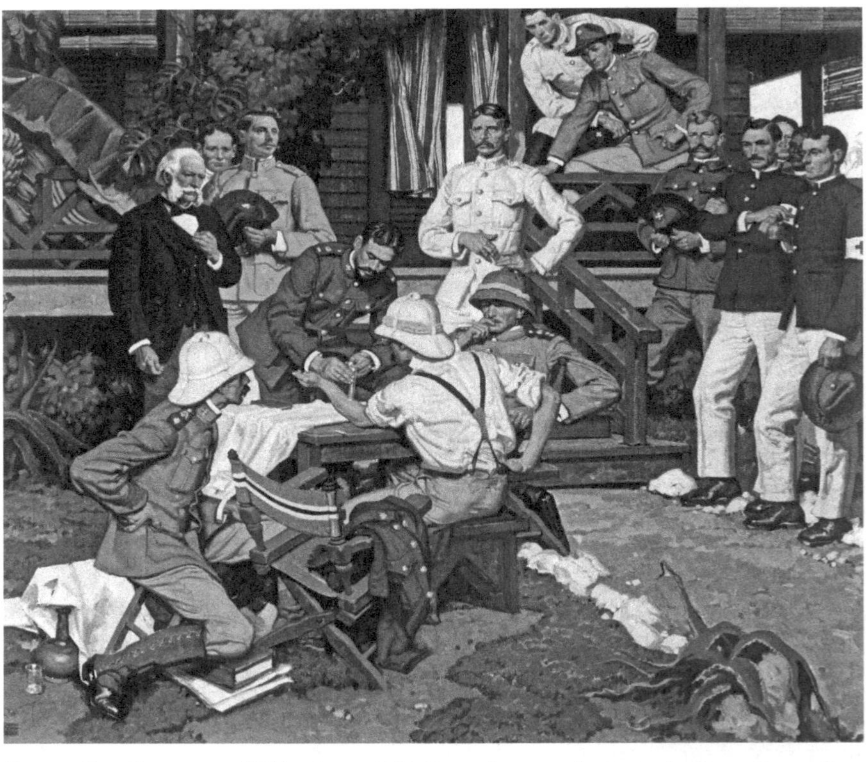

FIGURE I.1. *Conquerors of Yellow Fever*, 1939. Reproduction of painting by Dean Cornwell showing yellow fever experiments in which Dr. Jesse W. Lazear inoculated Dr. James Carroll with an infected mosquito at a US Army hospital, Havana, Cuba, in 1900. Gorgas is not in this portrayal. National Library of Medicine.

James Carroll with an infected mosquito, thereby inducing the first experimental case of yellow fever. It was allegorical because it had little to do with reality. The actual event took place in a laboratory on August 27, 1900, when Carroll and Lazear decided to give a female mosquito a blood meal on Carroll's arm to keep her alive. The artist, however, advised by Kean, set the event outside and populated it with fourteen men—including Kean—and featured Walter Reed, who was not even in Cuba at the time of the actual event. Gorgas is absent, because, Kean explained, "on the date celebrated in Cornwell's painting Gorgas was not a believer in the mosquito theory."[12] This is unfair and illogical, because at the moment of Carroll's infection, no one, not even Reed, believed Carlos Finlay's assertion that mosquitoes were to blame. They were doing the experiment to test that theory. But this painting has become iconic of the Cuban experiments. When Philip Hench, Nobel laureate of medicine and amateur scholar of the Reed experiments, unveiled the painting in 1941, he touted its historical accuracy, declaring that the public, "especially school children, may learn to know this painting and the men it memorializes and may perhaps come to regard it as the standard visual representation of the subject for years to come."[13] The Cornwell painting hung in the Walter Reed Army Hospital for years, and reproductions of it accompany many of the publications and websites about the eradication of yellow fever. A recent military textbook on preventive medicine includes the Cornwell painting and even identifies the figures in it as if it were an accurate depiction of events.[14]

The history of medicine has long favored scientific discovery such as the Reed Commission's over more pedestrian public health and sanitation work such as Gorgas's, but even the Arlington National Cemetery's website neglects Gorgas. It has a category "Medical Figures," which notes the gravesites of Walter Reed and Surgeon General George Sternberg, but more than one hundred years after his death, as of 2023, Gorgas's name is not on the roster.[15] It is therefore little wonder that few people have heard of the army doctor William C. Gorgas. His life story, however, should not be eclipsed, because it provides a lens to examine the most dramatic changes in the United States from 1860 to 1920: three wars that shaped the nation; industrialization and the modernization of the military and medicine; the transformation of the United States from a backwater slave state to a world economic and military power; and the changing fault lines of race, class, ethnicity, and gender in the country, the military, and the world. As he found himself at the fulcrum of history several times in his life, Gorgas was also a lucky man, born to well-educated and loving parents, with generous physical and mental gifts. The first to carry the mosquito theory of yellow fever transmission to many countries overseas, he was able to achieve seemingly miraculous eradication of a deadly scourge. But if Gorgas was lucky, he was also well equipped to seize these moments and bend them to the service of his country and its people.

But before we begin to explore this extraordinary life, it is time to introduce the most powerful and frightening characters in the story, yellow fever and its ally, the mosquito.

## YELLOW FEVER AND MOSQUITOES

Yellow fever is intimidating. Although outbreaks were infrequent, its high mortality rate and symptoms of high fever, delirium, and "black vomit" are terrifying.[16] The disease is caused by an RNA *Flavivirus* related to the West Nile virus and spread by the bites of infected female *Aedes aegypti* mosquitoes.[17] Mosquitoes drink nectar for sustenance, but females require a blood meal for reproduction. Only they, therefore, are the transmitters of disease. Most people bitten by an infected mosquito may not even know they are sick or experience only a mild illness, but for those who do get sick, symptoms begin three to six days after the bite. The initial symptoms include the sudden onset of fever, chills, severe headache, back pain, general body aches, fatigue, weakness, and nausea. Most people improve after the initial phase, but in roughly 15 percent of cases, after a remission of a day or two, a more severe form of the disease comes on, characterized by high fever, jaundice

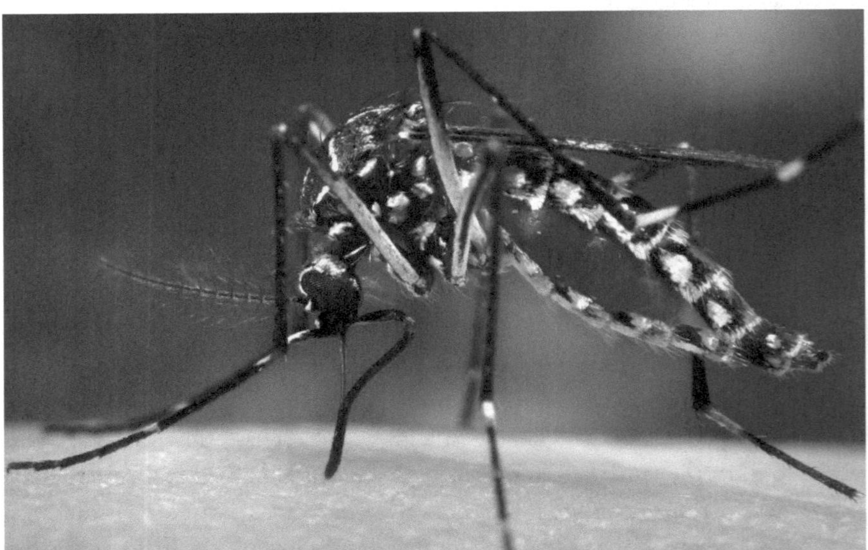

FIGURE I.2. Female *Aedes aegypti* mosquito after a blood meal. Public Health Image Library, Centers for Disease Control.

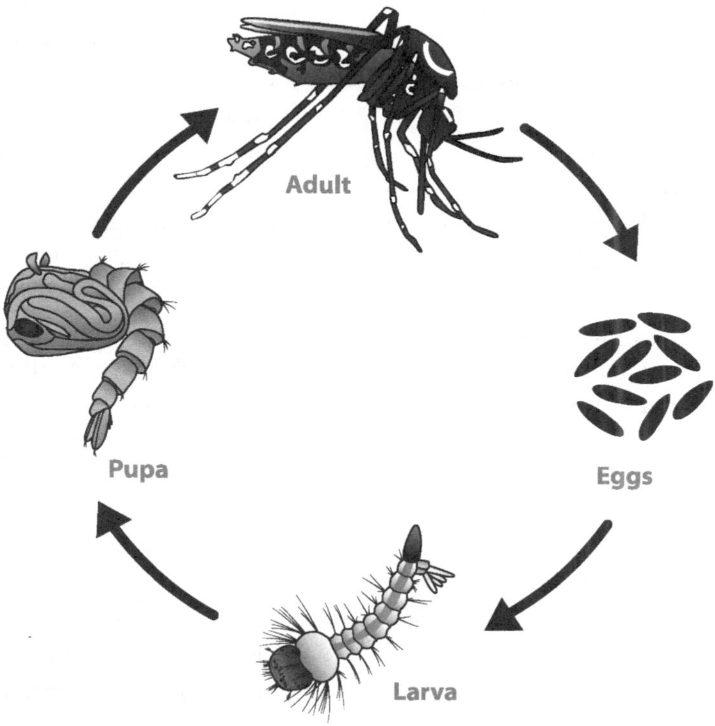


FIGURE I.3. Life cycle of the *Aedes aegypti* mosquito. The *Aedes* mosquitoes have four life stages: egg, larva, pupa, and adult, and the entire life cycle, from an egg to an adult, takes approximately eight to ten days. Centers for Disease Control.

(hence the name yellow fever), and, if the virus attacks the internal organs, hemorrhaging into the stomach and intestinal tract, causing the horrifying "black vomit," followed by shock, organ failure, and death.[18] Mortality rates in severe cases range from 30 percent to 60 percent, and death typically occurs between the seventh and tenth day of the illness.[19] People who survive yellow fever fortunately have lifetime immunity to the disease, but severe cases of the disease can damage the liver and the kidneys and weaken survivors for months or years. Today yellow fever can be prevented by a vaccine, but there are still no effective treatments other than managing the symptoms with rest, fluids, and pain relievers.

The origin of yellow fever is murky, but the most widely held theory is that it first emerged in Africa and came to the Western Hemisphere in the seventeenth century on ships bringing captives from that continent to the New World to work in the colonial sugar cane fields. The mosquitoes traveling on the slave ships could produce several generations that carried the disease. Adult mosquitoes could survive on sugar water, but females needing a blood meal to breed would feed on the humans on board and lay their eggs in the ship's water casks. Larvae then hatched, and the mature mosquitoes could repeat the cycle, transmitting the yellow fever virus from sick people to the nonimmune, contributing to the appalling mortality rates aboard the ships. As historians John Pierce and James Writer have so succinctly put it, "yellow fever was born of the meeting of slavery and sugar."[20]

The first recorded outbreak of yellow fever in the Western Hemisphere was in the Yucatán of Mexico in 1648, and the first confirmed outbreak in North America was in Boston in 1693.[21] The disease never gained a foothold to become endemic (year-round) in the United States because of the temperate climate. Mosquitoes are most active between 70 and 90 degrees Fahrenheit, will not feed below 60 degrees, become inert below 50, and die with freezing temperatures. They would arrive, however, in US ports during the summer and wreak havoc. Yellow fever has historically been confined to Africa and South America and is not found in Asia despite the fact that *Aedes aegypti* mosquitoes are common on that continent. One theory for the absence of yellow fever in Asia is that the prevalence of Japanese encephalitis and dengue fever viruses in the mosquitoes blocks the opportunity for the yellow fever virus to occupy the same niche in those populations.[22]

In tropical regions where yellow fever was endemic, the disease was rare among adults because the vast majority had immunity from surviving a childhood infection. Outbreaks occurred only when "nonimmunes" arrived in an area—such as when the Americans came as an occupying army to Cuba or to construct a canal in Panama. Yellow fever could ruin local economies. At the first word of yellow fever in a town, other cities and towns imposed quarantines against that location, halting travel and commerce for months and devastating cities and ports. For more than two hundred years, epidemics struck occasionally in port cities along the Gulf of Mexico and the East Coast. In 1699 Philadelphia and Charleston lost about 7 percent of their residents to yellow fever; in 1702 New York City lost 10 percent; and in 1793 yellow fever struck Philadelphia, then serving as the capital of the new nation, killing five thousand people, or 10 percent of its population. The city endured subsequent attacks in 1797, 1798, and 1799, undermining Philadelphia's chance to be the nation's capital. The worst yellow fever epidemic in American history began in New Orleans in 1878, moving up the Mississippi River, causing more than 100,000 cases and killing some 20,000. As a veteran of a dozen yellow fever epidemics, Gorgas observed the chaos that could ensue: "When this disease was announced in a town, everybody left who could." Yellow fever victims were treated like lepers and were "frequently left without care," he wrote. Businesses were "entirely paralyzed, the quarantines not allowing any communication between the affected districts and those not affected," and often, he added, "a great deal of cruelty and cowardice was shown."[23]

---

While Gorgas never served in combat, he fought on the front lines of yellow fever epidemics that threatened to halt the American enterprise. As a young lieutenant at a Texas fort, he survived a severe bout with yellow fever and met Marie Doughty, the woman who would become his wife. She survived yellow fever as well, and this lifetime immunity enabled them to go where others could not—into the deadly yellow fever epidemics and to regions where yellow fever mosquitoes terrorized the vulnerable. Dr. Gorgas would care for thousands of yellow fever patients during his career and see hundreds die. To yellow fever, Jefferson Kean observed, Gorgas "owed wife, opportunity, fame and great place, and the personal immunity which enabled him to walk without fear in the shadow of death."[24] Once he learned how to "conquer" yellow fever, Gorgas wanted to do so all over the world, and his methods of prevention rather than treatment, and mosquito eradication conducted with military thoroughness and discipline, would become a model for disease control in the twentieth century.[25] William Gorgas reveled in being a physician, an army officer, a public health official, and a mosquito warrior.

PART I

# TO MATURITY, 1854–1898

# CHAPTER 1

# A Young Witness to War and Defeat

Mother, isn't it solemn?

—William Gorgas, age six, April 12, 1861, Battle of Fort Sumter

WILLIAM GORGAS LIVED HIS WHOLE life in military worlds, but he was not a militant man. He was born to well-educated parents who provided both privilege and comfort, and as a small boy moved with them to army posts in Alabama, Maine, South Carolina, and Virginia. Their world embraced patriotism, prized the military, and adhered to a society based on enslaved labor. The Civil War, however, was the defining experience of his childhood. As a boy of six, Willie heard the first shots of the Civil War at Fort Sumter with his mother, and four years later he watched a battle at Appomattox Bridge with his father. He experienced the fall of Richmond as a boy of ten and would never forget it. His father was Josiah Gorgas, the Confederate ordnance officer responsible for arming the rebel army. His mother, Amelia (née Gayle) Gorgas, was the daughter of a former Alabama governor who nursed the Confederate wounded. But the defeat of the South swept their life away, and for the next ten years the family faced economic hardship and political and social insecurity. Josiah lost his profession, and Amelia her home, and their children faced uncertain futures as the family moved to four different towns across the South trying to rebuild. If Confederate Richmond was the crucible of William Gorgas's boyhood, the Reconstruction South was the stage upon which he came of age.

## JOSIAH AND AMELIA

William's parents were a union of the North and the South and a love match. The family name had deep roots in Spain, but the family was Pennsylvania Dutch. Josiah Gorgas was born in Pennsylvania in July 1818, the youngest of ten children.[1]

His parents were farmers who struggled to feed the family, but Josiah, determined to get a college education, won an appointment to the military academy at West Point. He graduated sixth in his class in 1841, choosing ordnance—the supply and storage of weapons and ammunition—as the branch of the military he wished to pursue. He showed such promise that the army sent him abroad in 1845 to study with the imperial armies of Europe. Traveling the continent, Josiah returned home with stories that would inspire his children to see the world.

Yellow fever entered the Gorgas family story in 1847 during the war in Mexico when Josiah joined Gen. Winfield Scott's expedition to Vera Cruz and encountered not only enemy soldiers but deadly disease. As yellow fever ravaged the US troops, Josiah suffered a mild case, which he survived, thereby gaining lifelong immunity. His next encounter with yellow fever came six years later when he met Amelia Ross Gayle. Josiah was thirty-five years old, a tall, vital man with black hair, sharp eyes, military bearing, and full beard. Amelia, twenty-seven, was the third of six children of the prominent Alabama jurist, former governor, US congressman, and owner of enslaved people John Gayle.[2] Amelia had a cossetted childhood, but her mother, Sarah Gayle, died in 1835 when Amelia was only nine years old. John Gayle remarried, but his second wife, Clarissa, had such poor health that when he was elected to Congress in 1846, twenty-year-old Amelia went to Washington with him to assume the family's social duties. There she moved in the highest political circles, living in the same boardinghouse as John C. Calhoun (D-SC), a leader of the antebellum South and an advocate for slavery and states' rights. Amelia was sympathetic, her family belonging to the fewer than 5 percent of Alabamians who held people in slavery, and her father supported the horrific system in his state and country as a lawyer, governor, congressman, and judge. Walking with Calhoun on the Capitol grounds and watching the Senate debates, Amelia learned about power and politics and developed social skills and political fervor that she would pass on to her oldest son.[3]

No photographs of Amelia in her youth remain, but Marie Gorgas later described her as "slight in frame, graceful and quiet, a slender dancer, a spirited horsewoman, yet she had a commanding presence—the kind that instinctively though unobtrusively becomes the center of things on entering a room."[4] Contemporaries remarked on her sympathy and ability to connect with people, characteristics that would be influential forces in William Gorgas's life. After her death in 1913, he told his sister Mamie that their mother, "more than any one I ever knew acted upon the believe [*sic*] that 'love is the principle of existence and its only end.' She felt sympathy for everyone with whom she came in contact and roused the same feeling in them."[5]

A yellow fever epidemic in 1853 brought Josiah and Amelia together. That year Amelia's sister Sarah, and her husband, William Bones Crawford, a prominent South Carolina physician, traveled to Europe in search of a cure for his tuberculosis, leaving their children with Amelia in Mobile. When yellow fever broke out in the city in July, she and the children escaped to the Mount Vernon Arsenal, where her brother Matthew Gayle was an army surgeon. Josiah Gorgas had volunteered to command the arsenal during the epidemic because of his immunity to yellow fever and moved into the officers' barracks next to the house where Amelia was staying with her family. In the heat of the day, Amelia would read to her nieces and nephews on the porch, and Josiah, enchanted by those afternoon sessions, asked for an introduction to the owner of the voice. The family story was that he fell in love with Amelia's voice before he met her in person. After a whirlwind romance,

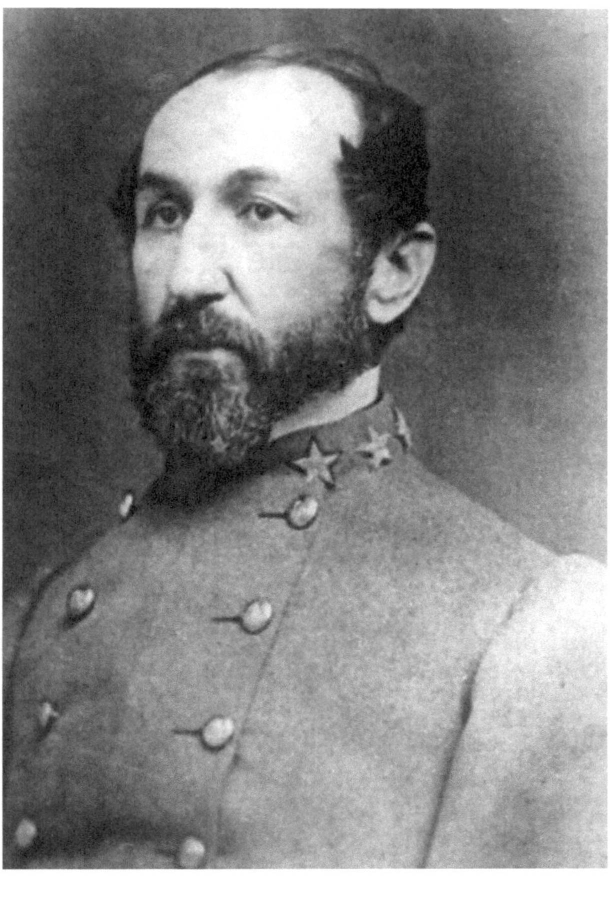

FIGURE 1.1. General Josiah Gorgas, c. 1863. Courtesy of the University of Alabama Libraries Special Collections.

Josiah proposed to Amelia, telling her that he wanted to hear her voice every day for the rest of his life.[6] They married the day after Christmas, December 26, 1853, at the Gayle mansion in Mobile. Josiah said it was the happiest day of his life.

Amelia soon became pregnant, and William was born October 3, 1854, at the Gayle mansion. They named him after Sarah's husband, William Crawford, who had died of tuberculosis in Spain just two days after Josiah and Amelia's wedding. In yet another yellow fever connection, the physician who attended the birth was Dr. Josiah Clark Nott (1804–1873), a prominent Mobile physician who had taken up the theory that mosquitoes carried malaria, and was one of the first to theorize that mosquitoes transmitted yellow fever as well.[7]

Josiah and Amelia had six children within ten years. The next baby was Jessie, born March 27, 1856; then Mary Gayle, "Mamie," born October 28, 1857; Christine Amelia, "Minnie," arrived June 4, 1859; and Maria Bayne, "Ria," was born in 1861. The final child and second son, Richard Haynsworth, called "Ritchie" or

FIGURE 1.2. Young William Crawford Gorgas, c. 1856. Courtesy of the University of Alabama Libraries Special Collections.

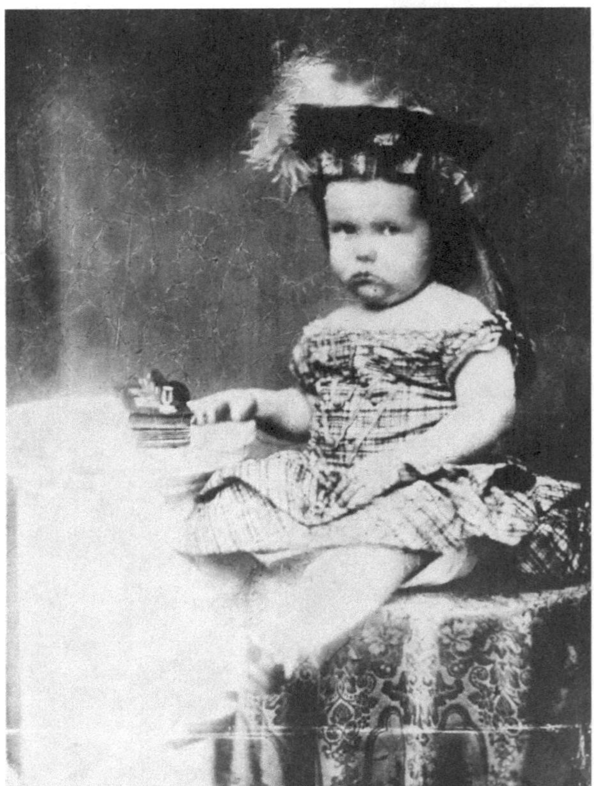

"Dick," was born during the war in 1864. Amelia and Josiah were very lucky in their child-rearing, because despite a 20 percent mortality rate for white infants in the nineteenth century, all their children survived to adulthood.[8]

## ANTEBELLUM DOMESTICITY

Josiah, the son of poor northern farmers, embraced the southern patriarchy into which he married. Not close to his own family, he devoted himself to Amelia, their children, and Amelia's extended family.[9] Josiah began to keep a journal in 1857, which he intended as instruction for his children, especially Willie. "Such a record from the hand of my father would command my reverence and affection," he wrote. "May this not be unworthy of theirs."[10] Marie Gorgas later wrote that Josiah, although a northerner, scorned abolitionists and "championed the extreme Southern view on the question of slavery."[11] The couple talked of having their own plantation and slaves, like Hugh Kerr Aiken, married to Amelia's sister Mamie, who had plantations in South Carolina of thousands of acres and three hundred enslaved people.[12] Josiah wrote in 1857 that Amelia would be happy if she could "see herself 12 or 15 years hence the mistress of 100 bales of cotton per annum and 40 or 50 ebony faces."[13]

The Gorgas family household included a maid, a cook, and Anne Kavanaugh, an Irish woman, who was the children's nurse. It is not clear how many people Josiah and Amelia held in bondage, if any. The Gayle mansion was staffed with enslaved African Americans, and Amelia may have brought an enslaved maid with her to the marriage. In 1858 Amelia asked Josiah about getting paid help, and the couple debated the merits of paid versus enslaved servants. Josiah had toyed with the idea of buying a child, reporting that "Hugh came within ten dollars of buying three little orphan darkies (Girl 10—boy 8—girl 6) – at $1250— I would have taken one of them." But, he reflected, ownership could be a burden. "I would rather <u>hire</u> the negroes we require than that either of us should own them. I find that the matter of <u>ownership</u> makes a difference in the sense of responsibility—both on my part and that of the negro." He preferred Black hired women to white women, telling Amelia, "A darkey would be preferable, they are so much less expensive."[14] According to Marie, Willie *owned* a boy as a playmate. "Like most Southern children, he possessed a piccaninny who was an inseparable companion, and there are some lively pictures of the fisticuffs in which the two boys frequently engaged."[15] There is no record, however, of William referring to this boy specifically, and we do not know his name. Gorgas would later contribute to an organization to build a monument to the "Slaves of the Southern Confederacy Monument Association," noting that "every Southerner who was old enough to recollect the house servants in antebellum days and the relation they bore to the members of their master's family will be glad to join in this movement."[16]

Josiah traveled often, from arsenal to arsenal, so letters were the means of keeping up with the health and welfare, loves and travails of an extensive and close-knit family.[17] Willie was the favored child, the eldest and the only boy for ten years, and appears in his parents' letters and Josiah's journal much more than the other children. The family lived in various army posts in Willie's early years, moving first from Alabama to the Kennebec Arsenal in Augusta, Maine, in 1856. Josiah observed his son closely, writing in his journal that his "temper improves as he goes out-doors more, not that he is ill-tempered, but confinement to the house worries him."[18] In Maine, Willie had a donkey named Beela and loved riding her and tromping about in the woods in the summer, and sledding and building snowmen in the winter.[19] He was obedient and "very bright," Josiah wrote, and took on a disagreeable task "like a little hero." He displayed good sportsmanship in games with his friends but could also be mischievous, stealing his sisters' dolls and hiding them in the trees. One time four-year-old Willie took off on a sled with such great speed that Josiah threw his cloak toward him to bring it to a stop.[20] A bundle of energy, the boy found it hard to sit still. One Sunday, Josiah wrote, "we went to church in the morning. Willie with us, behaved very well, & only fell off the bench once."[21] Willie was also an earnest boy. When he heard Josiah was coming home by train, he said to Amelia, "Tell Papa he must be sure not to put his head out of the window when he is coming on the train for it is very dangerous."[22]

Josiah continually monitored his family's health, at one point reporting that Willie fiercely resisted his medicine during his first bout with typhoid at age four. "We had the utmost difficulty in administering a dose of oil to him, the poor little fellow clenched his teeth firmly and for a time defied all our efforts," wrote Josiah with some admiration. When the boy saw his father looking for something to pry open his mouth, however, he gave in and "took it like a man."[23] Josiah also contemplated the best course in life. On the question of religion, he observed "it is Sunday and I thought of going to church, the bells for which are now ringing reproachfully, but I do not <u>feel like it</u>, a poor excuse I fear." Yet, he reasoned, "it is a good thing to have a day set apart for something besides making money, or doing work, something a little more intellectual, if not religious."[24] In 1860 Josiah began to abstain from hard liquor and wrote in his journal, "I trust if Willie ever reads this he will ponder over my example, and imitate it at an earlier period of his life." He also gave up cigars but, fond of wine, continued to drink it in moderation. He also advised Willie "never to eat so much as to feel that you have a stomach."[25]

In June 1860, the army ordered Josiah to the Frankford Arsenal near Philadelphia, a post he found agreeable. But he was tiring of the "wandering life" of the army. "I dislike to part with things, especially growing things, which I've collected about me." He wanted a home, "Where I could live and die, and where some of my children might live and die after me."[26] His next years would be anything but settled, however, as the family was about to enter the caldron of civil war that consumed all of their energies, wealth, and dreams, changing their world forever.

## A WARTIME CHILDHOOD

After the election of Abraham Lincoln in November 1860 on the Republican Party platform opposing the expansion of slavery in the West, the future of the nation hung in the balance. In early 1861, Alabama, with 435,000 people in bondage constituting 45 percent of its population, left the Union along with South Carolina, Georgia, Florida, Mississippi, Louisiana, and Texas. Josiah observed that "stirring events have taken place."[27] The Gorgases, like many other American families—Abraham and Mary Todd Lincoln of Illinois and Kentucky, and Theodore Roosevelt's parents, Theodore Sr. and Mattie of New York and Georgia—had to choose sides. For Amelia, a fervent Alabamian, there was no question of allegiance, but Josiah, the son of stern Pennsylvanians, was torn when the Confederacy offered him a promotion from captain to major of artillery and chief of ordnance. He at first declined but then reconsidered. He had frequently clashed with his superiors in the army hierarchy, and they had passed him over for promotion—so he relished the Confederate recognition. When the couple discussed the fateful decision at the dinner table with the children, Amelia told him to decide according to his conscience and assured him she would love him whatever choice he made.[28] Josiah chose the South, motivated by "my own sympathies & likings, & importuned by my Southern friends."[29] He resigned on March 27 and moved the family of four children under the age of six and Amelia pregnant with their fifth, to Charleston, South Carolina, to be with Amelia's sister Mary Aiken and her family.

At dawn on Friday, April 12, Willie and Amelia were startled by artillery fire. Fort Sumter in the Charleston Harbor was one of the main fortifications on the southern shore and of great importance to the army that controlled it. When resident Union forces had attempted to resupply the fort the day before, the South demanded that they instead surrender it. When they refused, southern troops fired cannon at the fort in response. Maj. Robert Anderson, commander at Fort Sumter, at first showed restraint but then returned fire at 7 a.m. As the two forces battled, Willie watched with Amelia from an open window of the Old Armory in Charleston with his hand in hers and commented, "Mother, isn't it solemn?"[30] It was. The battle resulted in few casualties, but the Union garrison surrendered the next day. Thus began the worst war in American history.

The Confederacy chose Richmond as its capital, and Josiah Gorgas spent most of the war there, managing the ordnance and munitions to supply the Confederate Army. He gained fame for his success, because despite the Confederate Army's lack of resources, he ensured that the South had sufficient munitions until the very last months of the war. Civil War historians credit Gorgas as one of the most effective officers of the Confederacy, and according to James M. McPherson, he "proved to be a genius at organization and improvisation. He almost literally turned plowshares into swords."[31]

Amelia's entire family joined the Confederate cause. Her brother Matthew served as a military surgeon; brother Richard Gayle was a blockade runner; brother-in-law Hugh Aiken, South Carolina plantation owner, was a cavalry officer; and brother-in-law Thomas L. Bayne, a lawyer in New Orleans, worked with Josiah as a supply officer. Amelia soon joined Josiah in Richmond and lived with her sister Ria Bayne and family. Willie at first remained in a boarding school in South Carolina but then attended Mrs. Anne Munford's Academy in Richmond. There he lived at the heart of the Confederacy and earned a reputation as a scrappy boy by paying little attention to his studies and fighting boys older and bigger than himself.[32] Willie courted disaster in many ways. Once he and a neighbor boy snuck into the arsenal and took some gunpowder, storing it in a shed behind Willie's house for some mischievous purpose. When a housemaid threw it out, they stole more powder to hide in the shed.[33] No explosions ensued, but Josiah knew that his son needed to work off his energy and, when he could, took him hiking or for early-morning swims in the river.[34] Despite his rambunctiousness, Willie managed to charm his elders. One of his Munford Academy schoolmates, Henry St. George Tucker, later a member of Congress from Virginia, said their teacher later told him, "You know, Harry, Willie Gorgas was always the favorite of everybody in the school, myself included."[35]

Willie also witnessed the bloodier consequences of war. Amelia, like so many army wives and mothers, worked in the hospitals, providing nursing care and comfort to the sick and wounded, and Willie sometimes accompanied her on her daily rounds. His interest in medical matters sometimes took a gruesome turn, though. One day a laborer was brought to the house with a leg crushed in an accident, and a doctor determined that it needed to be amputated. Willie and his sister Jessie were sent from the room but climbed up on a box outside to watch the procedure through a window and then followed the leg as it was buried behind the arsenal. It is unknown whether the man survived, but a couple of days later the children dug up his limb to inspect it.[36]

Disease thrives in both military and civilian populations during war, and in January 1862, an epidemic of scarlet fever struck the children of Richmond. The Gorgas children fell ill and recovered, but the family of Gen. James Longstreet, one of Robert E. Lee's most capable generals, was not so lucky. Three of his four children died. This deeply impressed Willie, because years later he wrote to Longstreet's widow, Helen, with memories of playing with her children in wartime Richmond, telling her he still had a "very distinct recollection of the severe epidemic of scarlet fever which affected your family so severely."[37] The Gorgas children did suffer toothaches, whooping cough, and measles, and submitted to smallpox vaccinations. Amelia's sister Ria gave birth to twin boys who did not survive the year. Such tragedies and uncertainties prodded Josiah and Amelia to join a church, and they were baptized in St. Paul's Episcopal Church in Richmond along with President Jefferson Davis in May 1862.[38]

In addition to being fascinated by medicine, Josiah's military career played an important part in Willie's vision of his future. He read military history and loved the ceremony and uniforms of his father's profession. Josiah fostered the children's support for the Confederacy, proudly noting, "Willie now boasts the personal acquaintance of two Generals (Lee and Bragg) three Lieut. Gens (Hood, Ewell & Hill, A.P.)."[39] He took Willie, Jessie, and Minnie to greet prisoners of war with baskets of food as they returned home after an exchange, and when Gen. Stonewall Jackson died in May 1863 from infection after a gunshot wound, Josiah took Willie and Jessie to see him lying in state.[40]

The stresses of war took a toll on family life. Amelia and her sister Ria began to bicker, so in the spring of 1864, the families separated, leaving Amelia and the children in the house near the arsenal.[41] In the fall of 1864, two more children in the extended family died, and Amelia gave birth to their last child in November 1864, naming him Richard Haynsworth after her youngest brother. Josiah marked the moment: "Two boys & four girls in a family will do very well. May Heaven bless & protect them all & bring them safely to years of maturity."[42] The family was now complete.

After three years as head of the ordnance department, Josiah had arsenals across the South and factories that were producing cannons, pistols, and ammunition to meet the demands of the Confederacy. Despite Josiah's organizational skills in arming their forces, the Confederacy could not produce enough to properly feed and clothe them and was failing the civilian population as well.[43] The North, with its strong economy, was better supplied and seemed to have an endless reserve of soldiers. When Josiah was promoted to brigadier general in November 1864, the Confederacy was in trouble. Lincoln and the Republicans had won reelection, Gen.

Ulysses S. Grant was punishing Confederate troops wherever he found them, and the Federal Army was moving through the South.

As conditions worsened in the South, Josiah had to sell some of his property to support the family.[44] Willie, too, made sacrifices, going barefoot one winter to show sympathy for the bedraggled soldiers he saw in Richmond.[45] In early April 1864, he and his father even saw some actual fighting when Union troops broke Lee's lines near Richmond, and they watched the Confederates drive them back at the Appomattox Bridge. "We could see smoke of the guns & the bursting of shells from the cupola of the War Department," wrote Josiah. "Willie saw & watched it with interest."[46] Another sacrifice was one Willie would never forget. A family friend had given Amelia a young turkey to raise for Christmas dinner in 1864. Willie took care of the bird and was looking forward to the holiday feast, but Amelia decided to send the bird to soldiers in the field at Petersburg. Willie was devastated, "I do not think anyone in the Confederacy made a much greater sacrifice to patriotism than I did in December, '64 in agreeing to part with my gobbler," he told one audience years later. "I went out and had a good cry on its neck."[47]

## WAR'S END

As Federal troops penetrated farther into the South, the family faced the prospect of having to flee. Amelia, fearing no reprisals for women and children, was determined to remain in Richmond, and Josiah agreed that with six small children it was "better than to fly."[48] He and Thomas Bayne, however, fearing arrest or worse, decided to escape south. As Josiah left at midnight, he beheld Amelia preparing to move the family, "still standing like a brave woman, over the remnants of her household goods." He wrote, "She had with her two faithful women of the neighborhood to whom she had been kind during the winter & Willie, who dropped off to sleep about this time."[49] Amelia had a different memory, writing that "my oldest child, a boy of ten years, remained at my side working all night." Arriving at Ria's house, "My son Willie assisted me to spread wet blankets over the flat roof of the house to protect us from the debris of the fires."[50]

In any case, Willie never forgot the events of that night. He remembered his father in full uniform waking him and directing him to help his mother get to the Bayne home and to take with them the family cow, the critical source of milk for the baby. Richmond was in flames, rife with looting and fear. Willie led the procession with the cow, followed by his sisters and Amelia with infant Richard in her arms. As they were making their way, the arsenal was torched and shells began to explode, sending out shrapnel. One piece hit the cow making her bolt and knocking Willie to the cobblestones. To his horror he had lost his charge.

When they arrived at the house, Amelia said, "Well at least the shell did not hit your baby brother." Willie, mortified by his failure, later wryly told an audience, "I thought at the time that women have a greatly exaggerated idea of the value of babies."[51]

As Josiah and Thomas Bayne fled south, they did not know whether they would be arrested, executed, or pardoned. News of Lee's surrender to Grant on April 9 at Appomattox reached them when they were with President Jefferson Davis in Danville. Josiah observed that Davis stood "thin, spare, erect, every inch the chief, so sorrowful but self-possessed, hopeless but self-reliant to the last."[52] While history now remembers the Union victory as one of "right over wrong," historian Elizabeth R. Varon argues that Confederates like Josiah Gorgas believed they had nothing to repent of and "survived the war with their honor and principles intact."[53] Days later Lincoln's assassination and the rise to power of Democrat vice president Andrew Johnson intensified the confusion and anxiety across the country. In the North the questions revolved around what form a new Union would take and how soon families would see their soldiers come home. In the South people faced immediate and searing questions concerning the future of four million emancipated men, women, and children. Half of the southern population had been enslaved. Now the question was, what would they do? Would they stay in the South? Would they work? And would the freedmen avenge themselves against their former enslavers?

Now, as the Confederacy failed, the balance in the Gorgas marriage and southern gender relations shifted as well. Men who had steeled themselves for battle now suffered injury, disability, and defeat; many of the men in Willie's world would never return to their previous mastery and vigor. From mid-1865 to mid-1866, Josiah and Amelia were separated—he on the run, she seeking safety, and each closely watched events. Josiah's health suffered from the stress of war, and he began to experience strokes in 1862. As an army officer on the losing side, he also lost his family's fortune and his ability to earn a living. In contrast, women found themselves running the households, farms, plantations, or businesses or working in hospitals as Amelia did. It fell to them to manage the finances, discipline the children, mourn their fallen men, and care for those lucky enough to come home.[54] As Amelia saw her way of life falling away, she stepped in to fill the gap and to support her family, recruiting her oldest son to her side. Willie in turn would adopt or seek to emulate many of her traits. Amelia, wrote Marie Gorgas, was "one of those women born to rule, but to rule through gentleness of manner and intention." She possessed "the quality of boundless patience and persistence—persistence of the kind that never irritates and never causes pain but almost as unconsciously to itself as to others, pursues the appointed course."[55]

Although the shift lay much beneath the surface, as Josiah faltered and Amelia rose to lead, Willie was old enough to observe and develop respect for the power of women.[56] And that power could be fearsome. Reflecting on the war decades later, Gorgas remembered how his mother had "impressed upon me that I would soon be old enough to go to the war." She even spoke of his baby brother as "another soldier for the Confederacy." He did not see this as bloody-minded, but high-minded. "War is certainly a terrible thing and debasing in many respects, but it also brings out strongly some phases of altruism." For his parents, "Everything was swallowed up in their devotion to the Confederacy."[57]

## RECONSTRUCTING THE GORGASES

### *Maryland, 1865–1866*

The postbellum society in which Willie developed his understanding of race and politics was different from that of his parents. Now, instead of experiencing the excitement and heroism of war, Willie and his family became refugees. Everyone in the South, regardless of their race, faced an uncertain future; the only promise was that of hardship. The Gorgases were better off than many. Josiah was able to sell some cotton and had funds from a blockade-running enterprise to finance the family for a while. Amelia was one of the lucky women, unwidowed, with a strong family network. She, however, feared possible retribution by the formerly enslaved people now moving freely in the South, and fled with the children to Cambridge, Maryland, as guests of family friends.[58] She told Josiah that if he needed to go overseas or to a border state in the North to find better opportunities, she would support him. She was no longer wedded to the Deep South; "I love my state but dread to reside there while the present status of the negroes remains unsettled," she wrote. Instead of revenge, however, freedmen were intent on reuniting their family members who had been sold far and wide, establishing their own farms or trades, building schools and churches, and creating new lives. But Amelia was bitter. "I do not feel as if it were my state or country while we are ground under the heel of Yankee despotism."[59] Josiah tried to be optimistic about the future and make peace with defeat and the fact that "the country has become one consolidated whole."[60] But Amelia still clung "fondly to some far-off hope of a resurrection of our poor country, a just retribution for the indignities & cruelties heaped upon us."[61] Josiah, however, cautioned "no more violence & bloodshed. If the blood already poured out so freely does not suffice, then God has otherwise decreed."[62]

The new president, Andrew Johnson, and Republicans in Congress heatedly debated the fate of the Confederate Army and political leadership. Johnson, a

Democrat from Tennessee, sought leniency, while Republicans were more vengeful. Confederate men lost their country and their citizenship, and Jefferson Davis was convicted of treason and spent two years in prison.[63] But after months of deliberations, most Confederate soldiers and government officials were pardoned or given amnesty upon swearing allegiance to the Union and the Constitution. Even the Radical Republicans of the North realized that vindictiveness and revenge would not make the country whole.

Free from arrest but without work, Josiah hated the idleness and uncertainty. In the meantime Amelia encouraged him to turn his attention to the children, especially Willie, and almost taunted him with their son. Willie, she wrote, "is so manly & obedient that I find myself growing quite dependent upon him." She added, "He is my escort to any part of the city at night . . . & we all think him a magnificent specimen of a rebel boy."[64] When Josiah asked her to send Willie to him, she declined, insisting that he instead come to them in Maryland.[65] She needed Josiah's help. "Willie loves me dearly & I control him entirely through his affection but I am too weak to insist upon duties repugnant to him." And, she confessed, "My rebellious feelings are I know sinful & I must begin to disguise them from the impressable children."[66]

Amelia was proud of Willie's political views. She reported to Josiah that when a Union officer offered to take their son for a ride in the country, he refused despite his love of horses. She encouraged him to go, saying he could "maintain his opinions & principles should the Com[mander] discuss them & not forget he was your son." Willie went on the ride and was true to form because the officer reported that he was "a splendid lad though an inveterate rebel."[67] Willie expressed his rebel sympathies in his first letter to his father. "I regret very much that I did not accompany you with my gun. I am extreamly [*sic*] anxious to use it well for I did not have my chance during this war."[68] He asked his father to excuse any errors in his letter, but with this first effort, Josiah began years of correcting and criticizing his son's spelling and penmanship. When Willie misspelled "Wednesday" in one letter, Josiah commented to Amelia, "Poor Willie has apparently done his best above but you see how terribly deficient he is in spelling."[69] William Gorgas did acquire a readable hand but throughout his life remained a poor speller.[70]

In November, Josiah joined the family in Maryland and approved of their Chesapeake Bay accommodations in an old country-house. "Good living but very cramped quarters, the children look well & for refugees the life is not bad."[71] But he soon moved them to Baltimore. There, Amelia found her old spirit when she attended a "grand Confederate wedding," with Willie, in her husband's absence, as escort. She told Josiah, "His grey suit shall be freshly trimmed with red and he shall appear as much as possible in the uniform of his lost but beloved Confederacy."[72] Fifty years later Gorgas told a Baltimore audience that he first came to their city "a ragged, barefoot little rebel, with empty pockets and an empty stomach." His family had lost everything with the fall of Richmond, leaving his mother, "stranded with six small children."[73] He always felt warmly toward the city due to the kindness and generosity with which they were received, but his remarks also show that the memory of his mother and her postwar struggles had eclipsed that of his father.

### *Brierfield, Alabama, 1866–1868*

By the end of 1865, Josiah was able to purchase a set of blast furnaces in the town of Brierfield, Alabama, south of Birmingham, and Amelia and the children joined him there in April 1866. Adjusting from the excitement of Baltimore and wartime Richmond to the slower, rural pace of Brierfield, Amelia and Josiah focused on educating their children. They dreamed of sending the girls to Paris to complete their educations as "young ladies," but with little family land or wealth, the boys needed to learn to make a living.[74] When Willie turned twelve years old, his parents sent him to a boarding school run by the Rev. Mr. Anastasius Menaeos near Greensboro, Alabama.[75] Before he left, Josiah pensively watched his son as he slept. "It is the natural desire of the parent to protect & watch over the offspring," he wrote in his journal, "to work hard, & bear the brunt of the struggle of life, that the child may be saved the same struggle in some degree."[76]

The family embraced country life, and in October 1867 Josiah observed "we are all living very comfortably here in our cottage—8 grown white people, and 10 children—with 4 colored Servants."[77] Amelia's widowed stepmother lived with them at times with her four children (Amelia's half-siblings) and would teach the younger children their lessons. When Willie was home, Josiah instructed him and Jessie in Latin. Willie also roamed the countryside on his mule, Beela, and took up hunting, shooting his first bird when he was twelve.[78] He enjoyed working outside, helping his father with a garden and an orchard, tending the cow, and raising a brood of two hundred chickens.[79] He also continued his mischief. When a playmate had to move away from Brierfield because her father remarried, Willie and a friend rode Beela to rescue her from her new home, and the three of them returned victorious to town astride the mule.[80]

Josiah struggled to adjust to the new economic realities of the southern iron industry as it restructured from slave labor to free. Defeated in war, Josiah now suffered humiliation in business failure as he encountered higher expenses for labor and supplies than he had anticipated.[81] In his desperation he could even understand why some people were driven to suicide. "To many," he wrote in January 1867, "annihilation must be the only thing left. Nothing is so terrible as despair."[82] That summer he was forced to shutter the furnace and pay off his workers, and Christmas that year was subdued. "Our holidays have been anything but merry," Josiah lamented to Amelia; "I cannot look the future into [*sic*] the face with equanimity. I have a dread of being poor & old together."[83] In 1868 he was able to reopen the ironworks, but the operation would soon again be idle.

After the war Thomas Bayne returned to his law practice in New Orleans, so in the fall of 1868, Josiah and Amelia took Willie out of boarding school and sent him to New Orleans to live with the Baynes. Josiah wanted Willie to study French, exhorting him to develop a good accent, as well as keep an account of the "little expenses" he made with his allowance. "You can not too soon learn the value of money for the prospect is very strong, my boy, that you will have to do as I did before you—make your own way in the world."[84] Willie did his part, receiving excellent grades at Marshall School in New Orleans, including a first in geography.[85]

As Willie studied, the nation struggled to remake itself. President Andrew Johnson's leniency toward southern white groups and hostility to freedmen angered Republicans in Congress. When he vetoed the Freedmen's Bureau bill and civil rights legislation in 1866, the Republicans passed articles of impeachment against him, and the nation responded in 1868 with the election of the "Radical Republican" Congress and Ulysses S. Grant as president. The new political leadership sought to reconstruct the nation with free labor and an industrializing economy. Congress passed the Fourteenth Amendment to the Constitution to ensure equal rights and due process under the law, and the Fifteenth Amendment to confer voting rights on African American men and impose martial law on the South. The latter measure divided the former Confederacy into sections, each governed by US Army troops, to enforce the new laws and protect freedmen and other Republicans from white supremacist violence.[86]

Amelia and Josiah chafed under Republican rule, and Amelia reported to her son on the violence of Reconstruction in the South as white elites battled with Black freedmen and poor white farmers for control of their government and economy. In one letter she told Willie that "Mr. Newl-Smith's distillery was burned a few nights since by a band of negroes and white men dressed in Yankee uniforms." She added that people were expecting the Ku Klux Klan to appear in Brierfield during the week.[87] Amelia also began to confide in Willie about family difficulties. The foundry was in trouble, and Josiah doubted that the Alabama Reconstruction government would help him. The destroyed southern economy had left few investors who could support the furnace, few customers to buy its products, and even fewer businessmen who could purchase the ironworks. By 1869 Josiah was $2,000 in debt (about $40,000 in 2021 dollars), and unable to collect even $1,500 his brother Solomon in Pennsylvania owed to him.[88]

### *Sewanee, Tennessee, 1869–1875*

The family was relieved when in 1869 Josiah took the position of department headmaster at the University of the South, an Episcopal liberal arts college in Sewanee, Tennessee. One historian described it as a "major institutional shrine to the Lost Cause," because the institution had deep roots in slavery.[89] Before the war, ten southern Episcopal dioceses had joined to establish a college free from northern antislavery influences and financed it in part with the fortunes of a former slave trader.[90] The cornerstone was laid in 1860, but the war interrupted construction until 1866, when building resumed and the board recruited several former Confederate officers to its faculty. (This was not uncommon. Robert E. Lee, for example, was president of Washington College in Lexington, Virginia, from 1865 to 1880.) Josiah arrived to take charge of one hundred students on July 1, 1869, and when he moved, he took Willie with him. They stayed at a boardinghouse until the family arrived, and while Josiah complained to Amelia about their accommodations, Willie was less critical, reporting that they ate well and had dessert twice a week.[91]

Amelia and the family arrived in June 1870, and Willie enrolled as a member of the second class of the university's preparatory school. Sewanee students wore Confederate gray uniforms to class, attended chapel services twice daily, participated in drills under former Confederate officers, and played for the athletic teams as the "R. E. Lees."[92] Willie slept in the dormitory and made a number of friends but got into fights with other boys and was a poor student. This ended, however, when, according to family lore, he heard his parents talking worriedly about his poor grades, and, alarmed and ashamed, he decided to study.[93] This paid off and the next year he stood first in his class. When Willie won a medal for scholarship from the State of Alabama in 1871, Josiah noted his accomplishment in his journal. "His mother & sisters are very proud of it & him, to say nothing of my feelings on the subject."[94]

Willie thrived at Sewanee. He developed into a healthy, handsome young man with twinkly eyes on which people would comment for the rest of his life. He pursued hunting and fishing with his dogs and riding the family horse Mollie (Beela's fate is unknown), activities he would enjoy as an adult. He excelled in sports, especially swimming and baseball, where he played first base. No longer prone to fighting, he spoke in subdued tones that belied a stronger character and, in one mark of maturity, joined the Episcopal church in town.[95] He also began to observe the world around him. When Jessie and Minnie went away to school in Columbia, Tennessee, Willie wrote to them about the news—the weather, his friends, and whether he could yet grow a beard. "I will be seventeen in a few days and begin to feel quite anxious about my upper lip," he told them. In the same paragraph, he described a lynching in a nearby town. "Three negroes burnt a house down in the valley the other day and were arrested and put in jail in Winchester but some men dressed in masks took them out and shot them."[96] These murders do not appear on the Equal Justice Initiative's list of lynching victims in the United States, but such violence and vigilante action occurred throughout the South during the Reconstruction and Jim Crow years.[97] Willie observed the racial violence around him, but absorbed in the fog of his teen years, he simply reported the deadly episode to his sisters without additional comment.

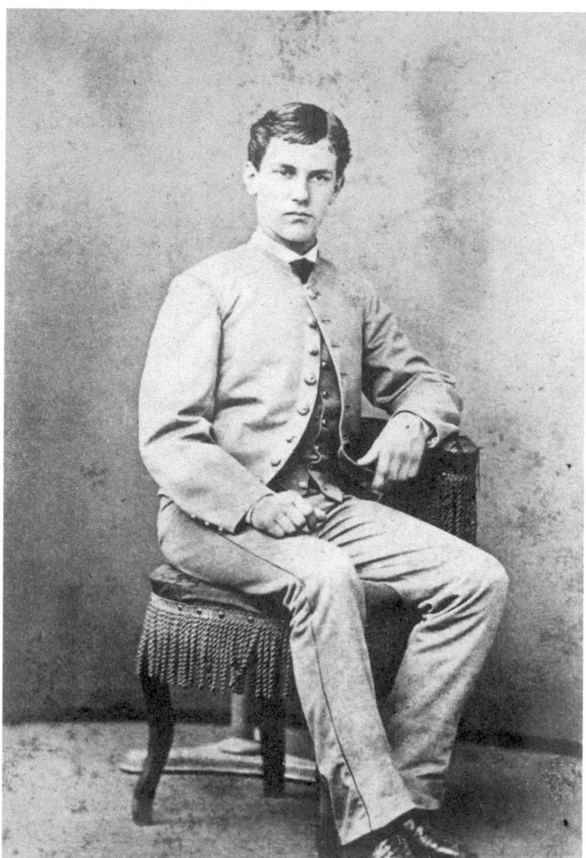

FIGURE 1.3. Willie Gorgas at Sewanee. Courtesy of the University of Alabama Libraries Special Collections.

When Gorgas returned to Sewanee thirty-five years later to give the commencement address, he offered a romantic, idyllic portrayal of the university of his day. Some may have thought it "old-fashioned," he remarked, but "you cannot find anyplace today a stronger, more forceful faculty, more motherly, cultivated, & refined ladies, prettier girls, & a more manly chivalric, honest & high-mannered set of young men than were collected here in the seventies."[98] For Willie Gorgas, Sewanee must have been an island of calm amidst the turmoil of the striving, violent years of Reconstruction. As one historian has written, "defeat, poverty, guilt, disillusionment, isolation, dread of the future—all have characterized the Southern past."[99] As his nation and his parents faced the future, the young man would have to find his own way, and that would lead him away from the South.

## CHAPTER 2

# The Making of an Army Medical Officer

If you have a deciding wish in any direction don't be influenced by anybody else to adopt some other course.

—William Gorgas to his brother, Dick, August 1881

ONE OF WILLIE'S STRONGEST MEMORIES from his youth was of a former officer in the Confederate Army who worked briefly with Josiah in the Brierfield ironworks. Years later, when he learned that the man had died, he told his son, Frank Polk, that his father "was my ideal. I fairly worshipped him." Gorgas remembered that when he was a boy of twelve, Polk's father arrived in Brierfield just out of the army, riding a beautiful horse. "He still wore his slouch hat, and I recollect him as one of the finest and most soldierly figures when mounted on this horse that I have ever seen."[1] That was Willie's aspiration, to be a military man on a horse. But in this quest, he faced his father's opposition. Josiah was not flattered that his son wanted to follow in his footsteps to West Point and an army career. When Willie was just a boy of five years, Josiah had written, "I do not want Willie to take or retain a commission in the Army. My great regret is the wandering life we are obliged to lead."[2] But the unsettled and impoverished southern economy and his father's struggles limited Willie's opportunities to make a living and intensified the pressure on him to find a career that would help support his family.

### THE WEST POINT CAMPAIGN

Willie continued to perform well in school and graduated from the University of the South in 1875. Josiah wanted him to pursue the law or engineering, so Willie dutifully returned to New Orleans to read law in the offices of his uncle Thomas Bayne's firm, Clarke, Bayne, & Renshaw. The agreement was that he would try the law for a year to see if it suited him. Amelia wrote, "Father & I feel so relieved that you take kindly to your office duties," but assured him that they would keep their promise "to release you at the end of the season if the profession is still repugnant to you."[3] But Willie did not take to the law and disliked being confined to an office and desk. When he turned twenty-one in October 1875, his interest in a military career had not waned, but time was running out. Candidates for the military academy at West Point had to be between the ages of seventeen and twenty-two and could only be nominated by a member of Congress or the president or vice president of the United States. Each elected official had several slots in the academy, which they could fill as they became open. The trick was to find a willing official with an open slot. With so many Republican officials in the South, it would be a heavy lift for the son of a Confederate general.

Admonished by Amelia, Josiah swallowed his pride and asked his former adversary, President Grant, to appoint Willie to West Point. He recruited Supreme Court associate justice John Campbell and former Union army officer C. C. Augur, to plead his son's case as well.[4] Augur's letter stated that Willie was "clever & well educated & with a fine physique. All his life he has been earnest & determined to get to West Point." Josiah, he assured Grant, was now working at a university and "entirely above & without the scope of politics."[5] Grant replied that his West Point slots had been promised years in advance, but he may also have been loath to promote the son of the man who had supplied the Confederate Army with the weapons and ammunition that had killed his Union soldiers. Trying another angle, Willie moved to Greenville, Tennessee, to establish himself in the district of Democratic congressman William McFarland in hopes of getting a nomination from him, but the congressman gave the appointment to another young man.[6] As the family watched the calendar and worried, Josiah told Amelia, "I hope as you say that he has made up his mind to failure at last."[7] Willie's twenty-second birthday on October 3, 1876, extinguished his dreams of West Point.

Knowing that he had to find a way to earn a living for himself and to help his family, Willie demonstrated the determination and perseverance that would get him through difficulties later in his life. If West Point was not the way into military service, he reasoned that medicine, an indispensable part of any military establishment, could be the route.[8] But as Willie contemplated a career as an army doctor, Josiah once again opposed his son's plan. The profession of medicine had not yet gained respectability. During the Civil War and before the emergence of germ theory, surgeons were sometimes known as "sawbones," because they often had to treat injured and infected limbs with amputation. But a family friend in

Sewanee, Dr. Hiram Bartholomew, encouraged Willie to apply to Bellevue Hospital Medical College in New York. He said it was the best school in the country and even offered to help pay for him to attend.[9] Willie was accepted to Bellevue and in mid-September 1876 departed Sewanee by train for the north to begin classes and a new life. Josiah resigned himself to his son's new path. "I am quite satisfied with his choice of a profession and am quite sure he will succeed. (D.V.) [Deo volente, God willing]," he recorded in his journal.[10]

Willie Gorgas arrived in New York amidst a national election campaign. He found lodging with other medical students from the South and told Jessie that the Democrats outnumbered the Republicans in his boardinghouse so that "the Democrats have things all their own way in any political discussions."[11] He supported the Democrat, Samuel J. Tilden of New York, who was backed by white southerners and northern immigrants who opposed government intervention such as the military occupation of the South under Reconstruction. The Republican, Rutherford B. Hayes of Ohio, ran on a platform that would continue Reconstruction policies but also spoke of restoring self-government to southern states, a message appealing to a nation wearying of the cost of military occupation. The election was a virtual tie. Tilden won the popular vote by three percentage points, while Hayes won the electoral college 185 to 184. Congress appointed a special committee to decide the election, and it produced the Compromise of 1877, whereby the Republican, Hayes, would become president but would appoint Democrats to his cabinet and withdraw the military occupation forces from the South. The compromise ended Reconstruction and freed southern Democrats of northern rule.

The end of Reconstruction had little immediate impact on Willie but meant that the army he wished to join had failed to defeat the Klan and the southern insurgency.[12] The military would instead turn to suppressing Native Americans in the West and labor protests in the North and West in support of the nation's nascent industrial empire. For their part, political elites in the South immediately began to rewrite their state constitutions, disenfranchising African Americans and many poor whites, and reasserting white supremacy and class dominance across the South.

That consequential fall, Willie began to think politically about his own interests. When one of their uncles was elected to Congress, he told Jessie, "It is a great thing to have a cousin so high up. He may be able to put in a word for me when I come up for the hospital." And now a medical student in New York City, living far from his parents' world, Willie claimed his adulthood. Instead of signing his letters "Willie," he began to sign them "W. C. Gorgas."[13]

## BELLEVUE HOSPITAL, NEW YORK

In attending one of the best medical schools in the country, William Gorgas put himself at the forefront of a revolution. Bellevue Hospital Medical College (now part of New York University Medical School) was a leader in medical science education, along with Harvard, the University of Pennsylvania, and Rush Medical College in Chicago, all seeking ways to combine clinical patient care and medical instruction with laboratory science to improve medical diagnosis and treatment. For centuries, western medicine had been based on Aristotelean and Galenic "humoral theory," the view that health was determined by the balance of the body's "humors"—blood, phlegm, and yellow and black bile. These humors were subject to environmental conditions of hot and cold, wet and dry, and individual bodies were prone to certain characteristics, giving them a "phlegmatic" or "choleric" nature. Illness, therefore, was the result of personal susceptibility to environmental conditions such as a cold, wet climate or "bad air," miasma.

Humoral medical treatment involved "heroic" methods of purging to induce bleeding, vomiting, urination, or defecation, or stimulants such as tonics or alcohol to restore an individual's humoral balance and health. Surgeons also cut out tumors, pulled teeth, sewed up gashes, and amputated limbs as they saw fit, treating pain with large doses of whiskey and opium. The single greatest killer in the United States during the nineteenth century was tuberculosis, and physicians could only offer sufferers "prayer and opium." Antibiotics would not be discovered for sixty years. Medical practitioners came from all backgrounds, men and women, Black and white, Chinese, and Native American, and those who brought their healing practices from the "old country" in Europe. They employed therapies that included faith healing, water cures, nutritional fads, and even electric shock. When William went to medical school, no one yet needed a license to practice medicine, and many doctors learned the trade through apprenticeship. Medical education and practice would not be regulated until the early twentieth century, and medical school curricula and courses of instruction varied from one college to another. Many schools were not connected to hospitals and did not offer students clinical experience.[14]

Josiah's skepticism about the medical profession therefore had some merit because it was not yet greatly respected or lucrative and until the late nineteenth century had little to offer the sick and injured. Many patients did not survive medical treatment of whatever type, and some health conditions were getting worse. Industrialization and urbanization were creating increasingly crowded and dirty communities, and without good public sanitation, clean water, and adequate nutrition, the nation suffered high infant and child mortality rates. These contributed to life expectancy in the United States in 1900 of forty-seven years at birth for whites and a disastrous thirty-three years for Blacks (compared to about seventy-seven for whites and seventy-two for Blacks in 2020.)[15]

After the Civil War period, physicians and scientists began to forge a new medical profession based on scientific research. Cities and towns began to vaccinate against smallpox and implement measures to ensure clean water, and scores of Americans traveled to Europe to study with scientists such as Robert Koch in Germany, a leader in the development of the germ theory of medicine.[16] Building on work by Louis Pasteur in France, who demonstrated that microbes, or "germs," promoted fermentation in wine and cheese and could cause illness in animals and humans, Koch theorized that a disease was caused by a specific pathogen that produced the same suite of symptoms from patient to patient. For example, people who had tuberculosis were not victims of a wet, cold climate or a "consumptive nature," but rather of bacteria that could be seen with a microscope. The same germs caused the same diseases from patient to patient whether they lived on a Virginia farm or in a Massachusetts city and could therefore be treated the same way.

William Gorgas was in the first wave of physicians who would employ the tenets and tools of this medical revolution, but when he graduated from medical school, germ theory was only emerging as an explanation for disease causation and prevention. What Gorgas learned in medical school from 1876 to 1879 was very different from what men and women would learn in the 1920s (due, in part, to his own work in public health), and Bellevue was at the forefront of much of that change. As William began his medical training, British physician Joseph Lister was touring the United States to promote his research showing that disinfection with carbolic acid could make surgical operations safer and more survivable, and instructors at Bellevue began to lecture on his methods.[17] Antisepsis, laboratory diagnostics, and new technology such as the stethoscope, thermometer, hypodermic needle, and the X-ray machine would by the 1880s and 1890s become powerful weapons enabling physicians to diagnose and differentiate diseases from one another, and to treat them with higher rates of success and with greater confidence. Epidemiological data also advised public health officials on the trajectories of infections in communities. This more scientific approach to health and disease and new technologies meant that physicians needed to acquire more formal education than simply working as a physician's apprentice.

Building on lessons from the Civil War, Bellevue was one of the first hospitals to have an ambulance service, so that by the time Gorgas arrived, seven horse-drawn ambulances brought the sick and injured to the hospital. Bellevue established one of the first nursing schools in the country in 1873, following Florence Nightingale's leadership in forging trained nursing as an occupation for middle-class women. In

1877 Bellevue opened an obstetrical service that practiced the recommendations of Hungarian physician Ignaz Semmelweis by requiring physicians to sanitize their hands before attending new mothers and babies, thereby quickly eliminating from its obstetrical wards puerperal fever, the historic killer of new mothers.[18] Gorgas attended lectures by Austin Flint, the author of a widely read medical textbook, and was instructed in the dissection room by William Henry Welch, who had studied with Koch and others in Europe.[19] Welch would become a leader in American pathology and bacteriology for the next five decades. Gorgas learned surgical procedures by observing the famed William Halsted perform some of the most skillful surgery in the country in Bellevue's "operating theater."

The work at Bellevue was not easy for William, and he later told Amelia, "I was more discouraged the first few months in New York with the difficulties of my profession than in New Orleans."[20] But he chose the more rigorous three-year course rather than the regular two-year curriculum at Bellevue and delved into his studies. He embraced New York as well. He found an affordable boardinghouse run by an Irish landlady not far from Bellevue Hospital and shared rooms with Nicholas Atwater of Memphis, two years ahead of him, and John Bowen of Kentucky.[21] The young men paid five dollars a week for room and board and saved money by sharing meals and acting as their own housekeepers. An earnest student, William eschewed many evenings of beer, poker, and gossip. He also read the Bible and said his prayers in front of other students with little self-consciousness. One fellow student remembered Gorgas's "delightful reading of the first chapter of the book of Ruth to several of us before we retired."[22] Another student, Benjamin J. Baldwin of Alabama, remembered that on the weekends the southern boys would go to the Bowery to "cast off the 'goblins' of the dissecting room, & forget the harassing, jaw-breaking names of muscles and bones." Gorgas would at times join them and became so adept at keeping them out of fights that his friends took to calling him "Old W. C." for his maturity. Gorgas also liked to go to the theater and spend as much time outdoors as he could. He went rowing on the Hudson and swam daily, even in the frigid waters of the Hudson and the East River after the ice formed. Baldwin said he would emerge out of the water "as red as an apple," but when they teased him about it, William said that Andrew Jackson used to swim in the Tennessee River every day of the year and "what Andrew Jackson did I can do."[23]

As his father advised, Gorgas kept records of his income and expenditures and accounted for every penny he spent. In 1877 he received irregular sums from home: fifty dollars in January, but only ten dollars a month later as his parents struggled to remain solvent. Expenses included postage, room and board, laundry, beer, ice, and cigars. He bought fruit to supplement his boardinghouse diet—melons, bananas, peaches, grapes, and his favorite, apples. He read the *New York World*, a leading national voice of the Democratic Party, and if he went to church, put ten cents in the offertory.[24] To Amelia's chagrin, her son saved money by not going home for Christmas or summer vacations. At one point he even considered dropping out of school for a year to replenish his funds.[25] When his Uncle Tom Bayne gave William ten dollars for Christmas, the young man bought trousers, shoes, and a hat suitable for the city.[26] Gorgas would worry about money and supporting his family for the rest of his life, but despite his early struggles, he told his brother, Dick, "I believe the four years I spent in New York were as pleasant as any I lived because I was constantly on stretch and trying to make both ends meet. I look back upon it with a great deal of pleasure now and feel very proud of my course there."[27]

## THE 1878 YELLOW FEVER EPIDEMIC

The budding physicians at Bellevue got real-life medical experience during the summer of 1878. First, in mid-July, New York and much of the country experienced an extraordinary heat wave with temperatures of 90 degrees and higher for ten days, something that would not happen again until 1952. The *New York Tribune* reported "fierce heat" of 97 degrees on July 19, and the next day listed the names of people who had been sickened or killed by heatstroke.[28] William and other medical students went out on the Bellevue ambulances to look for people who had heatstroke, and Gorgas treated twenty patients, two of whom died.[29] A few weeks later, an even fiercer scourge showed Gorgas its power to destroy: yellow fever.

The disease had been epidemic in Cuba during ten years of rebellion against the Spanish government's rule, and when the fighting ended in 1878, refugees began to arrive in New Orleans.[30] The *Emily B. Souder* from Havana brought mosquitoes and yellow fever to the city in May, and warm weather allowed the insects to thrive and spread the infection. Yellow fever took hold in the city, killing more than four thousand that summer. As the disease made its way north up the Mississippi with river commerce, local, state, and even the federal government tried to impose quarantines against traffic coming from infected countries and communities, but to little avail. Mosquitoes carrying yellow fever sickened and killed people in towns along the Mississippi as far north as St. Louis. Vicksburg, Mississippi, endured five thousand cases in a population of only twelve thousand, with more than 1,100 deaths, a terrifying case fatality rate of 23 percent.[31] Record-keeping was spotty at the time, but by November, when a hard frost killed off the mosquitoes, an estimated 120,000 people had fallen ill, and twenty thousand had died, with case fatality rates ranging from 55 percent in the Midwest to about 25 percent in the South. Financial losses were estimated at $200 million.[32] The epidemic so shocked the country that Congress created a National Board of Health (1879–1883), a short-lived effort to collect data about infectious diseases across the country. The board nevertheless appointed the first American yellow fever commission in 1879, which spurred investigation into the causes of yellow fever.

The worst yellow fever epidemic in American history both fascinated and traumatized William. Americans were subject to numerous fevers, including malaria, typhoid, influenza, typhus, and severe colds, but without bacteriology and germ theory, physicians could differentiate them only by observing symptoms. This gave rise to names such as "intermittent fever," "remittent fever," "break bone fever," or simply "ague." Yellow fever, however, with its dramatic yellowing of the skin and "black vomit," was distinctive and feared. William's professor Austin Flint's

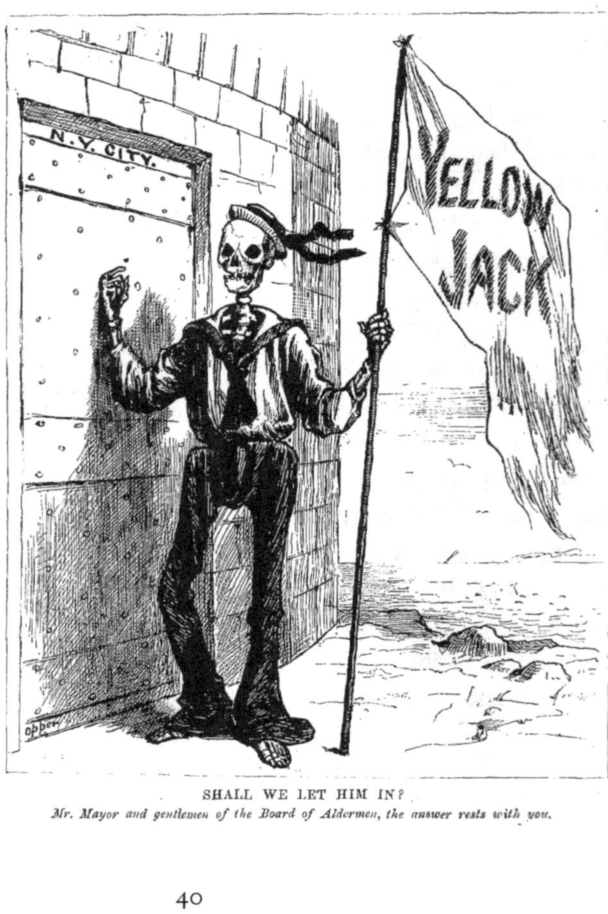


SHALL WE LET HIM IN?
*Mr. Mayor and gentlemen of the Board of Aldermen, the answer rests with you.*

FIGURE 2.1. "Shall We Let Him In?" *Frank Leslie's Illustrated Newspaper*, September 21, 1878.

textbook *Clinical Medicine*, explained that the disease "germs" came to southern ports from abroad, usually the Caribbean, and were carried on people's clothing, baggage, and other materials and cargo. Disinfection was key to preventing the spread of the disease, but "germs are reproduced only during the hot months of the year," Flint wrote, and then "destroyed or rendered inactive by frost." With mortality ranging between 10 and 75 percent, Flint noted, survivors acquired some immunity to yellow fever. He then stated ominously, "We have no knowledge of any remedy which will control this disease as quinia [quinine] controls malarial fever." To address symptoms, he prescribed treatments from milk with lime-water, pieces of ice, and cool baths, to the injection of opiates to ease pain and "alcoholics" to stimulate a feeble heartrate.[33]

Gorgas and his classmates tracked the disease as it moved up the Mississippi, and they became worried as it approached Memphis, where their friend Nicholas Atwater, recently graduated, now practiced medicine.[34] City leaders tried to impose a quarantine, but business opposition caused them to abandon the effort. The first case was reported on August 6, and deaths soon followed. By September more than half of the population of forty-seven thousand had fled the city. As he treated patients, Atwater wrote to William and his Bellevue colleagues about the epidemic and counseled that good nursing rather than harsh medicines would bring patients through successfully. Gorgas and his friends were eager to go to Memphis to get firsthand experience, but medical school officials would not allow it, because they were not immune. When he heard that Atwater had contracted the disease, however, Gorgas defied his instructors and traveled with John Bowen to Memphis to help his friend.[35] By the time they arrived, however, the young doctor had died, and city authorities barred the students from entering Memphis and becoming victims rather than saviors. Nicholas Atwater would be Gorgas's first loss to the cruel disease.

### *Trouble at Home*

In Sewanee, Josiah, who had once chafed under the control of his military superiors, now had trouble with the University of the South board of trustees. He had risen to the position of vice-chancellor, but after several disagreements the board decided that a cleric should lead the Episcopal university, a policy that made Josiah ineligible. To the family's great relief, Josiah soon found a new position as president of the University of Alabama at Tuscaloosa. In early September, while yellow fever still stalked the Mississippi Valley, Josiah arrived in Tuscaloosa to begin the new job. But within a week he sent a troubling message to Amelia. "I don't feel quite right about the head, in the place where the brain ought to be."[36] Unless he recovered, he told Amelia, "I doubt my ability to remain here and we may have to look for a house elsewhere and support ourselves the best we can."[37] The $500 they sent William for the year drained their funds. Josiah told Amelia that they would have to practice economy "until Willie is off our hands. You see $500 is a large hole in our salary. But we must not grudge it to him."[38] Yet in December 1878, along with a "a small Christmas check," Josiah told his son that he still opposed an army career for him. "I want you to accomplish more in life than I did."[39] He figured an army position would pay $1,000 a year, but a private medical practice in New York would carry a salary of $1,200. Amelia meanwhile pressured William to move closer to his father. "I made up my mind that you must settle some where near him."[40] William did not defy his parents outright but kept to his own course.

In February 1879 Gorgas received a tear-stained letter from Amelia saying that Josiah had suffered a severe stroke and was partially paralyzed. Their doctor said he would recover, but the future was uncertain.[41] She feared that Josiah would have to resign, and they would have to sell the house in Sewanee for funds. Writing to "My own darling big Dr. Boy," she described Josiah's frustration. "Yesterday he drew me down to him and said 'my poor darling, what will become of you if I do not recover' and for a moment was completely overcome." The pressure on William to succeed increased, for as Amelia told him, "Do what is best for your future, because your old Mother and Father may be your dependents."[42] A reprieve from disaster came when the University of Alabama Board of Trustees made Josiah the university librarian with a $400 annual salary, hired Amelia as hospital matron, and allowed the family to continue to live on campus rent-free.[43] Throughout these events William corresponded with Jessie, his closest sister, with optimism possible only through his distance from the family's woes. "As you say misfortunes seem at present to be falling on our family thick and fast," he wrote, but assured her that "having to take care of yourselves will be at first pretty hard on you girls and Mother, but with Mother's cheerful disposition and energy I feel quite confident that all difficulties will soon disappear."[44]

After he graduated from medical school in June 1879, William did help by contributing to his own support. Still intent on a military career, he turned down a chance to go to China as a physician with a Presbyterian missionary hospital.[45] Instead he won an internship at Bellevue Hospital, where he worked with William Welch and gained experience that would help him secure an army commission. Working in Welch's laboratory, however, Gorgas had difficulty in distinguishing among some of the bacteria on the specimen slides because he saw reds as grays. This meant he had red blindness, or color blindness, and, to William's shock, could not pursue laboratory science, because much of the work depended

Map 2.1. William Gorgas's United States. Cities and towns where he lived and army installations to which he was assigned.

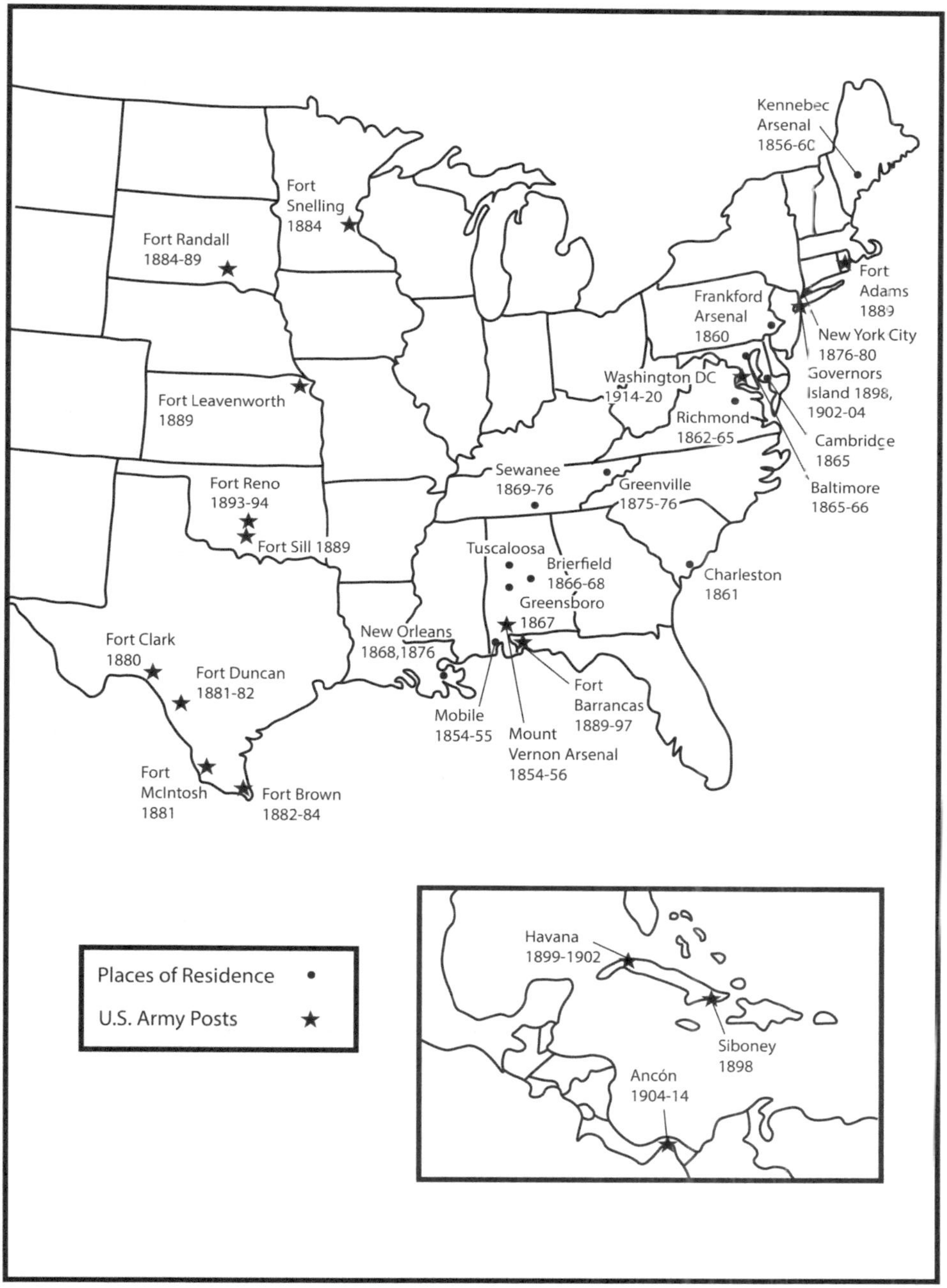

on seeing the colors of tissues.[46] Gorgas found another intern position on the staff at the City Insane Asylum on Blackwell's Island (now Roosevelt Island), just north of Bellevue Hospital. It paid no salary but gave him practical experience and room and board.[47] The asylum was a frightening place, though, in an era before the professionalization of psychiatry or psychology, and housed several hundred mentally ill patients, hiding them from the world. (Reform would not come until journalist Nellie Bly visited Blackwell's, and her 1887 exposé, "Ten Days in a Mad-House," spurred action.[48]) Amelia had not liked her son living at the asylum and was glad when he moved his lodgings to a seminary.[49]

## LIEUTENANT GORGAS

After graduation William immediately began to study for the Army Medical Corps qualifying examinations, while Josiah continued to caution, "It is not in the army that the sphere of a doctor is ennobling."[50] But William was not studying medicine to be a physician but to get into the army and a life outdoors. It would not be easy, though, because in the 1880s, the Army Medical Corps was at the forefront of the profession and held high standards for medical education and skill. Its qualifying examinations were among the most rigorous in the country. Medical officer candidates sat for five hours a day for six days: three days of general examination in fields including Latin, French, and German, mathematics, history, English and American literature, followed by another three days of written, oral, and practical exams on professional subjects such as medicine, chemistry, and physics.[51] But with his excellent preparation, in June 1880 Gorgas passed the qualifying exams in his first try and joined the ranks of the Army Medical Corps.

With his commission as a first lieutenant and assistant surgeon, Gorgas earned a salary of $133 a month, almost $1,600 a year, or just under $43,000 in 2021 dollars.[52] Despite Josiah's concerns, Army compensation was comparable to civil practice, allowing William to begin a lifelong practice of sending money home. The War Department also permitted medical officers to pursue private practice to supplement their income, both to keep them busy during the quiet times in the isolated posts and to serve the civilian population in a region. Gorgas embraced this practice for the income and soon learned that he loved caring for patients. Years later, after his successful military career, he still often went by the title "Dr. Gorgas."

The army that William joined was dramatically different from the Civil War armies of his youth. Congress had reduced national army strength from more than two million during the war to only 26,000 regular troops dispersed among far-flung posts on the frontier. With only 192 doctor positions in 1882, Medical Corps officers had to move from post to post to cover the health needs of the troops. The army supplemented the skeletal Medical Corps with about a hundred contract surgeons, physicians who had not taken the Medical Corps examinations and did not have commissions but were graduates of reputable medical schools and had passed qualifying examinations.

The horror of the Civil War, with its new rifling weapons, powerful artillery, and deadly diseases, had spurred the Army Medical Department to the forefront of American medicine. Medical officers gained experience and knowledge in the face of more than one million casualties—an estimated 750,000 deaths and 400,000 wounded. Yet some advances emerged amid the destruction. Appalled by the practice of leaving the sick and wounded on the battlefield for hours or days, medical officer Jonathan Letterman developed an army medical transport system of litter-bearers and ambulances to get the men more quickly to shelter, treatment, and possible survival. The Medical Department also established an Army Medical Museum to collect and study anatomical specimens from the dead and injured, and after the war produced the *Medical and Surgical History of the War of the Rebellion*, a comprehensive six-volume work published between 1870 and 1888. The project detailed thousands of surgical and medical cases with hundreds of charts, tables, and color illustrations of wounds, pathological specimens, and instrumentation, and represented the state of the art in American medicine. The Surgeon General's Library soon became the largest medical library in the country and the precursor to today's National Library of Medicine in Bethesda, Maryland.[53] This new knowledge would inform the practice of medicine by Gorgas and his colleagues in the 1880s.

In the first eighteen years of his military service during the waning years of the Indian wars, Gorgas was assigned to army posts across the West and the South. He was never engaged in military combat, however, and did not mention any such conflicts in his letters home. He was first deployed to forts in Texas: in 1880 to Fort Clark, in 1881 to Forts McIntosh and Duncan, and then in 1882 to Fort Brown, on the border with Mexico. "I am ambling over the plains of Texas at the head of my gallant column," he wrote Dick. But instead of regaling his brother with war stories, he sent game reports. As the troops traveled, they killed deer, partridge, and rabbits to supply the command. Setting up the camp, the men cooked their game and listened to howling wolves, and "all the officers would collect around the campfires and smoke and tell long yarns."[54]

As a military officer, Gorgas lived in a stratified community, a member of an officer corps of well-educated white men who enjoyed a better standard of living than enlisted men. The latter, most of them poor, many of them immigrants, some Native American "Indian scouts," and African Americans assigned to racially segregated units, earned only thirteen dollars a month.[55] Officers, with monthly salaries of more than one hundred dollars, also enjoyed decent housing, better rations, forage for two horses, travel accommodations, and one or two servants.[56] Gorgas enjoyed his comforts and told Dick that he and other officers lived "like fighting cocks," hunting, fishing, playing cards, and riding horseback. He could buy Parisian socks and high-quality liquors and cigars but joked that Dick should not be too impressed with his military status, because "it would be disagreeable to have one's brother saying 'yes sir' and 'no sir' and standing at attention."[57] William also failed to send home one of his monthly checks, because "one of my creditors unexpectedly dunned me and I have to pay up."[58]

V. H. Bridgman, an army engineer with Gorgas at Fort Clark, remembered that his colleague admired the good horsemanship, dancing skills, and discipline of West Point graduates and at times spoke of his regret in not having attended the academy. Gorgas, he found, was also more modest, less vain than other southerners he knew. He later told Marie, "Here to me was an anomaly; from a far southern state, Alabama, blind to self, inclined to exaggerate the importance of the other fellows." In addition to long yarns, officers often discuss politics and economics, and Bridgman was especially impressed by Gorgas's "acute sympathy for the unhappy and his desire to do something for them." Bridgman also remembered how Gorgas spoke so earnestly of wanting to learn how to dance that he began to give him lessons, whistling for music. The instruction, Bridgman said, continued until Gorgas was ordered to another post.[59] Gorgas continued practicing, but at one dance, he told Dick, "None of the ladies whom I met could speak English and I could speak no Spanish so communication is limited to a smile on your partner's part when you speak or step on her toes."[60]

That was not the young officer's only social setback. At one Texas fort, his pride was tested when Gen. William Tecumseh Sherman of the Union's "March Across Georgia" and now commanding general of the army, came to inspect their post. Gorgas was known for his mint juleps and, when asked to make one for the general, gladly prepared the drink. He gave it to Sherman, who took a big sip and then spat it out over the table and floor. Turning to Gorgas, the general barked, "Young man, are you from Georgia? Don't you know the war is over?" Gorgas, faint with embarrassment, replied, "No sir, I am from Alabama." Wiping his mouth, the general said, "Well, that is almost as bad." Gorgas in his nervousness had "sweetened" the julep with salt.[61]

After Josiah suffered the major stroke, William began to assume a fatherly role with Dick, age sixteen, assuring him that the family would provide money for his college education and advising that he would soon have to choose a path in life. "Some profession, law or medicine or anything that strikes your fancy," he counseled his brother. While business would be the only path to wealth, William would like to see Dick at West Point but added, "I believe that every man should follow his own tastes where he has any decided likes or dislikes." He also hoped Dick would wed, to carry on the name of Gorgas, because "if we should both go into the army I am afraid we would both have to die old bachelors."[62] But now William, happily an army medical officer and eager for what life held, would himself find a partner, a wife, with whom to share his life.

# CHAPTER 3

# Love in the Time of Yellow Fever

I spend a great deal of time that ought to be otherwise applied, just castle-building, always with you as the central figure.

—William Gorgas to Marie Doughty, January 16, 1884

William Gorgas's future niece, Aileen Lyster, fondly remembered Fort Brown in south Texas. They could swim, eat oysters, fish in the gulf, go to Padre Island, or cross the Rio Grande in a rowboat to Mexico and take the streetcar to the town of Matamoros. The streets there were narrow, and the houses had barred windows that made them look like jails, but a peek through an open door revealed courtyards full of flowers. Aileen liked to go to the opera in Matamoros, where the women wore veils and the men sported sombreros and high-heeled, pointed-toe boots. Between acts, she remembered, "the señoritas go out into the corridors and smoke cigarettes with the gentlemen. The most elegant ladies do it." The last sentence of Aileen's memoir simply stated, "While we were there, we had the yellow fever."[1]

When fever appeared in Matamoros in the summer of 1882, the medical director of the army's Southern Department went to Fort Brown to determine whether it was dengue, "break-bone" fever, or yellow fever. When he found it to be the latter, he imposed a quarantine and moved the Nineteenth Infantry fourteen miles up the Rio Grande to the town of Yturria to avoid contagion. He also sent additional medical staff to the camp, telling the commander, "I am sending you the most progressive young surgeon under my command."[2] It was William Gorgas. Thus began the most consequential experience in the young medical officer's life, for at Fort Brown he would gain immunity to yellow fever, and he would find love—both of which lasted a lifetime.

## FEVER AT FORT BROWN

Marie Cook Doughty of Cincinnati, Ohio, was visiting Aileen Lyster's parents, her older sister Martha ("Mattie") and brother-in-law, William Lyster, an infantry officer stationed at Fort Brown. Marie was the youngest of the eight children of William and Martha Doughty. Her father had a publishing business and was active in the Methodist Church.[3] Educated in Cincinnati public schools, Marie planned to go to college but, when her father died, traveled to Fort Brown to be with her sister.[4] On August 11, 1882, she was riding horseback with another woman at the fort when Captain Hewitt of the Nineteenth Infantry rode up to them with another man. They had a "spirited horse and smart trap from the post. By his side was seated a strange young officer about whose identity we girls were most curious."[5] Instead of introducing themselves, however, to the women's great indignation, the men just rode off. That may have been the first and last time William Gorgas was rude to Marie Doughty.

Gorgas thought his new post was the prettiest he had seen, but he told Jessie, "I had considerable difficulty in getting in as they had quarantined in every direction." Before he departed from Fort Duncan, his colleagues "looked upon me as a lamb sent to be slaughtered," and gave him all kinds of medicine for yellow fever, as well as whiskey, brandy, and cigars. "We left with flying colors," he reported, traveling by ambulance with two other medical officers. After they talked their way into Fort Brown, they found there were about a hundred cases in nearby Brownsville, but only two cases of yellow fever among the troops; one soldier had died, and the other was recovering.[6]

Fort Brown officers had orders not to visit the yellow fever ward if they were not immune. Gorgas, however, went straight to the autopsy room to dissect the yellow fever victim. When his superior officer arrived, Gorgas greeted him with, "Good morning, Capt.! Will you come in?"[7] It then fell to his roommate, Lt. Enoch Crowder (later the army's leading lawyer, the judge advocate general, from 1911 to 1923), to arrest the possibly contaminated and clearly insubordinate Gorgas and take him to quarters in the infected part of the garrison.[8] There he moved into rooms next to those occupied by the Lyster family. When William arrived, the Lysters were talking in the cool evening darkness of the porch. In echoes of Gorgas's parents' first encounter during the 1853 epidemic, Marie wrote, "I could not see the young officer's features distinctly, but I was pleasantly impressed by the musical tones of his voice and his soft southern accent." There were no further interactions until September 5, when Marie developed chills and a fever, and Mattie sent for Dr. Gorgas, now released from arrest due to the medical emergency. "I saw his face distinctly for the first time about 4 o'clock in the morning," Marie wrote.

"Col. Lyster was fanning me and my sister relates that no sooner had Dr. Gorgas entered the room than I, taking the fan from my brother, handed it to the doctor, saying you fan me. I have no recollection of this."[9] William later told her he said he was happy to continue fanning her, but, "you did not seem to care a snip whether it was Col. Lyster or I." He had just been glad to be of service. "I thought when I left you that day that it would be the last I should see you. I little knew then, how important a matter it was for me."[10]

Marie was deathly ill, vomiting dark blood, indicating that the virus was attacking her internal organs. The situation was so grim that soldiers had already dug her grave, and someone had asked Gorgas to read the Bible at her burial service. He was willing, but, Marie wrote, "To the amazement of all, I began to recover." Due to the severity of her case, including "heart complications," she was unable to sit up for two weeks.[11] Believing the disease was spread by air currents, the Lyster family carefully watched the garrison flag to see which way the wind was blowing so they could escape the bad air. Soon, however, nine out of ten of them, including the Mexican cook, came down with fever.[12] Gorgas tended them all, insisting on bed rest, careful nursing, and forbearance regarding the use of purges. Marie's nephew, Theodore Lyster, age seven at the time, credited Gorgas with saving his life, and grew to become a leading ear, nose, and throat physician and a pioneer in aviation medicine during World War I. He later wrote that he and Gorgas witnessed so many yellow fever epidemics over the years that they later realized that "we were more than fortunate not to have had a death among our family cases."[13]

Gorgas soon joined the sick rolls. On October 4 a colleague sent a telegram to their supervisor advising: "Dr. Gorgas taken down today with the fever case, rather serious."[14] He was sick enough to be off duty from October 4 to November 11, but not as sick as Marie and apparently had no lasting health effects. Now Marie, age twenty, and William, age twenty-eight, recuperated together. The isolation of quarantine nourished their relationship, because no one could enter or leave the camp, and there was little to do except get well. A nurse in the camp dubbed William "Gorgeous Doctor" and encouraged the couple by decorating his meal tray with a rose and telling him that Marie had put it there. Knowing that she was sensitive to the pronunciation of her name "Doughty," Gorgas sent his thank-you notes addressed to "Miss Tea and Toast," which pleased Marie. "Our little romance blossomed, though slowly," she wrote.[15]

The case mortality rate for Brownsville in 1882 was a terrifying 25 percent, and worsening the misery the Rio Grande flooded. The river left Fort Brown an island and flooded the cemetery, making it reachable only by boat.[16] One of William and Marie's early and memorable outings was when he rowed them out to the cemetery to what was to have been her grave but was now occupied by another young woman who had died.[17] Twenty-three years later Marie would tell a reporter their Fort Brown yellow fever story and how she "had the unique distinction of looking into her own grave after her recovery."[18]

William was so shy that Mattie noticed his interest in her sister before Marie did. When he brought them a gunnysack of apples, which were quite precious at the time, Mattie told Marie, "It is true, he doesn't seem to have much to say to you, but he looks at you all the time. And then – those apples!"[19] Marie was smitten as well, for she later conjured up a lovely portrait of Will, as she called him, as a young man. "Tall, slender, agile, extremely athletic, the saving grace of his baseball team, a swimmer who already had more than one saved life to his credit, a devotee of the rod and the gun, and an adroit horseman." She also remembered his dark hair, ruddy skin, and oval face. "His eyes too, quiet and twinkling, radiated the mildness and the gentleness which had made his mother so popular and influential." And there was his voice. "He possessed also his mother's soft cadences; he invariably talked in subdued tones; he seldom showed excitement, yet the persistence and determination that afterward became his most conspicuous qualities were already familiar facts to his close associates."[20]

By mid-November the cold weather had come, the epidemic waned, and Gorgas was back on duty, preparing for the return of the troops from Yturria and disinfecting everything at the camp to rid it of yellow fever contamination. At a dance to celebrate the return of the troops, Marie learned that despite his best efforts, William was not a good dancer and preferred to talk about politics and philosophy, in particular political economist Henry George's proposals to address poverty and Herbert Spencer's views on social Darwinism and "survival of the fittest." These topics were new to her, so the conversations were rather one-sided. "I listened," she admitted, "much mystified in my mind as to whether Herbert Spencer was the Spencer who wrote the 'Faerie Queene.'"[21] Gorgas stayed on at Fort Brown as post surgeon, and when Marie and the Lysters moved to Fort Clark up the Rio Grande, would ride the distance to see her. Captain Lyster had fought for the North during the war in such epic battles as Chickamauga and Sherman's March to the Sea, yet he and William discussed military history for hours with no sign of enmity. Marie played the piano and they sang, but the romance was slow to kindle. "He enjoyed this as far as it went," she wrote, but "there was no engagement."[22]

## COURTSHIP

In 1883, just months after he met Marie, William lost his father. Josiah suffered another debilitating stroke on May 4 or 5 and lingered on morphine until he died on May 15, with Amelia and his doctor at his bedside. William was at first unaware of these events; a letter to Marie dated May 9 indicates that he did not yet know about Josiah's final stroke. Amelia blamed the war's four years of strain and anxiety, and "the bitter disappointment of defeat [which] broke down his strong constitution and rendered him less able to bear the troubles of his life."[23] Reading over the letters Josiah sent to her over the years, she told William, "His love was so true and faithful that I feel almost humiliated to have been its object and to have inspired such feelings so noble in another."[24] William took leave in late May to go home to mourn and comfort his family.[25]

With his parents' model for love, Gorgas pursued his own. He was an earnest correspondent but felt the distance from Marie. "I am conscious of many disadvantages under which I labor in winning the place I wish in your esteem," he wrote. "Words are a poor means of expression or of winning regard. I think if I could be thrown with you from day to day and have you appreciate how dear you have become to me, it would be something in my favor." He did not want to be too forward but confessed, "The greatest object I have just now is to stand well with you." One of the first declarations of affection came from his dog, Duro. William wrote, "I know he wishes to send you his best love."[26]

William and Marie kept their letters light, often sharing news of their social activities. William told Marie of seeing a bullfight in Matamoros and attending festivals in Mexico, and reported on a picnic with friends, disclosing the less-than-charming detail that they all got "plenty of ticks."[27] William liked to share his doctoring experiences with Marie and at one point complained about mothers constantly consulting him about their babies' teething. He observed that mothers wanted their doctor to "express an opinion," about each tooth as it emerged, but "when you have six or seven babies to say something remarkable about every morning, you can well understand how a man of ordinary fluency is put to it to find an appropriate expression for his surprise and admiration at the particular developments of each individual baby." Wickedly, he told her, "I vaccinated them all the other day, thinking it might afford me some revenge."[28] After a trip to New York City, he reported to Marie that he and Crowder had done some shopping for Molly, the Black woman who cooked for them at Fort Brown. She had been saving money for a special gown and, when she heard that they were going to New York, asked them to buy one for her in black silk. After consulting another officer's wife, they got Molly's measurements and brought back a dress from the upscale store B. Altman and Company in New York. Satisfied, Molly wore the dress on Sundays and holidays.[29]

But William's romance languished. As he confided in Jessie, "I take it there is a wide gulf between being in love and getting married." Matrimony was "out of the question," though, for the time, "first and foremost because the young lady has not yet been brought to appreciate the many good qualities of your brother or does not desire to possess them." He also felt he could not afford to marry until he had increased rank and salary.[30] William courted Marie with flowers ($1.37), and a ring ($13.80).[31] He also tried to get transferred to the East to be closer to her, asking, "Will that please you?"[32]

Knowing that her son had found the woman he loved, Amelia nudged him toward matrimony. In 1884 William had malaria so severely that Amelia contemplated going to Texas to nurse him. She warned, "I want you to marry and have a good wife to take care of you, for you are not the sort of man to do it for yourself."[33] Therefore, when Marie took a job as governess for a family in Alabama, Amelia invited her to Tuscaloosa without consulting William. She then encouraged him to join them and explained that while she had not met Marie, she was sure to find her "a most sweet and attractive young woman."[34] Marie was surprised and embarrassed when William met her train in Tuscaloosa (with a sister and brother in tow), but she was charmed when she met Amelia on the portico of their home. "She captured in one second the obdurate heart that had withstood for two years the siege of her handsome son," Marie later wrote. Amelia suggested that the couple walk down to the river, and there, sitting on a fallen tree on the banks of the old Black Warrior River, William proposed. Marie always gave Amelia great credit for their engagement.

That October 1884, from his new post at Fort Randall in Dakota Territory, when he turned thirty years old, the now-engaged William told his mother that he felt like a sedate middle-aged gentleman and hoped to be married by his next birthday.[35] He asked Amelia to invite Marie and her mother to Tuscaloosa for Christmas so Mrs. Doughty could meet the family.[36] Months later, when they had still not set a wedding date, however, Amelia asked William what the problem was. It should not be finances, she said; even with what he sent them monthly, he earned enough to support a wife. And, she added, "Neither you or Marie are growing any younger."[37]

The next month William told Jessie his plans. When he was promoted to captain in June, increasing his annual salary from $1,600 to $2,200, he would request two months' leave so that Marie could set a September wedding date.[38] He had been worried that she would want a "swell wedding" but happily told Ria, "We will be married quietly from her brother's house. This is greatly to my liking."[39] Thus, on September 15, 1885, William and Marie were married in Cincinnati. Marie later told Mattie that she would always be grateful to Mattie's husband, William Lyster, because he had lectured her on the importance of marrying for love. "Bless his dear old heart!" she wrote. "I am glad I listened to his advice." She added, "I have always been more or less in love with Dr. Gorgas."[40] She would later credit another, writing, "It would be untrue to say that Yellow Jack was the best man at our wedding—but it would be perfectly true to say that in a sense he was an usher."[41]

## MARRIED LIFE ON THE FRONTIER

Having met on the southern border, William and Marie began married life on the northern plains. After a visit to Tuscaloosa, the newlyweds arrived at Fort Randall, in October 1885.[42] They were among the last generation of army families posted on the American "frontier," and over the next thirteen years they lived at Fort Randall, Dakota Territory (1885 to 1889), and then went south to Fort Barrancas near Pensacola Bay, Florida (1889 to 1898), interrupted by a stint at Fort Reno, Oklahoma Territory (1893 to 1894). During the 1880s special orders also sent William to posts as far east as Fort Adams, Rhode Island, and north to Fort Snelling, Minnesota, as well as to Fort Leavenworth, Kansas, and Fort Sill, Oklahoma Territory in the plains.[43] Fort Randall, established in 1856, was one of more than a dozen forts built in the northern plains during the Indian wars to "pacify" the Sioux who lived there and provide protection for westward-bound pioneers and settlers—to, in essence, extend European civilization across the continent. By the time William and Marie arrived, tensions with local native peoples had diminished—in large part because most of them had been driven off their land and confined in reservations—and army troops were responsible more for police work than Indian fighting. Fort Randall had become quite domesticated, with a school, a church, an amateur theater group, and dances, but would be abandoned when the land was opened for settlement in 1892.[44]

Gorgas was happier in the West than Marie was. He loved life in the army and retained his admiration of West Point, often turning the conversation to the military academy and military heroes. He had little interest in heavy drinking and gambling but enjoyed hunting and fishing around the post, and riding his horse Traveler (who had the same name as General Lee's horse!) or Mollie, his parents' horse, whom he had adopted when Amelia could no longer afford her.[45] Gorgas told a colleague that the winters at Randall were "excessively cold" but that in the fall the climate was perfect. "If it were not for the fact that Marie suffered so much there I would like my next tour at Randall if I have to go to a cold climate at all."[46]

Marie found life on the army post isolating and made no secret of her unhappiness. Fort Randall stood on a bluff overlooking the Missouri River, a strategic position from which to watch for Indian attacks, but was seventy-five miles from the railroad and surrounded by prairie. "No neighbors, except for a few red men and half breeds," Marie wrote in the racist language of the time. Except for extended visits from family, and some "cultivated and entertaining colleagues," she found little society. "Cities, towns, diversified society, theaters, clubs, libraries, and the like—formed no part of this existence." Post life was a routine of dinner parties and "listening to the same stories, laughing at the same jokes," she wrote. Card parties, however, were entertaining, while "the affable quarrels of such a small society added a little spice, and a faint whiff of scandal came as an occasional godsend."[47]

William and Marie saw improvements in army life during their time on the frontier. Some of it was simply due to the consolidation of garrisons as the Indian Wars wound down from 175 posts in 1870 to 80 in 1894, leaving the remaining posts larger and better supplied. As railroads, manufacturing, and the timber and mining industries offered new employment opportunities for young men, Congress had to make army life more attractive to compete. It therefore passed reforms to encourage enlistment and retention and to counter problems with desertion, alcoholism, and general misconduct. It also created a retirement program for soldiers with thirty years' service and even legislated an increase in the vegetable ration for enlisted men.[48]

## FRONTIER MEDICINE

Marie later wrote that while her husband was working in isolated and desolate army posts, "the science of medicine was still in the dark ages." But, she continued, "When he emerged as a commanding figure in 1900, medicine had developed into a mighty force, destined to become more powerful than armies or navies for statecraft in directing the course of the world."[49] The years from 1880 to 1900 did witness some of the most dramatic changes in the history of medicine, but William Gorgas was not a passive observer. He had studied with the leaders in medicine, and when new surgical techniques, medical tools, and sanitation methods became available, he put them into practice. Physicians became able to distinguish between lung ailments such as tuberculosis and lung cancer, or between typhoid and malaria fevers, and scientists identified the pathogens causing tuberculosis, cholera, leprosy, surgical infections, tetanus, typhoid fever, malaria, amoebic dysentery, and diphtheria. This knowledge enabled them to develop specific treatments and interventions, launching the medical profession into a new era of effectiveness and prestige. The Medical Department was building one of the best medical libraries and museums in the world, and medical officers kept up with developments through journals such as the *Journal of the American Medical Association*, the British *Lancet*, and the *Journal of Experimental Medicine*, and in 1891 the Association of Military Surgeons of the United States began to publish its annual meetings transactions, a publication which became by 1907 the monthly journal *Military Surgeon*.[50]

Each army fort kept a medical log, and post surgeons submitted detailed monthly reports—what amounted to a public health report for the army installation—to the commanding officer.[51] Categories included the sanitary conditions of the buildings and grounds, the quality of the water supply and the food and its preparation, the sufficiency and suitability of clothing for the weather, and whether the men's habits were "good," that is, not too much drinking or fighting. Officers also reported epidemics or injuries of interest and made recommendations for improvements. In 1885 Gorgas recommended more blankets for prisoners at Fort Randall and that the guard house be enlarged to alleviate crowding. The suggestion was apparently ignored, because he reiterated it the following year. In 1887 Gorgas recommended that laundry workers be given more privies, because there was only a one-hole privy for six families.[52] When in 1890 he traced the source of twenty-nine cases of typhoid fever to the most popular well at Fort Reno, he worried that people there would resist abandoning a source of water they found "clear, cool, and palatable."[53] He was learning that a good sanitarian had to be adept at public education and politics as well as medical science and needed to explain to post residents the dangers of infection in order to shut down the well.

In 1884 Congress passed legislation authorizing medical officers to provide medical care to the families of service members, army retirees, and people in the community if it did not interfere with regular duties. Gorgas kept ledgers of his medical work and had a true general practice, treating all kinds of maladies and accidents.[54] He lanced boils, removed tumors, set broken bones, treated the scrapes and cuts of people thrown from horses and wagons, and fixed up a laborer who "struck himself with axe on right temple."[55] Gorgas cared for pregnant women and delivered their babies. He treated patients with measles, mumps, tuberculosis, typhoid, cholera, syphilis, alcoholism, and hemorrhoids, and an Indian child with whooping cough. He gave quinine for fevers and bad colds, and opium for cramps, and applied Vaseline to sore eyelids. Gorgas also practiced dentistry on the frontier, including tooth extractions. "I flatter myself that I became exceedingly skillful in this," he once told a group of dentists.[56] At Fort Randall his patients included members of a local Indian nation, the Lakota, and Marie passed many winter nights alone as he rode out on patient calls. At times the temperature could be thirty below zero when Gorgas, clad in buffalo robes and earmuffs, ventured out. Once he lost his way home and almost died in a blizzard.[57]

If Gorgas did not experience combat in the army, he surely saw pain and suffering. One of his first deaths as a medical officer was that of Pvt. Thomas Pratt, of the Twenty-Second Infantry, who arrived at Fort Duncan in August 1881, weak and with a temperature of 103 degrees. Gorgas put him to bed on a liquid diet and quinine. Pratt seemed to improve, but three weeks later Gorgas "found him suffering profoundly from shock. Cold at the extremities, pulseless, anxious face, delirious." Pratt died within the hour. Mystified by the deadly turn, Gorgas did an autopsy. In the absence of the internal imaging and diagnostic tests of modern medicine, physicians often conducted autopsies to learn how internal lesions or other damage compared with the symptoms they observed in living patients. In this case Gorgas found a perforated intestine and internal bleeding, indicative of typhoid.[58]

Marie admired her husband's skill and demeanor as a doctor, writing that he "rapidly developed the rare medical virtue of feeling, and showing that he felt a deep personal interest in every patient and had an uncommonly intimate knowledge of and sympathy for others' personal troubles."[59] She also noted that he was an "advocate and believer" in the use of animals in scientific research—medical officers, like other scientists, had guinea pigs, rabbits, and other animals in their laboratories that they used for various experiments.[60] But Gorgas also had a great fondness for animals, especially horses and dogs. In 1895 he kept a complete medical record for Old Scout, "one of the best dogs I ever knew." When Scout became ill, Gorgas tried to treat him, even operating at one point, seeking a tumor or blockage to explain the dog's illness. After Scout died Gorgas conducted a necropsy and found that his kidneys had failed.[61]

Gorgas paid great attention to Marie's medical needs. She suffered gastrointestinal problems for much of her life, perhaps due to the damage yellow fever waged on her internal organs, and he would mention in letters to his family that Marie had her "old dysenteric trouble."[62] He also worried about the effect pregnancy would have on her heart. According to biographer Robin Lampson, Marie first became pregnant in early 1886 at Fort Randall and had a baby boy who lived only a few hours. She almost died after the birth and was bedridden for several months. The couple did try again, though, and had another baby on September 10, 1889. William took leave to accompany Marie to his mother's home in Tuscaloosa for the birth of their daughter.[63] They named her Aileen Lyster Gorgas, in honor of Marie's sister Mattie's daughter and husband. With dark eyes and black, curly hair, Aileen "so closely resembled her father—in particular she had his dark eyes—that she was known on the post as "Little Doctor." Marie told Mattie, "I don't think very young babies are pretty but this baby is as good looking certainly as the majority." She added that Will was "sitting by me, holding baby on a pillow on his lap and after all his talk of discipline is doing his level best from the start to spoil her."[64] It took Marie weeks to recover from the birth, and she and William did not have any more children.

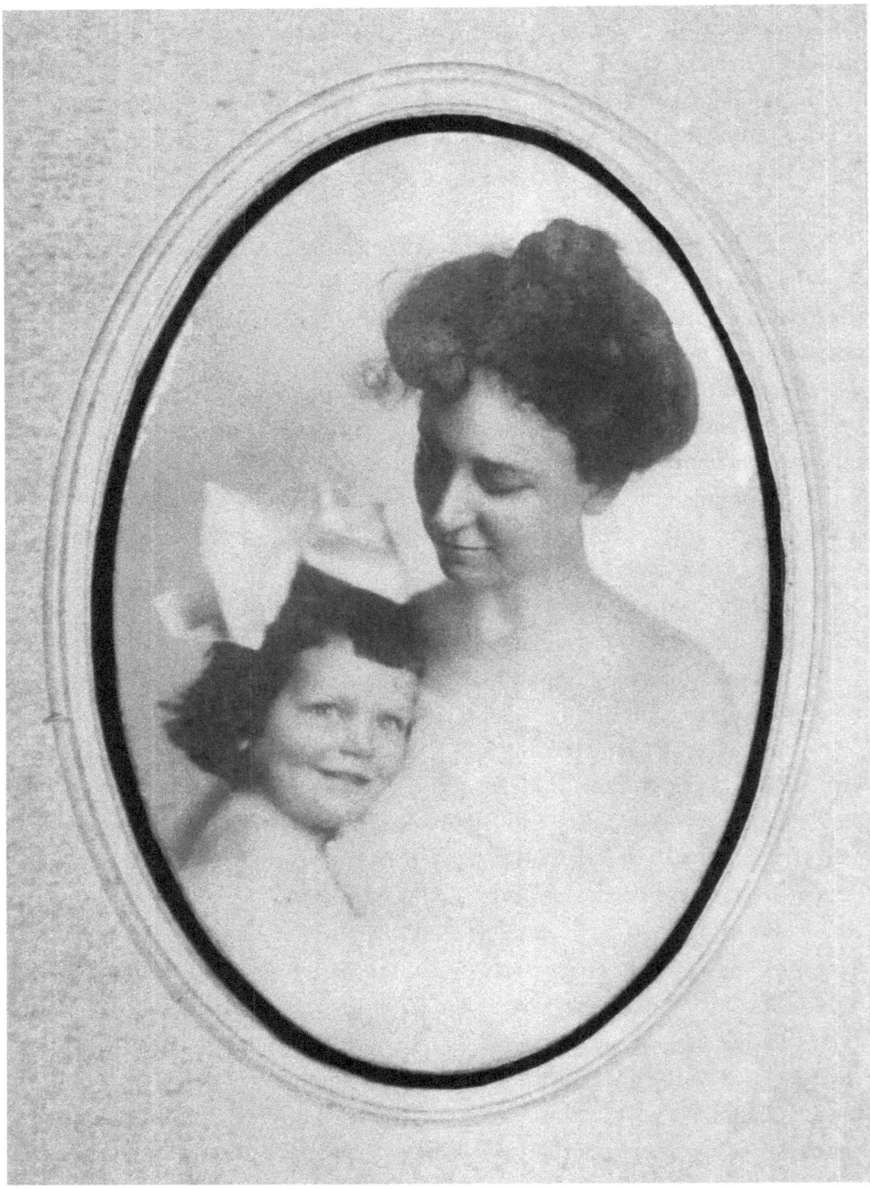

FIGURE 3.1. Marie and Aileen, c. 1891. Library of Congress Prints and Photographs Division.

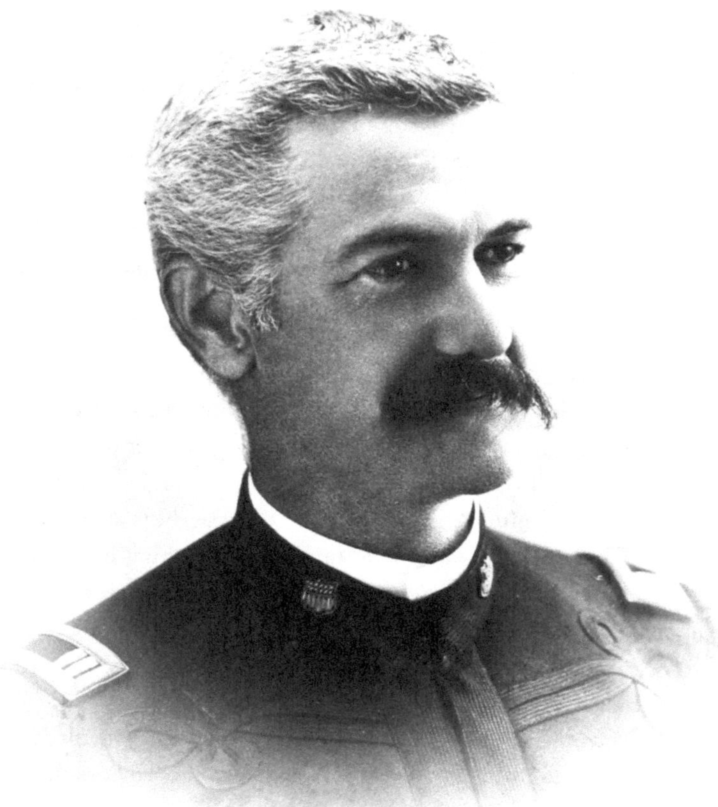

FIGURE 3.2. Captain William C. Gorgas, MC, age thirty-nine, at Fort Reno, Wyoming, 1893. Courtesy of the University of Alabama Libraries Special Collections.

## FORT BARRANCAS

As a medical officer, Gorgas was a general practitioner, but as a southerner he was especially interested in yellow fever epidemics, and his immunity to yellow fever caused the army to call upon him when a case was suspected at an army installation. Fort Barrancas, near the Port of Pensacola, was often exposed to yellow fever, so the surgeon general assigned him there in 1889. In Barrancas, Gorgas met John R. Ross, a US Navy surgeon who would become a lifelong friend. Ross and Gorgas were the first physicians in the area to employ antiseptic surgery, and together they cleared up myriad surgical problems that had accumulated among the civilian community. Many procedures were done without remuneration and involved the removal of benign tumors and long-standing sites of infection in people's bodies, including two amputations on people dying from infection, who then recovered.[65] Gorgas published his first medical article in 1891 on the surgical treatment for abdominal wounds.[66] He also sent some medical specimens to the Army Medical Museum, including the heart of a young man who died of a laudanum overdose, and the stomach of a woman who succumbed to a perforating ulcer.[67] Gorgas and Ross also oversaw the cleanup of weeds and underbrush and the drainage of pools of water around Fort Barrancas to enable salubrious breezes to reach the encampment, but the measure had the added advantage of eliminating mosquito habitat several years before the insects were discovered to be yellow fever perpetrators.[68]

Fort Barrancas was Gorgas's favorite post. It was just a train ride from his mother in Tuscaloosa and afforded him plenty of deep-sea fishing. As he told one colleague, "with a heavy rod and reel and a 21-strand line there is nothing in the world to equal it."[69] But he worried about Marie's health. If the winters in Fort Randall were too cold, the summers in Fort Barrancas were too hot, so when in September 1897 the Medical Department assigned Gorgas to be the attending surgeon for the army in New York, the couple was happy to move.

One of Marie's favorite stories about her husband at Barrancas involved Henrietta, an African American woman who did their laundry, and provides an example of Gorgas's soft touch with his patients. When Henrietta's legs were crushed in a train accident, she called for Gorgas to examine her, and when he advised that her legs needed to be amputated above the knee to save her life, she insisted that only he perform the operation.[70] The surgery went well, and Henrietta recovered, but she could not pay for the operation, and Gorgas paid for her artificial legs as well so that she could continue to earn a living. The next time he took his laundry to her, therefore, he was surprised that she had increased her prices. When he asked why, she explained that not just anyone could get his laundry done by a lady with wooden legs![71] V. H. Bridgman, who had been with Gorgas in Fort Clark, Texas, also served with him at Fort Barrancas and told another story of Gorgas's benignity. He attended the birth of the Bridgmans' baby and became the child's godfather, so they carefully heeded his advice. Gorgas, Bridgman said, had long counseled mothers to not pick up their babies when they cried, because it would encourage them to cry more often. One day their newborn was on the porch crying loudly, and when the crying suddenly ceased, they rushed to the porch, afraid their child been kidnapped or killed. Instead they found Dr. Gorgas with the infant in his arms.[72]

Another officer attested to Gorgas's bedside manner. Champe McCulloch succeeded Gorgas at Fort Barrancas and inherited his private practice. McCulloch's disparaging remarks about the people in Pensacola contrasted with Gorgas's gentler, more patrician approach. McCulloch called the patients "Florida crackers" and used racist language to describe the Black servants who worked for him. With no sense of irony or curiosity, he could not understand Gorgas's popularity. "I used to complain that the confounded people would rather die and be buried under Dr. Gorgas's care than get well under mine."[73]

## YELLOW FEVER, FORT BARRANCAS

Gorgas would soon rejoin McCulloch at Barrancas, because yellow fever outbreaks in towns along the Gulf Coast near Mobile, Alabama, threatened the fort and caused the commanding officer, Capt. Junius W. MacMurray, to seek Gorgas's advice.[74] Gorgas arrived on September 18 and over the next weeks reported to his superiors almost daily on the epidemic. The outbreak was remarkable enough that he published a report, and his description and analysis illustrate how public health officials had to maintain a delicate balance between public safety on one hand and panic and economic ruin on the other. Standard army practice was to move troops from an infected location, but that was expensive and time-consuming, and alarmed everyone involved. Now, Gorgas and MacMurray decided instead to monitor reports of yellow fever cases in the region, consult with the state health officials, and hope for an early frost. Unaware of the role of mosquitoes, Gorgas and others reasoned that "the actual freezing of water and formation of ice in the houses [was] supposed to kill every trace of yellow fever germs."[75] No cases appeared in the fort until an army private vomited blood and died, on November 14. Gorgas and MacMurray ordered the command to remove to the pine woods away from the coast, and when four more cases appeared, Gorgas called in immune male nurses to care for them.

Businessmen in Pensacola, fearful and angry that an epidemic could interfere with commerce, blamed the army for the outbreak, charging that soldiers had released the toxin when they tore down an old yellow fever hospital that summer.

MacMurray called on the War Department to counter the charges and defend the national government against what he saw as commercial avarice and local selfishness.[76] Meanwhile, Gorgas cared for the sick with the help of the immune nurses. Two nonimmune corpsmen volunteered to help him bury the victims. To prevent contagion, they wrapped each corpse in a white shroud and filled the grave with quicklime. Gorgas then read from the Bible at the head of the grave.[77] When frost finally arrived and halted the outbreak, it left only five cases and two deaths in its wake. Gorgas and MacMurray had averted a disaster. Gorgas wrote up commendations for the corpsmen who assisted him. Caring for yellow fever victims, he wrote, "requires as much courage and gallantry as in battle, and should be recognized in some way, just as acts of bravery in the field now are."[78]

Fighting yellow fever made Gorgas feel "useful." In his 1897 holiday letter home, he said that the years at Barrancas had been the happiest of his life, and "that is saying a good deal because I have had a pretty jolly good life of it."[79] He did not know that just weeks later the USS *Maine* would explode in Havana harbor, and his life would take a dramatic turn.

# PART II

# NEW PURPOSE, 1898–1904

# CHAPTER 4

## Trial by War and Disease, 1898

We would have both been buried in the same coffin.
The one the chaplain used for the public ceremony. . . .
It was the hardest worked coffin that I know of.
—William Gorgas to Theo Lyster, March 1915, describing events of 1898

GORGAS FOLLOWED THE NEWS, ESPECIALLY war news such as the ongoing civil war in Cuba, but like many Americans he was shocked when the USS *Maine* blew up in the Havana harbor on February 13, 1898, killing 268 American sailors and marines. The disaster set off a firestorm in the press against the villainy of Spain. In just a matter of weeks, under the pretense of securing the liberation of Cuba, "*Cuba Libre*," the United States entered the Spanish-American-Cuban War to protect its economic interests and domestic sugar industry, and to prevent yellow fever and other diseases from spreading to the mainland.[1] Now, instead of just reading the news, William Gorgas would witness it firsthand. Soon he would be on a hospital ship steaming to Cuba and a new yellow fever epidemic. This new venture would expose him to untold suffering and death, and test him as only war and disease can.

### DISEASE AND HISTORY

Deadly disease was intimately tied to the history of the Caribbean. As early as 1492, the "conquest" of the Americas was achieved less by superiority of arms than by the smallpox, measles, bubonic plague, and influenza pathogens that Spanish explorers and conquistadores brought with them.[2] Early explorers reported epidemics among the indigenous populations on every island they encountered. Gonzalo Fernández de Oviedo y Valdés, a Spanish soldier and historian who traveled with Columbus, observed a smallpox epidemic from 1518 to 1520 "so virulent that it left Hispaniola, Puerto Rico, Jamaica, and Cuba desolated of Indians." It seemed, he wrote, "a great judgement from heaven."[3] Historian David Cook has traced this collapse of the Amerindian population, writing that on "the islands of Hispaniola, Cuba, and Puerto Rico, for example—destruction was virtually complete."[4] In one of the best-documented cases, the population of the island of Hispaniola, what is now Haiti and Santo Domingo, plummeted from an estimated 500,000 to only 2,000 by the early 1500s.

Yellow fever came late to this devastation, with the first recorded cases in the Americas in the 1640s.[5] When the Spanish brought Africans to work the fields and mines on the depopulated islands, the slave ships introduced *Aedes aegypti* mosquitoes harboring the yellow fever virus. The disease so ravaged colonial populations—Amerindian, European, and African—that it became a factor in geopolitics. When the English seized Cuba from the Spanish in 1762, they were soon run off by fever and consequently returned the island to Spain in exchange for Florida (a yellow fever story Gorgas would often tell[6]). Napoleon had a similar experience when his army in Haiti and St. Dominique lost fewer than a hundred soldiers in suppressing a slave rebellion but then watched as fifty thousand troops succumbed to yellow fever and other diseases in 1802.

Revolutionary wars swept much of Latin America during the early nineteenth century, but Spain held on to Cuba by letting Cuban elites, sugar growers, and mill owners maintain control over workers and profits from sugar and tobacco in exchange for deference to Spain. By the mid-nineteenth century, Cuba was the world's largest sugar producer, sending much of it to its close neighbor, the United States. Afro-Cubans, however, continued to press for economic and political power, and restive Creole (Cuban-born) landowners rebelled against Spanish rule in a failed ten-year war, 1868 to 1878. By 1886, when Cuba finally abolished slavery, American businessmen were so invested in Cuban sugar and tobacco plantations that the United States was Cuba's largest trading partner.

Resistance to colonial rule, however, smoldered, and in 1895 Cuba's founding father, José Marti, led another rebellion against Spanish rule. Spain sent the ruthless general Valeriano Weyler, known as the "Butcher Weyler," to quell it. He led 100,000 troops to forcibly relocate 400,000 *campesinos*, or peasants, almost a third of the population, from their rural homes to urban camps to cut them off from the Cuban rebel army. Without adequate shelter, food, or water, at least 150,000 Cubans—9 percent of the population—died in those camps. In the chaos American landowners and business owners in Cuba sought military protection, and in January 1898 the US Navy moved ships, including the *Maine,* into Havana harbor to protect Americans in case the violence escalated.[7]

Many people in the United States were torn about their country assuming the role of a colonial power. Democrats, many of whom rejected government control in their own states, objected to an expansion of American power overseas, and white supremacists were loath to bring people of color into the national body politic. Imperialists and many Republicans, however, viewed the projection of American economic power overseas as vital to economic growth and military security. Some even dreamed of building a canal across Central America to facilitate global trade and military movement, and influence over Cuba as a gateway to the Caribbean was critical to this plan. A number of government officials also viewed Havana as a source of yellow fever infections in the United States, and imposing public health measures there such as a maritime quarantine would help them prevent epidemics while maintaining trade.[8]

After the sinking of the *Maine,* the issue of American involvement was no longer theoretical. The source of the explosion, whether internal or external to the ship, is still debated, but bellicose press coverage and an indignant Congress blamed the Spanish.[9] American papers, especially William Randolph Hearst's *New York Journal* and Joseph Pulitzer's *New York World,* urged the United States to retaliate against Spain and to "Remember the Maine." Congress passed legislation to increase the regular army's strength from 26,000 to 200,000 and pushed a reluctant President William McKinley to declare war on April 25, 1898. To appease anti-imperialists and ensure that the island's sugar would not compete with the US sugar beet crop, Congress added language to the war resolution stating that the United States would not annex Cuba. It also disclaimed any intention to exercise sovereignty over the island and promised that once pacification was achieved, the United States would "leave the government in control of the island to its people."[10] On the other side of the world, shortly after the United States declared war, US Navy vessels in the South Pacific moved to assist rebels in ousting Spain from the Philippines in hopes of advancing American interests in the region. In late April they quickly destroyed the Spanish fleet, and several weeks later US troops were marching on Manila.[11] Deployment took longer in the Caribbean. American troops planned to sail to Cuba and Puerto Rico, also in rebellion, in June. The timing, however, alarmed the army surgeon general.

## STERNBERG

Even before war was declared, George Miller Sternberg, the army surgeon general, sounded the alarm about the risks of deadly disease in the Caribbean. A leading bacteriologist, Sternberg knew what he was talking about.[12] Born in New York in 1838, he received his medical degree from the College of Physicians and Surgeons in New York City in 1860 and then served as a surgeon in the Union Army, earning commendations for his courage. After the war, during quiet times on army frontier posts, he conducted scientific experiments and became an expert in photomicroscopy, photographing the "germ" of tuberculosis in 1881 just months after it was identified by Robert Koch. A prodigious scholar, Sternberg wrote the first bacteriology textbook published in the United States, *A Manual of Bacteriology*.[13] When he was named army surgeon general in 1893, he already had extensive experience with yellow fever epidemics. He had even survived the disease in 1875 while posted at Fort Barrancas but lost so much weight that when he was reunited with his wife, Martha, she hardly recognized him. After the disastrous epidemic of 1878, the National Board of Health named Sternberg to its yellow fever commission and sent him to Havana to investigate the epidemic's origins. There he met leading scientists in the field, Cuban physicians Carlos Finlay and Juan Guiteras, beginning decades of cooperation.[14] Sternberg ultimately wrote more than forty papers on yellow fever.

Gorgas was delighted when Sternberg was named surgeon general. He had met him at Fort Barrancas and told his sister that the new surgeon general was "about the most fit that could have been selected."[15] Sternberg proved him right, quickly moving to professionalize and modernize the Medical Department and the Medical Corps, intent on making them the most advanced medical institutions in the country. He updated the hospital system, improved the dental services, designated specialized tuberculosis hospitals, and established an Army Medical School to train medical officers in modern bacteriology and laboratory science.

As the United States prepared for war in Cuba, Sternberg wrote an urgent memo to the secretary of war warning against a military campaign during the rainy summer months—yellow fever season. He reviewed the deadly history of the disease in Cuba, beginning with the epidemic of 1648, detailing death rates in Cuban ports and towns. Typhoid fever, malaria, dysentery, and parasitic diseases could also infect the troops, he cautioned.[16] Gen. Nelson Miles, the highest-ranking general in the army, supported Sternberg's recommendation to delay the invasion until the fall, but Secretary of War Russell Alger and President William McKinley overrode him.

US Army troops therefore sailed in early June from Tampa for Cuba, approaching the island from the south to avoid the Spanish stronghold at Havana. After a short battle, they captured Guantánamo Bay and landed troops at Daiquiri and Siboney. From there the famed "Rough Riders" commanded by Col. Leonard Wood and Theodore Roosevelt, the irrepressible and influential New Yorker and recent assistant secretary of the navy, planned their attack. On July 1 the Rough Riders and the "Buffalo Soldiers" of the Twenty-Fourth and Twenty-Fifth African American infantries charged the San Juan heights and drove the Spanish from the field of battle. Only ten days later the fighting was over, and the last American soldier died in combat. On July 16, after US naval ships defeated the Spanish fleet in the Santiago harbor, Spain agreed to unconditional surrender in Cuba. American troops then sailed to Puerto Rico and marched to San Juan virtually unopposed.

In defeating a force of almost 200,000 Spanish troops, the 16,000 Americans and 50,000 Cuban rebels had a powerful ally: disease. Mosquitoes and yellow fever preyed on the thousands of nonimmune soldiers newly arrived from Spain, sparking an epidemic that hobbled the Spanish Army, killing some 41,000 troops, compared to 3,100 men killed in combat. Cuban rebels, largely immune to yellow fever through childhood exposure, lost only 1,300 men. Yellow fever season was on their side. The rebel leader Gen. Máximo Gómez said that his best generals were "June, July, and August."[17]

But if the fighting had stopped in Cuba, disease was still on the offensive. Malaria and dysentery were weakening American troops, and on July 6 the first case of yellow fever appeared in Siboney. George Sternberg was ready. Knowing the acute risk of yellow fever, he had hired several Cubans to supplement the Medical Department's staff.[18] One of these was physician and scientist Aristides Agramonte, who had trained in the United States and was now chair of the University of Havana Department of Bacteriology. Born in Cuba, Agramonte had lived in the United States since age three and had been a bacteriologist with the New York State Health Department before returning to Cuba. Sternberg also brought on his Cuban colleagues Carlos Finlay and Juan Guiteras, who had both left the island during the conflict. Finlay was retired and living in Tampa at the time, and Guiteras was teaching at the University of Pennsylvania, but they returned to Cuba for the war emergency to advise Sternberg on yellow fever.[19]

## THE *RELIEF*

William Gorgas arrived in Cuba just one day after the first American case of yellow fever. With the declaration of war, the Medical Department had converted several passenger ships into hospitals, and Gorgas was aboard one of the first such ships—the USS *Relief*.[20] Workers created hospital wards by removing stateroom walls and bolting 250 iron-framed patient bunks to the floor, furnishing them with cotton mattresses, side rails, linen sheets, blankets, and horsehair pillows. Each ward boasted two toilet rooms, a bathtub and sink, and even hot and cold water.[21] The ship had electric fans, a small laboratory, a surgical ward with a steam sterilizer, and

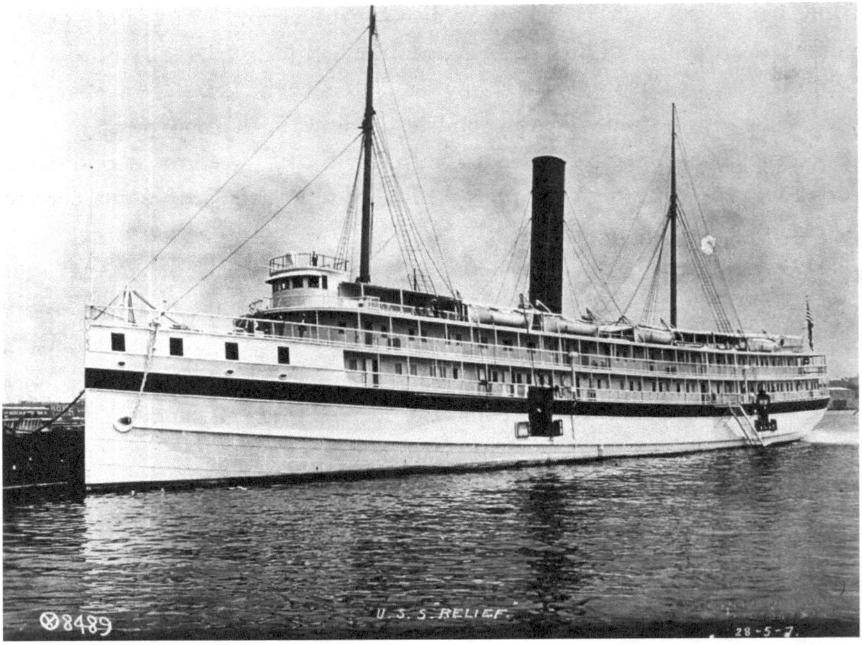


FIGURE 4.1. USS *Relief* (hospital ship): port side view. National Library of Medicine.

one of the first x-ray machines in the country. "We are a kind of floating hospital," Gorgas told his mother, "taking aboard the sick and wounded and bringing them to the nearest American port."[22] Sternberg knew Gorgas was immune and familiar with yellow fever so he promoted him from captain to major to serve second in command under Col. George H. Torney. The medical team included several other medical officers, two chaplains, numerous male hospital attendants, and six female nurses. One of the nurses, Ester V. Hasson, declared the ship a beauty, with "her fresh coat of white paint, the green stripe of the Medical Corps encircling her hull, Stars and Stripes and Red Cross flags flying."[23]

Gorgas was joined on the *Relief* by Theodore Lyster, Marie's nephew, whom he had treated for yellow fever as a boy in 1882 at Fort Brown. Theo, already in possession of a PhD, was in medical school at the University of Michigan, and consulted his Uncle Will about joining the war effort. Gorgas recommended the Hospital Corps, adding a fatherly note: "I would like you with me. So let me know before you take any positive steps in the matter."[24] When Theo left medical school to volunteer, Sternberg obligingly put him on the *Relief* because he, like his uncle, was immune to yellow fever.

The hospital ship departed New York Harbor on July 2 with seven hundred tons of medical supplies, more than two weeks after combat troops had sailed. Arriving at Siboney on July 7, Gorgas and his colleagues encountered a chaotic scene on the shore. Maj. Louis La Garde was in charge of a hospital with a thousand patients so poorly provisioned that the sick and wounded were lying on the ground with few blankets or tents to protect them.[25] Supplies were short because although the Medical Department prepared adequate field hospital sets and medicines for the Fifth Army Corps, including 7,500,000 quinine pills for malaria, many of the supplies arrived after men had fallen sick and wounded.[26] The *Relief* was therefore very welcome, and the ship staff immediately went on shore to evacuate the most seriously wounded to their hospital. Gorgas wrote that while they were a "stone's throw" from the shore, the water was so rough that they could take on patients only in the morning.[27] They were in "pitiable condition," nurse Esther Hasson wrote, but "a bath, clean bed, and plenty of nourishment worked wonders."[28] In four days they were able to take on and treat all of La Garde's patients and transfer them to ships going North.[29]

The Spanish-American-Cuban War would demonstrate the value of both hospital ships and female nursing. Women had of course long been caring for the sick and wounded, but they were often family members or "camp followers," women of ill repute, and the prevailing view was that it was unseemly for women to see men naked and vulnerable.[30] Since the mid-nineteenth century and the Crimean War, however, Florence Nightingale had been promoting in Britain the education and employment of trained female nurses whose skill and behavior were beyond reproach. In the United States, Clara Barton and others had cared for the sick and wounded in hospitals across the North and South during the Civil War, but these women, like William's mother, Amelia, were never part of the Union or Confederate armies. Some civilian hospitals like Bellevue did begin to employ nurses after the war. In medical school, in fact, William had told Amelia that doctors preferred female nurses to male attendants "both because you are better served and because my head nurse is quite pretty."[31]

But the US Army was reluctant to put women in uniform. The creation of the Hospital Corps in the 1880s had provided a dedicated, trained cadre of male hospital attendants, which improved the care in army hospitals. New medical knowledge and technology, however, were requiring an increasingly well-trained staff, and thousands of middle-class women across the country were entering nursing schools to acquire those skills. Recognizing the need for trained nurses and foreseeing the burden on the Hospital Corps, Sternberg sought their help when the wartime emergency came.[32] His office recruited nurses immune to yellow fever and arranged with the Daughters of the American Revolution to enlist female nurses for the Medical Department. The department contracted with 1,563 female nurses during the war, all of them white and unmarried; the government barred Black women and married women from service.[33]

The *Relief* was anchored off Siboney for three weeks and then returned to New York with 254 patients on board. From there it made several trips to Puerto Rico and by some stroke of luck avoided carrying anyone infected with yellow fever. But troops on shore were not so lucky. Sternberg's predictions came true as yellow fever ripped through the Thirty-Fourth Michigan Volunteer Infantry Regiment, with 794 of 4,500 troops sick by July 20.[34] La Garde's hospital on the beach was so overwhelmed that he had to establish a new yellow fever isolation hospital, and Gorgas was ordered on July 15 to leave the *Relief* to help set it up.[35]

## SIBONEY

Yellow fever became a leading cause of death during the Spanish-American-Cuban War, and when a postwar investigative committee asked Louis La Garde if the army should have expected this, he said yes, and that Sternberg's words "read like a prophecy and everyone should have understood."[36] The lion's share of yellow fever cases were at Siboney, and their care fell to La Garde, Gorgas, and their colleagues. The prevailing theory in 1898 was that yellow fever was spread by filth and fomites, bits of soiled material, so that medical officers, including Gorgas, believed that buildings could become infected if they housed people who had yellow fever. When one of the commanding officers learned that nonimmunes were entering buildings that had been inhabited by yellow fever patients, the army command ordered that every such habitation be burned to the ground. The commander of the Cuban forces argued that there had been no recent cases of yellow fever and that burning the village "might seem like wanton destruction of property."[37] The Americans nevertheless evicted the residents and sheltered them in army tents, promising to rebuild the village after the war.[38] They then constructed two new hospitals, a detention hospital in Siboney to care for the sick and wounded and monitor them for yellow fever, and a dedicated yellow fever hospital located two miles up the rail line from Siboney, with La Garde in charge and Gorgas second in command.

Gorgas moved quickly to rework the hospital's yellow fever treatment protocols, writing out instructions by hand to ensure that physicians serving with him did not continue with the centuries-old "heroic" measures of purging and heavy dosing with medicines. With his appreciation of skilled nursing, he understood that complete bed rest and warmth were the most effective treatments and that such care required careful and prolonged nursing. Upon the first sign of a chill, patients should be "put to bed at once, give[n] a hot toddy, hot-mustard foot-bath, hot bottle to feet, till patient ceases to complain of cold." He kept patients with fevers on a liquid diet, offering a tablespoon of medicinal tea or milk every hour. He treated headaches with cool cloths, and back pain with flannel sprinkled with turpentine or with a flaxseed plaster to the kidneys. After three or four days, most fevers would subside, and many patients would recover. But for others, "fever will return though not as high as before & patient usually dies within a few days of this second rise either of black vomit or suppression of the urine." In all cases, he wrote, "Insist upon the patient keeping strickly [*sic*] recumbent. Use bed pan & urinal."[39]

Gorgas's most famous patient was Victor C. Vaughan, renowned epidemiologist, public health expert, dean of the University of Michigan Medical School, and now a surgeon with the Thirty-Third Michigan volunteers. Theo introduced his dean to his uncle, and the two men quickly became friends. Only a week after the hospital was set up, though, Vaughan became a patient in it. Gorgas was his doctor, and Theo his corpsman. Vaughan hated being in bed, but Gorgas told him, "You must understand that your pulse is 44 and your temperature 106 degrees. You cannot move without endangering your life. Your heart may stop if you lift your arm." As the virus attacked his internal organs, Vaughan endured black vomit and

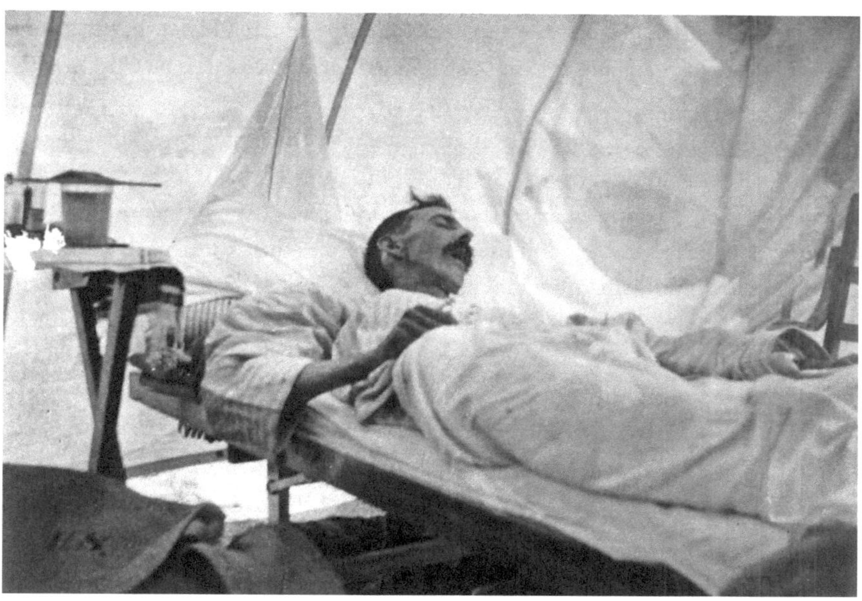

FIGURE 4.2. Yellow fever patient in hospital at Siboney, Cuba, July 1898. National Library of Medicine.

great pain, and did not eat for eight days. Then, on the ninth day his fever broke. He soon saw Gorgas at his bedside, with "the beloved twinkle in his eyes." The doctor said Vaughan could now have some beef tea, and when Vaughan asked how much, Gorgas answered, "All you want. Have the orderly roll in a hogshead." But the weakened man's first sip was from an ounce cup.[40]

Vaughan lost 60 of his 210 pounds from his illness and credited Gorgas with saving his life.[41] Gorgas told the story more modestly and morbidly. "I gave him my sympathy, but very little else," he explained. "The only real thing I did for the Doctor was to get a dead man moved out of his cot." Vaughan was sharing a bed with a patient who had died, and he had feebly asked to have a cot to himself for the for short time that he had left to live. Gorgas obliged, "particularly as it would not inconvenience his bedfellow to any great extent."[42] Vaughan's admiration of Gorgas's skill in managing yellow fever cases was supported by the fact that while the army-wide death rate for yellow fever was 12 percent, Gorgas lost only 8 percent of his cases.[43] But it was a struggle, because Gorgas and La Garde began with 150 patients and only five men and few supplies to care for them.

William began to keep a journal when he got to Cuba, as his father had during his war. Mail service, already unreliable, stopped completely after the postmaster caught yellow fever, so William wrote to Marie in the journal as a way to stay close to her. It provides a glimpse of his desperate war with disease. In mid-July, he told her, "I write hastily as I scarcely even have a minute to spare." Patients arrived continuously, he wrote on July 21, so "everything is in more or less confusion—the camp not having gotten into running order and 25 or 30 patients being pushed in daily—we have about 400 patients now in camp." When twenty-five male nurses and eleven female nurses arrived, Gorgas noted, "This will be of great assistance to us, but the greatest thing we need is organization. Being second in command this falls to me in great part." He confided, "I much prefer the treatment of cases." The generally sunny William complained, "I have had quite enough of Cuba for the present. I do not mind the hardship and the heat so much [as] the discouragement of trying to take care of the sick with only inadequate supplies and help of every kind and the impossibility of getting anything organized." On the last day of July, he reported, "We have buried at this camp 125 men."[44]

The hospital at Siboney ultimately had six hundred beds, and on August 5, La Garde, not immune to yellow fever, fell ill himself. Before he was evacuated, he turned the hospital over to Gorgas and Dr. George McCreery, who had worked together at Bellevue.[45] McCreery took charge of administration, and Gorgas devoted himself to patient care. The camp had about four deaths a day, and William told Marie that when he was making an inventory of the effects of a deceased lieutenant, what hit him the hardest was reading letters from the man's wife about their daughter's fifth birthday and how they were looking forward to his return home. That could have been himself, he wrote; "I want to get home to my wife and baby."[46] But when McCreery came down with yellow fever, Gorgas was put in charge of the yellow fever hospital with no prospects for going home soon.

In recognition of the danger of tropical disease in Cuba, the War Department had created ten "immune regiments," segregated combat units of Black and white soldiers, one thousand men each, from the southern states. The assumption was that southerners would be more resistant to malaria and yellow fever because they had survived childhood infections or, in the case of Black Americans, because they were erroneously believed to be immune due to their race. Many African Americans did have genetic resistance to malaria by virtue of the sickle cell trait (receiving a sickle cell gene from one parent), as did some people who lived in malarial zones of the Mediterranean, Africa, or the Middle East. But in an era before fevers could be specifically diagnosed and differentiated, people mistakenly believed Black people were resistant to other fevers as well.[47] The War Department designated the Seventh through Tenth Immune Regiments as Black units and, in an unusual step, assigned African American officers to them. Only one of the Black immune regiments went to Cuba, the Ninth Volunteer Infantry, recruited largely from Louisiana. Hardly immune, the Ninth alone lost seventy-six men to disease in Cuba, many of them at Siboney.[48]

The Siboney hospitals treated Black and white patients alike, because while the army in 1898 was racially segregated, it was not practical (to say nothing of humane) to segregate the field hospitals. Although the Medical Department barred African American women from contracting as nurses, Black nurses made their way to Cuba anyway, and shorthanded hospitals hired them to care for Black patients. Denied admission to most nursing schools, they were often less well trained than white nurses, but Gorgas needed them. "We got 18 new female nurses last night," he told Marie on August 4. "This will be a great help to us. Nearly all of them have no training, are just Negro women picked up in New York, but they can help."[49] But when two Black lieutenants came to Gorgas asking to visit some nurses at Siboney, their courteous behavior so favorably impressed him that he told Marie, "I must confess that the negro nurses seem more respectable than the white."[50]

Gorgas, however, showed his racial prejudices when it came to considering his next assignment. He knew that his immunity meant that he might be ordered to remain in Cuba with the occupation army, but when the chief surgeon of Santiago, Col. Valery Havard, asked Gorgas if he wanted to stay in Santiago, Gorgas demurred. He had heard that the Ninth Volunteer Infantry—one of the immune units—had arrived and, in one of his most overtly racist statements, told Marie that he declined because, "They have as part of the garrison a Negro regiment with all Negro officers and it will make a very disagreeable complication."[51] The southern paternalist was willing to care for Black patients, but the white supremacist would find it "disagreeable" to work with their officers as equals. Gorgas did not, however, object to having Black men serve him. In early August he told Marie, "We are so shorthanded that I've had to look after myself so far."[52] Then he found Jim Robertson, a Black soldier he knew from Fort Barrancas, in the hospital with an illness. Gorgas got him transferred to the Hospital Corps so he could work as his and Theo's servant.

Living conditions in the Siboney camp were awful. The Cuban heat was so oppressive, Gorgas told his family, "I feel very chirpy and energetic until about 8 o'clock [a.m.] when the sun wilts me. I never felt anything like it. After 8 o'clock I stay in my tent and transact all my business from there." Water was piped in from a spring below the camp, and people used a hose to bathe. "Of course it has to be done in public, but nobody seems to care what clothes they have on or whether they have any at all."[53] When the pipes broke, Robertson had to bring water in buckets up to the camp.

Although the fighting had ended, troops languished in Cuba, and Roosevelt's 1,100 Rough Riders, who had only twenty-five men killed in action, began to fall ill with dysentery and malaria. By late July more than 80 percent of his men were unfit for duty. The future president sent a letter of alarm to Washington, DC, reporting that there were 1,500 cases of malaria in the Army Fifth Corps and that the whole command was "so weakened and shattered as to be ripe for dying like rotten sheep." A yellow fever epidemic, he warned, would be devastating. "To keep us here," he wrote, "will simply involve the destruction of thousands."[54] When the letter was released to the Associated Press, the *New York Times* broadcast, "Nine Men Out of Ten Sick: Col. Roosevelt Declares the Whole Army Is in Danger Unless Moved North at Once." The *Chicago Tribune* reported, "Tide of Misery Still Flows."[55] Within days, the War Department leased five thousand acres on Montauk Point at the end of Long Island for an isolation camp to which they could evacuate troops without endangering the general population. Roosevelt's men were among the first of the twenty-two thousand men to arrive.

In Siboney news that the army was ordering men home acted as a tonic, but it would take time and ships to evacuate the troops. William longed to leave. Writing to Marie on August 9 from a perch overlooking a forest of royal palm trees and the harbor, he watched the transports going to and from the ships. "Those going I know are filled with happy men," he wrote.[56]

As the medical staff became increasingly depleted, Gorgas was called back down the hill to run the field hospital there, and Theo was left in charge of the yellow fever hospital. By mid-August, the patient flow had slowed, but Gorgas was still under tremendous strain. "I have the unenviable job of picking out those who are able to go." And, he confided to Marie, "Those who are left feel personally agrived [*sic*]."[57] Gorgas worried that his patients, convalescent from yellow fever, could now die of dysentery or typhoid while waiting for transport. Five or six men a day were dying of gastrointestinal disease. When the transport officials in Santiago said there was no room for his patients, Gorgas went to Santiago himself and found a ship that could take several hundred. "You would be surprised to see grown men as utterly broken and demoralized as these men are. Doctors & all," he told Marie. "They are childish about going home."[58] The next day he was able to get 375 patients off, but the new nurses were beginning to get sick. "It is a scuffle from morning till night to get the men fed and waited on. I am trying to get another ship and if I succeed, I will get on with the rest of my hospital."[59] His hastily written letters had a desperate tone. He still had 443 patients on August 16 and was telegraphing regularly for transport but four days later still had no news. "This is all we think of or talk about now."[60] On August 26 William told Marie, "The whole of the 24th infantry got off this morning, leaving our camp pretty desolate."[61] But worse was to come. One of the nurses, Carolina M. Anthony, later told Gorgas, "There isn't a page in my life as sad as the last 10 days I spent in Siboney."[62]

## TYPHOID

The Spanish-American-Cuban War may have been a "splendid little war" to Theodore Roosevelt, but it was a humiliation and disaster for the Medical Department. On August 6, as the Fifth Army Corps was being evacuated from Cuba, the *New York Times* broke the story of typhoid fever raging in the US training camps. Camp Thomas at Chickamauga, Georgia, housing eighty thousand men, was the worst; almost 10 percent of the men had contracted typhoid. It was scandalous because typhoid was known to be a waterborne bacterial disease transmitted through the oral-fecal route, that is, poor sanitation.[63] Sternberg had failed to realize that many of the volunteer medical officers were not well informed on modern sanitation.[64] Typhoid is a disease caused by *Salmonella typhi* bacteria, and symptoms include a sustained fever, headache, abdominal pain, and extreme weakness. The illness lasts for several weeks and in severe cases damages the intestines, liver, and spleen. Unlike yellow fever, an attack does not induce immunity and can recur; some people retain and can transmit bacteria for years without symptoms. Today typhoid vaccines are available, but there are still ten to twenty million cases worldwide and more than 150,000 deaths annually.[65]

While Cuba was the source for yellow fever in the United States, typhoid was traveling in the other direction, with soldiers from the training camps bringing typhoid to Cuba. Soon medical officers came to dread typhoid more than yellow fever, because, as La Garde later told Congress, "yellow fever meant a sickness of about a week, whereas typhoid meant a sickness of weeks."[66] The army did not have supplies or personnel to care for people that long.

In late August, Gorgas became one of typhoid's victims. After not writing for a few days, he told Marie on August 29, "I am laid by the heels at last and have been in bed yesterday and today." A few nights before, he had experienced chills but felt well enough to go to dinner at the home of the nearby mine superintendent. He soon went home to bed, however, with a temperature of 100, cared for by Jim Robertson. Gorgas took quinine daily, believing that it prevented other fevers in addition to malaria. "Now I think I will call Jim, drink a bottle of ginger ale nicely iced, take two quinine pills, and luxuriously snooze till it gets cooler." He teased, "Don't you wish you were here and [could] have some of the good time?"[67] But he also confessed, "I am having trouble in my camp since I have been sick." He had to reprimand one of his doctors for getting drunk; Robertson had gotten into a fight; and the nurses were in an uproar. What the uproar was about, he did not say, but he trotted out the old prejudice against women nurses, saying that most of them were "no better than common prostitutes."[68] When Theo soon came down with typhoid too, both men had temperatures of 100 degrees for several days.[69]

Finally, Gorgas had a chance to go home on the hospital ship *Missouri*, but the officer in charge of transport, Valery Havard, would not put Theo on the same boat. When Gorgas refused to leave without Theo, Havard revoked Gorgas's order of evacuation. The medical officer on the *Missouri*, however, Maj. William H. Arthur, so strenuously insisted on taking both men that Havard changed his order and put them on board.[70] Gorgas later told Arthur, "I think that both Lyster and I are at present living in this world due to your efforts at that time in getting us away from Siboney." Staying there would have meant his death. "I could never have gotten through such an attack of typhoid as I had with such care as they could have given me at the abandoned hospital in Siboney." He and Theo would have been buried in the same coffin they had used for so many funerals there.[71] The *Missouri* brought 256 sick men back from Cuba to Long Island, arriving on September 12.[72] McCreery, Gorgas's colleague, was less fortunate. He had boarded an earlier transport but, weakened by yellow fever, died of dysentery on the way home.[73]

Marie sped to Long Island to bring William home, carrying a letter from a West Point medical officer authorizing her passage through quarantine. It stated "Mrs. Mary D Gorgas [*sic*] not only comes from this northern town direct but she is also an immune having had a most severe attack of yellow fever at Fort Brown Texas in 1882."[74] The couple immediately went to the Presbyterian Hospital in Manhattan, where William was admitted with a temperature of 104. He had already been through the worst of the illness, though, and after a week in hospital, went home to recuperate. He had lost some thirty pounds.[75]

## AFTERMATH

In addition to the trauma of yellow fever, for Gorgas and his Medical Corps colleagues, typhoid fever was the "signature event" of the war, with more than twenty thousand cases and almost 1,600 deaths.[76] The disease scandals in the training camps and Cuba prompted several investigations into the causes of the epidemics. Final death statistics of 345 deaths from wounds and 2,485 deaths of disease presented a 1:7 ratio of combat deaths to disease deaths, far worse than the 1:2 rate of the Civil War.[77] Advances in medicine such as the introduction of first-aid packets, radiology, and antiseptic/aseptic surgery gave battle-wounded servicemen a far better chance of wound recovery than ever before, but epidemics signaled the War Department's failure to care properly for its men. Angry and embarrassed, Sternberg appointed a typhoid board of three scientists, Maj. Walter Reed, US Army, and E. O. Shakespeare and Victor Vaughan, with the US Volunteers, to investigate the causes and modes of propagation of typhoid in the training camps. From August to October 1898, they visited every camp and collected one thousand pages of testimony. The board's report proved to be a scientific breakthrough. They determined that contaminated water was not the primary means of spreading typhoid, but rather that flies acted as carriers of the infection as they swarmed over fecal matter and then onto food. People could also carry germs on their hands and clothing. The board recommended more rigorous sanitation, especially regarding latrines and kitchens, but concluded that typhoid could not be eliminated without some form of immunization.[78] The report thus prompted increased sanitation in both military and civilian spheres and spurred the search for a vaccine.

To address broader problems during the war, President McKinley appointed another body to investigate the conduct of the war; it was known as the Dodge Commission, after its chair, former Union general and US representative Grenville M. Dodge.[79] The commission, composed of members of Congress and prominent citizens, heard from scores of witnesses on the problems and failures in the conduct of the Spanish-American-Cuban War. Sternberg, exhausted by the war, stung by the medical disasters, and conscious of his own miscalculations, nevertheless adamantly blamed the epidemics on the War Department's haste in troop enlistment and training, overcrowding of camps and transports, and the failure of military commanders to consult with medical officers about sanitation and the location of camps. He told the Dodge Commission that until inspectors reported the dire camp conditions to the secretary of war, "practically nothing was done to make the men comfortable or to remedy the insanitary conditions."[80]

The Dodge Commission largely exonerated the Medical Department and instead blamed the War Department leadership for not following the Medical Department's advice and not grasping the need for sanitary efficiency and discipline. It also faulted Congress for not granting sufficient funds for medical and sanitary needs, and recommended a number of reforms, including improved medical transportation and procurement systems, medical training for line officers, better medical personnel/troops ratios, and the professionalization of the Medical Department.[81] It was especially forceful about trained nursing. It found that the hospital personnel, both regular and volunteer, were inadequate throughout the summer of 1898 due to the failure of Congress and the War Department to recognize "the value of women nurses and the extent to which their services could be secured."[82] Over the next decade, Congress enacted legislation to implement all of these recommendations, but medical officers, including Gorgas, would long remember the humiliation of the scandal.

The Spanish-American-Cuban War was short but consequential for the country as well as for the Army Medical Department. In December 1898 Spain and the United States signed a peace treaty establishing the independence of Cuba, ceding Puerto Rico and Guam to the United States, and allowing the United States to purchase the Philippine islands from Spain for $20 million. The war had cost the United States $250 million and almost three thousand lives, but it also acquired control of new territories. As for Gorgas, after his sick leave, he returned briefly to duty in New York, but Sternberg called on his battle-tested yellow fever expert to return to Cuba to help protect the occupying American army from disease. William and Marie spent Christmas 1898 in New York with Aileen, and after delivering her to boarding school, sailed to Havana to take part in a new American enterprise—empire building.

# CHAPTER 5

## The Terror of Yellow Jack in Havana

> Since December 1898, I have been in Havana, continually and daily in contact with this disease, . . . I have had ample facilities for observing the disease, and for controlling the treatment in a large number of cases.
>
> —William C. Gorgas, "Notes on the Treatment of Yellow Fever at Las Animas Hospital," 1903

THE WRECKAGE OF THE USS *Maine* was still visible above the waterline when William and Marie steamed into the Havana harbor on New Year's Eve, 1898. They checked into the Inglaterra Hotel on the central park, and William immediately went to work at Las Animas, the main yellow fever hospital in Havana. He would attend hundreds of yellow fever patients there from 1899 to 1901 and recorded each case in a large journal, creating two leather-bound volumes, "Yellow Fever Cases, 1899" and "Yellow Fever Cases, 1900." Each patient had a paragraph with his or her name, age, occupation, and symptoms such as temperature, albumin in the urine (which indicated kidney trouble), tenderness in the stomach, jaundiced skin, and black vomit, as well as a notation of whether the patient died or was discharged. Gorgas took a smaller diary with him on home visits to quickly record patient information that was later transferred to the journal. Some entries noted "not yellow fever," while others recorded the ominous symptoms and then simply "yes." These records of hundreds of yellow fever cases reveal the extensive suffering and death that William Gorgas witnessed during those two years in Havana, perhaps more than any other officer in the US Army. He kept the journals for the rest of his life.[1]

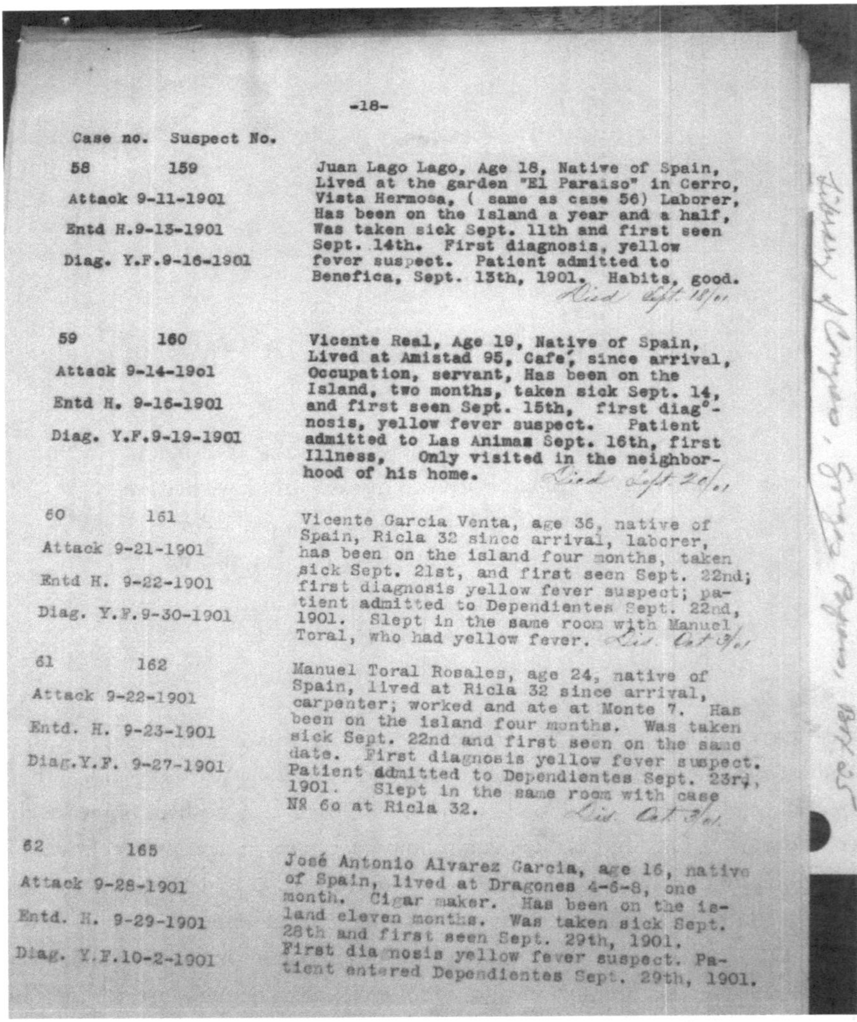

-18-

Case no. Suspect No.

58 159
Attack 9-11-1901
Entd H.9-13-1901
Diag. Y.F.9-16-1901

Juan Lago Lago, Age 18, Native of Spain, Lived at the garden "El Paraiso" in Cerro, Vista Hermosa, ( same as case 56) Laborer, Has been on the Island a year and a half, Was taken sick Sept. 11th and first seen Sept. 14th. First diagnosis, yellow fever suspect. Patient admitted to Benefica, Sept. 13th, 1901. Habits, good. Died Sept. 18/01

59 160
Attack 9-14-19o1
Entd H. 9-16-1901
Diag. Y.F.9-19-1901

Vicente Real, Age 19, Native of Spain, Lived at Amistad 95, Cafe, since arrival, Occupation, servant, Has been on the Island, two months, taken sick Sept. 14, and first seen Sept. 15th, first diag°-nosis, yellow fever suspect. Patient admitted to Las Animas Sept. 16th, first Illness, Only visited in the neighbor-hood of his home. Died Sept. 20/01

60 161
Attack 9-21-1901
Entd H. 9-22-1901
Diag. Y.F.9-30-1901

Vicente Garcia Venta, age 36, native of Spain, Ricla 32 since arrival, laborer, has been on the island four months, taken sick Sept. 21st, and first seen Sept. 22nd; first diagnosis yellow fever suspect; pa-tient admitted to Dependientes Sept. 22nd, 1901. Slept in the same room with Manuel Toral, who had yellow fever. Died Oct 3/01

61 162
Attack 9-22-1901
Entd. H. 9-23-1901
Diag.Y.F. 9-27-1901

Manuel Toral Rosales, age 24, native of Spain, lived at Ricla 32 since arrival, carpenter; worked and ate at Monte 7. Has been on the island four months. Was taken sick Sept. 22nd and first seen on the same date. First diagnosis yellow fever suspect. Patient admitted to Dependientes Sept. 23rd, 1901. Slept in the same room with case Nº 6o at Ricla 32. Died Oct 3/01

62 165
Attack 9-28-1901
Entd. H. 9-29-1901
Diag. Y.F.10-2-1901

José Antonio Alvarez Garcia, age 16, native of Spain, lived at Dragones 4-6-8, one month. Cigar maker. Has been on the is-land eleven months. Was taken sick Sept. 28th and first seen Sept. 29th, 1901. First diagnosis yellow fever suspect. Pa-tient entered Dependientes Sept. 29th, 1901.

FIGURE 5.1. "Yellow Fever Cases, 1900." A page from William C. Gorgas's personal journal of the yellow fever cases he treated in Havana, 1900. Manuscript Division, Library of Congress, Washington, DC; photographed by the author.

## AMERICAN OCCUPATION, AMERICAN GOVERNANCE

As her husband began his work at Las Animas, Marie began to get her bearings and enjoyed taking in the scenes around her. "The streets are filled with Americans and the hotels—especially the Inglaterra—brilliant with uniforms," she told Amelia. Havana looked dilapidated and dirty, but their accommodations were fine. "Our room is very large, has a marble floor—two huge windows with no glass—only outside wooden shutters." With two beds, easy chairs, and a rug, it offered "a great deal to be thankful for."[2] People in the hotel were singing and dancing, celebrating their independence, and she wanted to join, but did not feel she could without speaking the language. She therefore immediately started Spanish lessons, telling her mother she studied "every spare moment."[3]

But if Cubans were celebrating, their country was in disastrous condition after decades of war and brutal Spanish rule. Havana, long a power center for the Spanish Empire, was a grand capital of the Western Hemisphere. The vegetation was lush, and the Morro Castle, one of the oldest and largest forts in the Americas, protected the harbor, which Marie called "one of the most beautiful harbors in the world."[4] Much of Havana's architecture included grand structures such as the Plaza de Armas, the Catedral de la Habana, and palatial colonial mansions with Carrera marble floors. But now, in the early months of the American occupation, evidence of the carnage was everywhere—unburied corpses, plundered farms, and formerly prosperous plantations and the peasants' homes alike burned to the ground.[5] Roads and railroads were destroyed, as well the cattle and coffee industries; only one-third of the agricultural land remained under cultivation. In 1899 the island produced only one-sixth of the tobacco and one-half of the sugar that it had in 1894, and of 1,100 sugar mills operating in 1894, only 207 survived the war.[6]

The Treaty of Paris stipulated that the United States would assume control of the country on January 1, 1899, and prepare Cuba for self-governance. When the Gorgases arrived, some seventeen thousand Spanish soldiers remained in and around Havana. The US Army sent forty-three thousand troops to ensure order and prevent further violence between the Cubans and the departing Spanish. The transfer of government proceeded on New Year's Day without major incident, and the United States assumed the role of an occupying force. The last Spanish troops left Cuba on February 6, and once it was clear that there would be little Cuban retribution against the Spanish or resistance to the American takeover, American troops went home as well. By the end of October 1899, only about eleven thousand American troops remained on the island.[7]

As Cubans set about dismantling the centuries-old Spanish colonial rule and constructing their own national identity and institutions, the United States was initially supportive. In fact, the first two laws governing the US occupation were intended to curtail American imperialism in deference to congressional Democrats' distaste for empire. The Teller Amendment to the war resolution of 1898 barred the colonization of Cuba, and the Foraker Amendment to the 1899 military appropriations bill discouraged economic exploitation by preventing American companies from acquiring concessions and franchises in Cuban enterprises. The plan was to help the island restore its economy, control disease, build a viable political system, and then leave Cuba to govern itself.

President McKinley appointed Maj. Gen. John R. Brooke as military governor of Cuba, and he divided the island into three departments, each overseen by an army general. Maj. Gen. Leonard Wood was the most successful of the three. A medical officer who gained fame as a soldier during the Indian wars and led the Rough Riders in battle, Wood moved to clean up the Santiago Department, quell the violence, restore the economy, and demonstrate how important public health was to social order and economic health. When smallpox broke out in Wood's sector in the fall of 1898, his group extinguished it by vaccinating six hundred American military personnel, who then cared for 1,200 smallpox patients and vaccinated more than thirty thousand Cubans.[8] Wood was also adept at assuring the Cuban generals that it was the American government's policy to work for Cuban independence. He and other US officials encouraged the Cuban insurgent military to disband, with payments of $3 million and millions more in loans to rebuild, and a promise that their occupation would be temporary.[9]

Many among Havana's elite considered themselves European and were contemptuous of "Yankee interlopers" who now sought to govern them. Three sectors in the Cuban power structure vied for control as they sought to modernize their nation in the postcolonial era: well-connected Cubans returning from New York, where they had fled during the war; insurgent military officers who controlled the diminishing army; and an ad hoc assembly of Cuba's businessmen and professionals. Race also divided Havana, because many rebels were Afro-Cuban, while virtually all of the loyalists to Spain were white.[10] The Gorgases were fascinated by this complex, transnational, transcultural blend of Afro-European culture, food, music, dance, and politics. Like most white Americans of their time, they considered themselves superior to people of color, but Marie and William were both very social and shared a sense of adventure and curiosity about their new post. William enjoyed the tropical fruits and smoking Cuban cigars in the evenings; for years after he left Havana, friends shipped him cartons of cigars from the island.[11] His close working relationships with Cuban physicians and Marie's study of Spanish enabled them to negotiate the social politics of Havana and engage with Cubans more comfortably and freely than did many other members of the American occupation.

## HAVANA CLEANUP, 1899

If Havanans were proud of their culture, Americans considered the city one of the pestholes of the Western Hemisphere. Improved sanitation with clean water and sewerage had vanquished diseases such as typhoid, plague, cholera, and dysentery in most American cities by the end of the nineteenth century. Vaccination controlled smallpox; swamp draining was diminishing malaria in the South; and careful inspection of incoming ships for infectious diseases was reducing other outbreaks as well. Now the country faced public health threats from overseas. After her first blush of excitement in Havana, Marie Gorgas found Havana "little better than a huge cesspool." She later wrote, "Unspeakable odors assailed; streets were filled with decaying vegetables, dead animals, miscellaneous sewage, and refuse of all kinds." The hospitals were so overcrowded that sick people were lying in the streets, she wrote, and "children wandered homeless, the existing government being unable to provide for them, and everywhere beggars with livid sores pleaded pitifully for alms."[12] William and Marie, immune to yellow fever, remained in the city to be close to Las Animas Hospital, but the army command set itself apart from this scene. Mindful of the disease scandals of 1898, the War Department now generously funded the Medical Department for the construction and supply of hospitals in the occupied territories of the Philippines, Puerto Rico, and Cuba to protect Americans as well as to assist the local populations. Selecting a garrison site west of Havana in the healthier neighborhood of Marianao, within weeks soldiers had constructed Camp Columbia, Havana's largest military post, complete with a sewer system, bathhouses, barracks, and storehouses.

Sanitarians had also gained a new weapon in their public health efforts. British scientist Ronald Ross, working in India, had published research in 1897 showing that *Anopheles* mosquitoes transmitted malaria, and in response to Ross's findings, Leonard Wood ordered hospitals in his jurisdiction to put net screening around malaria patients to keep the insects off them and prevent the spread of the disease to others.[13] Surgeon General Sternberg, however, did not immediately follow suit. His focus was on typhoid, and, arriving in Havana the second week of January, he was alarmed that typhoid had appeared in an army camp outside of the city. Sternberg had no misgivings about Gorgas's yellow fever wards but left orders to inspect all army camps, clean up the Cuban villages to eliminate typhoid, and investigate all fevers and transfer yellow fever cases to isolation wards as soon as possible. He did not, however, recommend the general use of mosquito nets in the barracks against malaria. Ronald Ross had sent him a copy of his article, but mosquitoes were not yet Sternberg's enemy.[14]

The American occupation government set out to clean up Havana in the belief that filth was the cause of most diseases, including yellow fever.[15] Gorgas, as sanitary officer, was involved, but in 1899, the massive project was directed by the army chief engineer, Col. William Black. Most of the work was done by Cubans and financed by Cuban revenue, under the direction of American sanitary engineers. In one particularly wise policy, former soldiers could trade in their weapons for brooms to work in the clean-up crews.[16] The early work involved sweeping garbage from the streets to eliminate rats and stray animals and throwing the offal into the harbor for sharks to devour. One American remembered how the giant predators could "seize like a flash every man who fell off the barges, and he would disappear in an instant."[17] A workforce of 260 cleaned individual houses in the city, and another crew conducted routine inspections to ensure that residents kept them clean. In July a team of doctors began to vaccinate fifty thousand Havanans against smallpox, and in the fall, sanitary officers inspected markets, stables, and slaughterhouses to improve drainage and clean them up in order to protect the food and milk supply. Such sanitation work reduced typhoid, dysentery, and smallpox infections, and cut the death rate in Havana by a stunning three-quarters, from 99 per thousand in 1898 to 24.4 per thousand in 1900. It did nothing, however, to reduce yellow fever.

## YELLOW FEVER IN HAVANA

Yellow fever was not rampant in early 1899, because most Cubans were immune, but as thousands of nonimmune people came to the island looking for work, they offered fertile ground for the disease. This danger was revealed in the early days of the occupation when President McKinley sent George Waring, a public health specialist from New York, to investigate the sanitary conditions in Havana. Soon after Waring returned home in October 1898 to write his report, he fell ill with yellow fever and died.[18] This caused many officials to become wary of the island and reinforced the view that immune people like Gorgas should conduct the work of the occupation. He consequently served in increasingly responsible positions in Havana: first as head of the Las Animas Hospital, January to May 1899; then as chief sanitary officer, with oversight over all of Havana's hospitals, May 1899 to April 1900; and finally as chief surgeon of Havana, overseeing all of the health facilities in the city, including the hospitals and general sanitation of Havana from April 1900 to May 1902.[19]

One duty Gorgas maintained throughout his time in Cuba was serving as the only American on the Havana yellow fever board, with physicians Carlos Finlay, Juan Guiteras, and Antonio Diaz Albertini. Fevers were difficult to distinguish for physicians and laymen alike, so the board's job was to positively identify yellow fever cases and then isolate and treat them at the patient's home or in a hospital. If the case was treated at home, the Department of Sanitation deployed guards to ensure that only physicians and nurses were allowed to pass. When the case was completed, workers scrubbed the room with bichloride solution, sterilized all fabrics in the room, and disinfected the entire house with formalin, a formaldehyde mixture. This process became very unpopular because it was disruptive and could damage people's property.

Given the disease threat, the military command told the men to stay out of the cities, but in August 1899, fever broke out anyway across the harbor in the Cabana barracks, near the Morro Castle. When Gorgas recommended that the army move the garrison out farther into the countryside, men and officers alike resisted the idea. "It took all the urging I can do to get General Ludlow to move them," William told his mother. Many of the sick ended up in his hospital, and he ultimately had twenty-three cases and eight deaths at Cabana, "all of which could have been avoided had they moved when I advised," he wrote. Key to patient survival was to begin treatment within the first three days of illness, so new cases were sped to the hospital. "You can imagine the impression the Las Animas ambulance makes coming down the Prado," he wrote. It was "a big Army ambulance, and the driver appreciates his importance. He has to fly a yellow flag, and with Mrs. McManus [a nurse] in uniform . . . the mules going as if life hung on its early arrival, they make such an impressive appearance that everyone turns out-of-the-way for a block ahead."[20]

These patients would end up in Gorgas's wards, and his yellow fever journals show the youth and varied backgrounds of his charges. Cases from October and November 1899 include Zacon Lanker, a Swiss photographer, age thirty-three, who had been in Cuba for eighteen months when he fell ill. He delayed going to the hospital and died the day of his admission. Gorgas noted that he "had black vomit, albumin, turned yellow after death." Francisco Blanco Carballista, age seventeen from Spain, was admitted October 20, 1899. He had been in Cuba one year, and was admitted with pain, vomiting, albumin in urine, eyes tinged, and gums swollen and red. "Yes," wrote Gorgas. "John Curry, America, Negro," age twenty-two, arrived at the hospital unconscious on October 9 but had few yellow fever symptoms other than albumin in the urine. Gorgas's diary stated, "no diagnosis," but when Curry died the next day, he did an autopsy, and noted, "gave clear case of yellow fever. Did not see it." Most of his cases were men, but Mrs. Daisy Harlee, a twenty-three-year-old American, was admitted for yellow fever in late October and survived a mild case.

Before the mosquito theory of yellow fever transmission, Gorgas and his staff took patient histories to get clues as to why they had caught the disease, such as if they had bad habits likes drinking or visiting houses of prostitution, or had been in "infected" buildings, like those at Siboney. William L. Wallace, thirty, an American carpenter, was admitted on October 22, 1899, and died within hours. His record noted, "Was a hard drinker. Loafed at Casa Blanca. Where he spent most of his time. visited Havana frequently." Eley Rodriguez Terrano, age twenty-two, from Spain, never drank alcohol, "not even with his meals," because his uncle told him that if he did, he would get yellow fever. He recovered. Poor little Pedro Garcia y Garcia, twelve years old, had been in Cuba for only twenty days when he fell sick. His record noted that he had good habits, except for overeating the day before he was admitted to the hospital vomiting blood. He died on November 22. The longest entries are for Cecilia Wyman, age twenty-six, and Paul Mackjon, just six months old, on whom Gorgas conducted autopsies, perhaps to understand how and why the disease had killed such innocents—a young woman and a baby.[21]

Las Animas had three yellow fever wards averaging thirty-five patients daily, one for suspected cases, another for acute cases, and a third for convalescents. Here, Gorgas could employ his treatment regime of bed rest, assiduous nursing, and a liquid diet under much better conditions than at Siboney. As he explained in an article for the *Military Surgeon*, "a desperate case stands better chances of pulling through if the patient is carefully nursed, supplied freely with water and nothing put into circulation that could possibly irritate the kidneys."[22] Unlike most physicians, Gorgas gave as little medication as possible. He might prescribe five grains of phenacetin, one of the first synthetic analgesics, or some other analgesic for headaches or muscular pain, but little else.[23] Patients who were accustomed to more rigorous treatments such as purging with mercury-based medicines or stimulating with strychnine did not welcome this simpler approach, but Gorgas reasoned that as new patients saw how others recovered under his care, his reputation and that of his hospital would benefit.[24]

Understanding that nursing was important to saving lives, Gorgas encouraged other hospitals to increase their expenses for nursing care. His department established the first nurses' training school in Cuba, at Mercedes Hospital in Havana. Las Animas nurses, however, could be overwhelmed, working twelve-hour shifts, with an additional hour for record-keeping. One of the night nurses, a Miss Turner, later recounted how one of her duties was to total all fluids a patient consumed and excreted in twenty-four hours and to keep the test tubes of urine in a rack on the patient's nightstand. Each morning, while Gorgas and the other doctors were making rounds, she would boil the newest sample so they could compare it with the previous tubes and see whether albumin was increasing or decreasing. Years later she still remembered with regret one night when she had seventeen acute patients and could not prepare all of the samples. But Turner wrote glowingly of Gorgas and how he worried that the nurses were overworked and might get yellow fever, but "he never spared himself." On his daily rounds he carefully noted the condition of every patient and seemed to have time to look into everything, "no matter how trivial it might be." Turner told one story of a Cuban intern who refused to go out in an ambulance to retrieve patients, so the chief nurse had to go. When someone mentioned this to Gorgas, he nodded vaguely, but the next day rode himself in the ambulance with a yellow fever patient—and the Cuban intern in tow. That settled the matter, and the head nurse could thereafter stay in the wards.[25] With time Americans began to trust Las Animas over other hospitals, because while the yellow fever death rate in all Havana hospitals was about 24 percent, Gorgas lost only 9 percent of his patients at Las Animas.[26]

Despite his success, Gorgas was frustrated working under the military governor General Ludlow, who had not heeded his advice on the yellow fever outbreak at Cabana barracks and failed to give Gorgas the authority he felt he needed as chief surgeon. In mid-1899 he told Marie that he was thinking of asking to be relieved from his position, and that he declined to join a party of uniformed officers to receive Ludlow when he returned to Cuba from Washington. "I have neither the time nor the inclination for such capers. It savors to me too much of bootlicking," he said. "While I like Gen. Ludlow personally, I feel no obligation whatever."[27] By the end of the year, during a holiday visit in Tuscaloosa, Gorgas told John Ross that he wanted to continue his work on yellow fever but was reluctant to return to Havana. "I do not think there is much chance for improving the civil hospitals to any great improvement under Ludlow. He does not appreciate the importance of the work."[28]

## HAVANA CLEANUP, 1900

Gorgas did go back to Havana in 1900, though, because Ludlow left. The new secretary of war, Elihu Root, appointed Leonard Wood governor of Cuba, and in December 1899 Wood began to organize Havana with a more direct and vigorous drive toward Cuban independence, launching a series of sweeping economic, social, and political reforms. Regarding sanitation and health, he appointed Gorgas chief sanitary officer in February and gave him more support than Ludlow had, including control of Havana's hospitals. William told Marie that he did not think Wood knew much about his work. "He gives me very much more authority, though, than Ludlow did, and the position is much pleasanter."[29] Gorgas's department continued the rigorous sanitation begun in 1899, cleaning more than a million square meters of streets daily, applying 8,500 gallons of disinfectant to sewers, streets, and latrines, examining more than a thousand premises and removing 534 carloads of disinfected material from houses and streets in just one month alone.[30] There was little resistance to these measures by Havanans, perhaps relieved to be at peace and eager to rebuild their country. According to Cuban historian Mariel Iglesias Utset, public health and sanitation would even become viewed as jettisoning the "dirty" habits of life under Spanish colonial rule, replacing them with "sanitizing" customs introduced during the US occupation.[31]

With his broader purview, Gorgas and his staff conducted statistical studies of Havana's public health. Using mortuary records from 1884 to 1900, they adopted the modern epidemiological method of tabulating the cause and place of death for thousands of people in the city and mapping the location of all yellow fever cases. This revealed that more than twenty thousand people had died of yellow fever in Havana during the thirty years between 1871 and 1900, and that from 1856 to 1897, only one month recorded no yellow fever cases. Most Havanans were immune to the virus, having contracted it as children, so the heavy mortality largely came with the arrival of the Spanish military personnel and their families. It was so bad in 1895 that immigration nearly stopped altogether and did not resume until August 1899.[32] Under American occupation, some twenty-five thousand immigrants had arrived during 1899 and 1900, primarily from the United States and Spain, as well as sixteen other countries, including Italy, China, Turkey, Korea, Russia, and Norway.[33] They had to pass through a rigorous quarantine protocol managed by the Public Health Service (hereafter, PHS).

Gorgas managed the stress of the daily life-and-death struggles by embracing a domestic routine and finding pleasure in everyday events. He brought the family horse, Mollie, to Cuba and rode in the country when he had time.[34] He and Marie were torn about whether to bring Aileen to Cuba, because she was not immune. She therefore stayed in boarding school in New York City or visited her grandmothers in Tuscaloosa and Cincinnati, and Marie shuttled between Cuba and New York. The family continued to stew about the separation. William told Marie in September 1900, "I dislike being separated from Aileen, but I do not think it wise to bring her down here if we are having much Fever in October."[35] When Marie was not in Havana, William lived in the Florida Hotel and shared his meals with other officers, having "a pretty jolly time in a dignified sort of way."[36] But he missed Marie and wrote of his love. Their wedding day was, he told her, "the most fortunate day of my life, and I shall never cease to thank the good Lord for giving me such a helpmate."[37]

William also devoted time to writing to his family and discussing politics and foreign affairs with his mother. As the federal government sought to advance democracy in Cuba, southern states were rolling back the rights of African Americans with Amelia's full support. She remained an unreconstructed Confederate to her last day, serving as historian to the Tuscaloosa chapter of the Daughters of the Confederacy, and maintaining antebellum views on race, religion, and politics. Amelia told William that the constitutional convention in Alabama "will practically eliminate the negro from election politics in our state," and that Dick "cast his vote rightly considering white control of vital importance." A ceremony memorializing the "Lost Cause" awarded her the Southern Cross of Honor as the widow of a veteran, which would then be passed on to the oldest living son. This, she knew, would be "an anomaly in your case as you wear the US uniform but you can hide the dear 'Con. Cross' upon your breast."[38]

William responded with a declaration of his own deeply held beliefs. "Let me have the Confederate cross," he told Amelia. "I will wear it on the outside of my full dress coat. Because I wear the blue now does not make me any less an ardent Confed." Asking for photographs of Generals Lee and Jackson and of Josiah in his Confederate uniform, he told her that he regretted the failure of the Confederacy. If the South had not lost the war, he wrote, "We would have been one of the world powers, would gradually have abolished slavery, and our people have gone on increasing their wealth." Instead, "the intelligence of the country has been impoverished & everything that our people can save is taken away for the benefit of the Northern states." Those who had won the war, however, had "lost all patriotism" and instead "have banded together purely for the purpose of plundering the treasury." Protective tariffs, especially, had caused the concentration of wealth in a few and the "impoverishment of the masses." The matter, however, was settled, he concluded in a rare show of bitterness, and "it seems hopeless to think of setting up a republic of our own now, & we just have to drift with tied hands to the destruction which it seems to me our country is plunging."[39]

As Gorgas lived among northerners, he rarely revealed such resentment or anger. His anti-northern views were based more on economics than on virulent racism or states' rights. Perhaps after seeing the impoverishment of so many white southerners after the Civil War, he was drawn to economic reforms and critiques of wealth and class divisions in the United States. He embraced the Lost Cause critique of the North as materialistic and mercenary, and blamed northern businessmen and the industrialized economy for the poverty and suffering in the country much more than he advocated white supremacy and the violence of Jim Crow. And, ironically, although a member of an occupying force, William opposed the United States' involvement in Western competition for territory in China, because it would lessen the chance of economic and tax reform to assist working people, the sick, and the poor. "I am an anti-imperialist," he told Amelia. "These foreign wars distract the attention of the people from internal affairs."[40]

## CRISIS

After a year and a half of US occupation, city government agencies were up and running, the economy was recovering, Havana was no longer filthy, and many diseases had been controlled. But yellow fever continued unabated. In 1900 some 1,500 cases were reported in Havana alone.[41] An outbreak began May 19, 1900, in Quemados, a village close to the Camp Columbia barracks, producing thirty-two cases with eight deaths, and three cases with no deaths in the barracks. In July eighteen more soldiers got yellow fever, and four died. By the end of July, five of Leonard Wood's staff and forty-eight civilian employees had fallen ill as well. Health authorities were at their "wits' end," Gorgas wrote, "I believe that Havana was cleaner than any other city had ever been up to that time," but "we evidently could not get rid of Havana as a focus of infection by any method we then knew." The Cubans even "twitted" them because yellow fever rates were highest in the cleanest parts of the city.[42] Governor Wood was losing his patience. Gorgas tried to explain that the increase in cases was due to the number of nonimmunes arriving, but he, too, was frustrated and told Dick that Americans are getting "very uneasy and frightened." The result was that "they press Wood, and Wood punches me."[43] Wood then urged Sternberg to appoint a special commission to solve the riddle of yellow fever.[44]

The yellow fever outbreak and American deaths attracted national press attention. As Havana's chief sanitary officer, Gorgas began speaking to reporters about health conditions using the statistics his office had developed to argue that things were improving. "I've been talking to reporters so much that I have these things down," he told Marie. "I can just prove anything from my statistics." He noted, for example, Havana had 518 yellow fever cases in July 1900, down from 577 the previous July, and that was "the best criterion of general sanitary conditions." He was so confident that he could protect his loved ones from yellow fever that he told Marie that some of the family should visit Havana in the winter, during low fever season. "There is no use having relatives on foreign service unless you visit them," he said. "Well," he jauntily closed his letter, "I must go to stamping out Yellow Fever."[45]

But such confidence (or cockiness) did nothing to stem the epidemic. Cases spiked with 175 cases and thirty-nine deaths in the first half of October.[46] The most dramatic episode came after the wife of Maj. Matt R. Peterson, chief commissary officer in Cuba, who had been stricken by yellow fever, rushed to Cuba to be at his bedside. Gorgas was the officer's doctor and was with him when he died three days later. He tried to comfort Mrs. Peterson, but she threw herself upon her husband's body in despair. When a nurse led her away, she asked for some medicine and went to her quarters. There, however, instead of resting, Mrs. Peterson shot herself in the head with her husband's revolver, shocking the camp. The couple were buried side by side in Camp Columbia's growing military cemetery.[47] When a member of Wood's staff and an American hospital superintendent died of the fever a few days later, it seemed that the American mission in Cuba was under attack.[48]

Gorgas tried to calm the panic, and the *New York Times* seemed to follow his lead, reporting that according to "Señor Gorgas," no attempt was made to suppress fever information; all cases were being reported and going to the hospital, where the best treatment was available.[49] Naturally optimistic, however, Gorgas could at times be too sanguine. He told one reporter that since 525 city blocks out of 857 had no cases of yellow fever, and 184 blocks had only one case, it was a "misnomer" to call ten cases a day in a population of 242,000 an epidemic.[50] That cannot have comforted anyone.

## CHAPTER 6

# War against Mosquitoes Begins

> This work was so brilliant in its execution and so positive in its results that, as I look back now, I am surprised that I was not at once convinced.
>
> —William Gorgas, *The Lancet*, 1902

HAVANA AT THE TURN OF the twentieth century was one of those times and places in which reputations were made; lives were saved, lost, and ruined; and some people found fame and even glory. The story of how an army board discovered that mosquitoes transmit yellow fever has become overly simplified with time, largely because American scientists made it an American story, overstating the contributions of army bacteriologist Walter Reed and diminishing those of Cuban scientists, Spanish volunteers, and even William Gorgas.

This simplified version is that after the Spanish-American-Cuban War, Walter Reed headed up a commission that came to Cuba in 1900 and conducted a series of elegant experiments on human volunteers to prove that the *Aedes aegypti* mosquito was the vector of yellow fever. Reed introduced the use of informed consent documents for the volunteers who risked their lives for science, and, according to this telling, only one man, scientist Jesse Lazear, died, martyred for humanity.[1] William Gorgas then put the findings into practice by eradicating mosquitoes from Havana, and within months yellow fever vanished from the city. It was a triumph of American science, modern medicine, in the "age of bacteriology," and Walter Reed joined the pantheon of medical heroes with the likes of Edward Jenner, who introduced smallpox vaccination, and Louis Pasteur and Robert Koch, who developed germ theory. As the story of the Reed Commission was told and retold over the decades, it became increasingly simplified in its hagiography of Walter Reed.[2] But scientific discoveries are rarely the act of one person, and the single focus obscures the rich scientific and cultural aspects of the story.

A broader, more accurate view of the yellow fever triumph includes six phases of the story that fundamentally involved American and Cuban scientists, Spanish volunteers, women volunteers, and tragedy and jealousy, as well as victory. Such a view begins with a decades-long search for the causative agent, or "germ," of yellow fever by scientists of several nations. The second phase introduces the 1900 Reed Commission, which narrowed its search from causative bacteria to the mosquito as a vector for the pathogen. The Reed experiments, 1900–1901, then proved the mosquito theory and disproved the fomite theory, and while none of the volunteers died, several suffered lifelong disability from their illness. In the fourth phase, Gorgas's 1901 mosquito mitigation efforts in Havana showed the correctness and the power of the mosquito theory, but a subsequent effort to develop a yellow fever vaccine ended in tragedy. The sixth and final episode in this revised yellow fever story involves the 1902 demonstration by a member of the Reed Commission that yellow fever was caused not by bacteria but by a "filterable virus," a discovery that stood as an important precursor to virology. This broader story takes little away from Walter Reed and brings to light the contributions of at least a score of courageous men and women, including William Gorgas, Cuban scientists, and Spanish volunteers.

## THE SEARCH FOR THE GERM

Yellow fever is a messy disease, producing all kinds of effluvia—vomit, blood, mucus, feces—so people reasonably believed it was a disease of filth, transmitted by fomites on soiled linens or other materials. In the late 1800s, bacteriologists were feverishly looking for disease germs, including one that caused yellow fever. Between 1879 and 1898, Surgeon General Sternberg participated in three yellow fever commissions seeking to identify the yellow fever germ without success. The race heated up in 1897 when Italian scientist Giuseppe Sanarelli announced that he had found the offending bacterium, *Bacillus icteroides*, and a few months later, Sternberg published his own work, naming a different bacterium, which he called *Bacillus X*, as the causative agent.[3]

Sternberg wanted to settle the controversy and hopefully prove his own theory right, so he turned to his protégé, Walter Reed, to settle the matter. Reed, born in rural Virginia, had been a prodigy as a young man, graduating from the University of Virginia and medical school in his teens.[4] He was a physician at Bellevue Hospital several years before Gorgas arrived, and like Gorgas served as a medical officer on frontier posts, conducting research in his spare time. In 1890 he got an opportunity to study bacteriology at the new Johns Hopkins Hospital, where he flourished, so that in 1893, Sternberg made him one of the first instructors at the Army Medical School. In 1898 Sternberg appointed Reed to the army Typhoid Board to investigate that epidemic in the US camps, but as that work was wrapping up, directed his best bacteriologist toward yellow fever. Reed and his research associate, English-born James Carroll, a bacteriologist and medical officer, began investigating yellow fiever in the army's laboratory in Washington, working with Aristedes Agramonte, the scientist whom Sternberg had hired as a contract surgeon in 1898.[5] He was in Havana conducting autopsies on yellow fever victims and sending tissue samples to Reed and Carroll.

In May 1899, with no amount of sanitation controlling yellow fever in Cuba, and under Leonard Wood's urging, Sternberg formalized the work of Reed, Carroll, and Agramonte into a special board to study infectious diseases in Cuba and named a fourth member, Jesse Lazear, from Johns Hopkins Medical School. He had studied malaria and mosquitoes in Italy, and as a contract surgeon had been running the hospital laboratory at Camp Columbia near Havana. Sternberg verbally instructed Reed to "give special attention to questions relating to the etiology and prevention of yellow fever."[6] Reed and Carroll arrived in Cuba on June 25, and what became known as the Reed Commission quickly met at Camp Columbia to organize their work.

One of the first things Reed did upon arriving in Havana was visit his friend Jefferson Kean, a medical officer for the US Department of Cuba, who was in Las Animas Hospital with yellow fever. It was the first case of yellow fever Reed had ever seen.[7] Gorgas was Kean's doctor. The men had arrived in Havana at the same time, and in one of the ironies of this story, before Kean became ill, the Medical Department had offered both Gorgas and Kean the assignment of chief surgeon for the US Department of Havana. Kean declined the position and instead took the job of overseeing improvements for hospitals, asylums, and other charitable institutions on the island. Gorgas took the job, and this decision put him, not Kean, on the path to fame.[8]

## FROM A GERM TO A BUG

Mosquitoes were literally in the air in Cuba, especially during the rainy season, which created more breeding habitat for them. Theo Lyster, newly commissioned in the Army Medical Corps, had come to work in Las Animas with his Uncle Will. Writing to his mother, he had to stop to light his pipe to create a smoke screen to keep the mosquitoes at bay. "I don't know how we would live here without tobacco and mosquito bars [nets]," he told her.[9] This ubiquity of mosquitoes and spikes of yellow fever during rainy season had given the Havana doctor and scientist Carlos Juan Finlay much to think about. Born in 1833 in Cuba to a Scottish physician and his French wife, Finlay grew up on a prosperous coffee plantation.[10] Educated

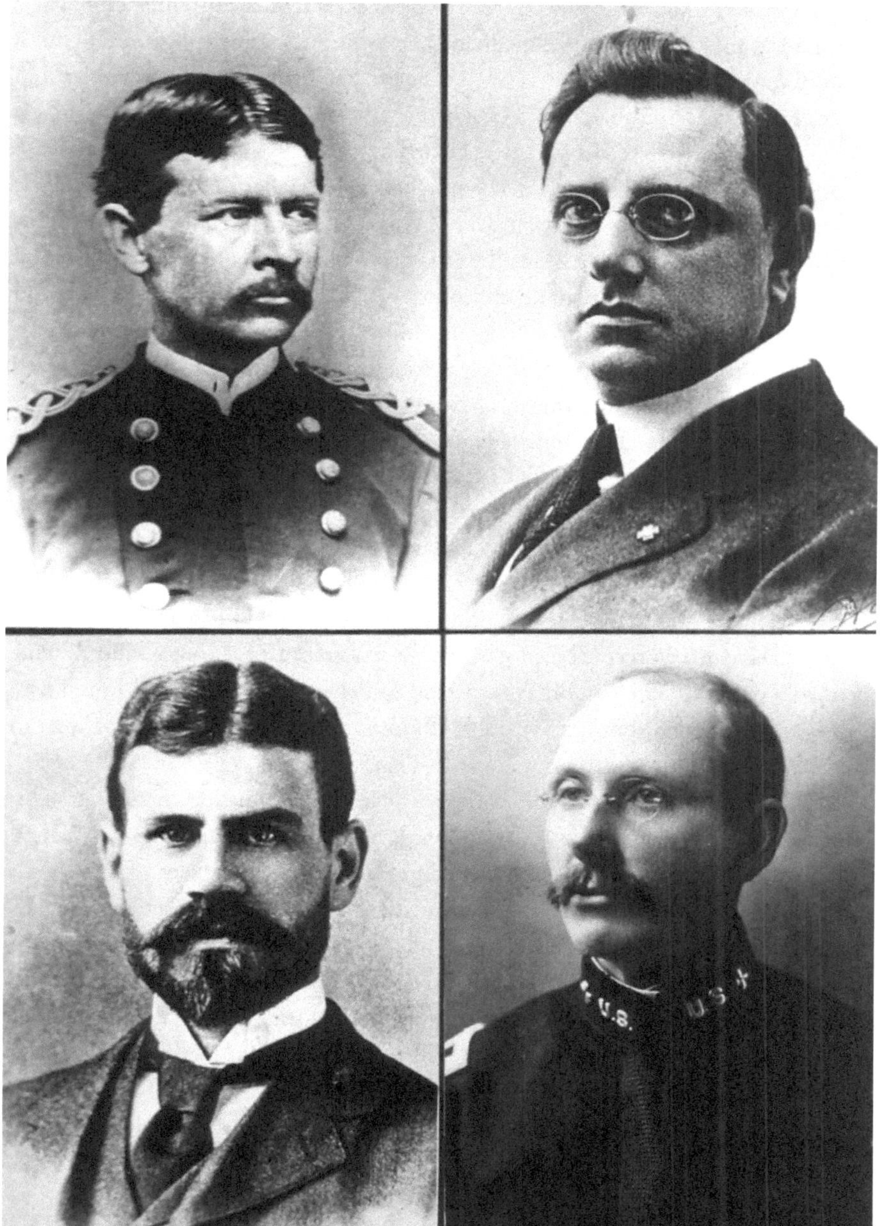

FIGURE 6.1. Members of the US Army's yellow fever commission clockwise from top left. Walter Reed, Aristides Agramonte, James Carroll, and Jesse W. Lazear, undated. National Library of Medicine.

in Europe, he earned an MD from Jefferson Medical College in Philadelphia and returned to Havana to practice medicine and continue biological research with a powerful new microscope. Fluent in English, French, German, Spanish, and written Latin, Finlay met Sternberg in 1879 when the first American yellow fever board came to Cuba. After reading in the scientific literature that yellow fever weakened blood vessels, causing them to hemorrhage, Finlay theorized that some agent other than "miasma" was infecting people. "To inoculate [introduce] yellow fever it would be necessary to pick out the inocuable material from within the blood vessels of the yellow fever patient and to carry it likewise to the interior of a blood vessel of a person who was to be inoculated," he reasoned. And such conditions "the mosquito satisfied most admirably through its bite." Only females had mouth parts capable of biting (male mosquito mouth parts were suited for nectar gathering), and out of six hundred mosquito types, Finlay correctly identified the female *Stegomyia* (today, *Aedes aegypti*) as the culprit.[11] He first announced his theory in 1881 and thereafter published scores of scientific papers on the matter and developed plans for mosquito mitigation. Finlay could not, however, reliably transmit yellow fever from one person to another. He tried by having mosquitoes bite yellow fever patients and then bite healthy individuals but could induce only three cases of the disease in 104 recorded efforts. He thus faced great skepticism and ridicule as the "mosquito man."[12] Gorgas respected Finlay as a physician and found him "a most lovable man" but later wrote that most scientists "were rather inclined to make light of his ideas, and none more so than I."[13]

But something was causing yellow fever. The Reed Commission's first order of investigation was to dispense with the notion that Sanarelli's *Bacillus icteroides* caused yellow fever. Within weeks of studying tissues from the yellow fever victims in Las Animas Hospital, Reed, Carroll, and Lazear showed that Sanarelli's bacterium was actually a variety of the hog-cholera bacillus and only a secondary infection to yellow fever. They also determined that Sternberg's *Bacillus X* did not cause the disease either.[14]

But if Gorgas and Reed Commission members dismissed Finlay's ideas, other scientists were beginning to substantiate the role insects could play in disease transmission. A Scottish physician, Patrick Manson, had shown in 1878 that a small worm, *Filaria sanguinis hominis,* could be injected into a person's body by the bite of the mosquito and cause filariasis (elephantiasis), a disease that causes grotesque swelling in the lower limbs. A French army surgeon, Alphonse Laveran, found a parasite in the blood of malaria patients in the 1880s, and theorized that it caused the illness by feeding upon red blood corpuscles. British scientist Ronald Ross then isolated this parasite in *Anopheles* mosquitoes and in 1898 showed that female mosquitoes could inject it into humans with their bite.[15] During the 1890s scientists had also shown that ticks transmitted Texas cattle fever and that flea bites spread bubonic plague.

Meanwhile, the Reed Commission was making other observations that undermined the fomite theory. For one, Havana was now as clean as many American cities, yet yellow fever persisted. In addition, nonimmune nurses and other medical staff who cared for yellow fever patients, handled soiled bedding, and conducted autopsies, did not get sick in greater numbers than people with no contact with yellow fever patients. And everyone knew that yellow fever "season" ended with a frost, which would eliminate mosquitoes. Commission members thus began to consider all methods of infection, including Finlay's mosquitoes.[16]

A pivotal observation came in late June when thirty-six soldiers contracted yellow fever and ten died at an isolated camp in Santa Clara, and commission members could not identify an "infected building" or individual as the source of infection.[17] Then in July they investigated an outbreak in Pinar del Rio Barracks that had been misdiagnosed as pernicious malaria. Despite the error in diagnosis and failure to disinfect bedding or clothing, yellow fever had not spread by contact with patients.[18] Commission members were especially intrigued by a case of yellow fever in prison whereby an army private confined in the guardhouse for several weeks had no exposure to yellow fever patients but fell ill with the disease. None of the other eight prisoners in his cell got sick, which raised the question of how the disease reached the hapless private. Reed began to conjecture that a mosquito had entered through the cell window to deliver the infection.[19]

A final building block in their thinking came with work by PHS scientist Henry Rose Carter. Before he joined the occupation forces to run the quarantine station in Havana, Carter had investigated an 1898 yellow fever outbreak in Mississippi and observed that after a first case of yellow fever appeared in a locality, subsequent cases did not emerge for ten to seventeen days. He theorized that the first sick person conveyed the disease to the environment, but only after a week or more was it transmitted to another person. He called this time interval "extrinsic incubation," and this helped explain Finlay's failed efforts to transmit the disease.[20] A mosquito could not simply bite a yellow fever patient one day and transmit it the next. The germ had to first incubate in her gut. Carter had published his findings just weeks earlier in May 1900 and gave Reed a copy of his paper. It was now time for Reed to meet the "mosquito man."[21]

## TESTING THE MOSQUITO THEORY

When Reed and his commission members finally visited Finlay at his home in Havana on August 1, the Cuban scientist eagerly reviewed his experiments with them, shared his research notes and publications, and, most importantly, gave them a porcelain dish containing eggs of a mosquito that had bitten a yellow fever patient.[22] This meeting was memorialized by Cuban artist Rafael Lillo just weeks later, portraying the Reed Commission, Finlay, and Gorgas peering into a beaker containing an enormous mosquito. Given his work with Finlay on the Havana yellow fever board, Gorgas may have introduced Reed to Finlay, but he never mentioned that he was at the meeting.[23]

Reed realized that he would need to experiment on human beings to prove definitively the mosquito vector theory. Sternberg concurred.[24] Commission members discussed experimenting on themselves, a practice not uncommon in nineteenth-century science, but before they developed test protocols, Reed had to return to Washington to finish the Typhoid Board report. While he was gone, Carroll and Lazear cultivated Finlay's mosquito eggs to adults in the Las Animas Hospital laboratory, feeding them banana and even letting them bite their arms for a blood meal. They learned how to coax adult females into test tubes so they could be transferred to Gorgas's yellow fever wards, where the researchers could "load" the mosquitoes with pathogens by letting them bite yellow fever patients. Between August 11 and August 25, Lazear, Carroll, and Agramonte inoculated nine volunteers through the bites of infected mosquitoes that had incubated the virus but were unable to induce yellow fever. On August 27 Carroll and Lazear were worried that one of the mosquitoes had not taken any blood and would die, so in the laboratory Carroll let her feed on his arm. (This is the event erroneously

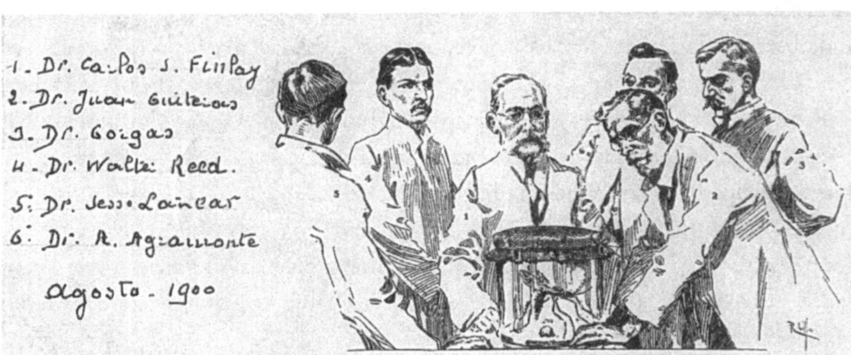


FIGURE 6.2. Photograph of a sketch of Carlos J. Finlay, Juan Guiteras, William Crawford Gorgas, Walter Reed, Jesse W. Lazear, and Aristides Agramonte, by R. Lillo, August 1900. Philip S. Hench Walter Reed Yellow Fever Collection, Courtesy of the Claude Moore Health Sciences Library, University of Virginia.

memorialized by the 1939 Cromwell painting placing fifteen men in an outdoor setting). Four days later Carroll was feverish and in bed—the first experimental case of yellow fever observed to be caused by a mosquito bite.[25] It was not a scientifically rigorous case, however, because Carroll had been in the yellow fever wards and about Havana and could have otherwise been exposed. Agramonte and Lazear therefore decided to try to infect another nonimmune. That afternoon American William H. Dean of the Seventh Cavalry walked into the laboratory, curious about their work, and allowed the same mosquito that had bitten Carroll to bite him. Six days later he too fell sick. Agramonte and Lazear wired the news to Reed.[26]

Gorgas was called to care for the men at Camp Columbia and told Marie that their cases excited "a great deal of interest." Carroll was asking specifically for Gorgas's attendance to his case, which, he admitted, "tickles me in my weak spot." Although Carroll had a serious case, under proper care he would probably survive, William wrote, adding, "I am getting quite a reputation on account of my success at Las Animas."[27] Then tragedy hit. As Carroll and Dean were recovering, Jesse Lazear was bitten by an infected mosquito, becoming the third experimental case. It is still unclear whether he allowed this or was bitten accidentally, but he developed the ominous symptoms of high fever, delirium, and internal hemorrhaging. Gorgas and others did what they could but were unable to save the young bacteriologist. He succumbed on September 25, just weeks after his wife had given birth to their second child.[28] In his condolence letter to Mabel Lazear, Gorgas told her that he had gotten to know her husband during his illness and had "formed the highest opinion of him in every way."[29]

When Reed returned to Cuba on October 4, the situation was grim. During September Havana had its worst yellow fever toll in two years, 269 cases with a 20 percent death rate. But recognizing that the team had made a scientific breakthrough, Reed made plans to present the findings at the American Public Health Association conference in Indianapolis later that month and went to Leonard Wood to ask for funding for human experiments to demonstrate mosquito transmission of yellow fever. Wood supported their efforts with alacrity and authorized $10,000 for the work, adding, "If that is not enough, I will give you $10,000 more."[30] Funding secured, Reed left to share the commission's findings with the world, reporting that "the mosquito serves as the intermediate host for the parasite of yellow fever, and it is highly probable that the disease is only propagated through the bite of this insect."[31]

On the strength of this evidence, under Wood's command, Jefferson Kean issued Circular No. 8, October 15, ordering army camps to use mosquito bars in all barracks and hospitals and to destroy mosquito larvae in the water: "The evidence is now perfect and conclusive that malaria, as well as filarial infections, are carried by this insect [the mosquito], and there are reasons to suspect that it may be connected with the transmission of yellow fever also."[32] But the epidemic drove on, with October worse than September.

While Reed was gone, Agramonte kept the mosquitoes alive, found an isolated location for an experimental camp, and began to recruit volunteers from nonimmune American and Spanish workers for the experiments.[33] When Reed returned, workers set up hospital tents for staff and volunteers and constructed two experimental cabins. The "Infected Mosquito Building," was carefully screened, while the "Infected Clothing Building," was tightly enclosed to prevent any mosquitoes or fresh air from entering and had a stove to maintain tropical temperatures. Completed on November 20, the experimental site was named Camp Lazear after their martyred colleague.

Given the risk involved with the proposed inoculation experiments, Reed had volunteers sign documents of "informed consent" in English or Spanish acknowledging the dangers they could encounter, and that they would receive $100 for their participation and another $100 if they contracted yellow fever.[34] Participation, however, was not as suicidal as it might seem, because many people survived yellow fever, and volunteers were assured of excellent medical care. Hospital corpsmen and nurses often sought immunity so they could get additional pay and status for yellow fever duty; others figured they would get yellow fever anyway and might as well do so for science and the money. Volunteers, most of them men in their twenties, stayed in quarantine for twenty-four days to ensure that they were in perfect health before the experiments. Then, in the following weeks, from December 5, 1900, to February 7, 1901, the Reed Commission induced twenty experimental cases of yellow fever. Medical officers and hospital corpsmen monitored the volunteers and cared for them when they became sick. The Havana yellow fever board of Gorgas, Finlay, Guiteras, and Albertini confirmed each diagnosis and assisted in treatment.[35]

The first experiment involved the Infected Mosquito Building, whereby a small group of men entered each of two sleeping rooms that had been sanitized and supplied with fresh linens and nightshirts. Researchers kept one of the rooms free of mosquitoes and released fifteen infected mosquitoes into the other. The first yellow fever case developed on December 9 when a volunteer, John Kissinger, fell sick after receiving more than a dozen mosquito bites on three separate occasions. Gorgas confirmed the diagnosis, and it was a severe case. "My spine felt twisted and my head swollen and my eyes felt as if they would pop out of my head," Kissinger later wrote.[36] He survived but never fully recovered and was invalided the rest of his life.[37] Other volunteers in the mosquito room also developed yellow fever. One of them, John Moran, remembered that Gorgas visited him daily and "was deeply interested in the experiments and plied me with questions."[38] Men in the room free of mosquitoes, meanwhile, stayed perfectly well. On December 15, Reed cabled Sternberg, "Experimental station established November 20, three cases already diagnosed, confirmed by Guiteras, Finlay, Albertini and Gorgas, theory conclusively proven. Reed."[39]

Even before the conclusion of the experiments, the Americans celebrated. On December 21, Gorgas attended a gala to honor Finlay, with Juan Guiteras as the master of ceremonies. The Americans gave Finlay a bronze statue and accorded full and equal credit to the Cuban physicians and scientists for the success.[40] The same day Kean and Wood expanded the mosquito-net order to all military units in Cuba, stating, "It is now well established that malaria, yellow fever and filarial infection are transmitted by the bites of mosquitoes."[41]

The Reed Commission's research continued with the aim to discredit the filth theory. During December and January, in the Infected Clothing Building, three groups of stalwart volunteers slept in pajamas and bed linens soiled by yellow fever patients' vomit and diarrhea, for twenty nights each. None of them developed the disease. In a third set of experiments, Reed's team used hypodermic needles to inject blood from yellow fever patients into volunteers to see whether the disease was transmitted through the blood and did not necessarily have to go through a mosquito. Several of these men developed the disease, including two Army privates who were injected with filtered blood serum, but they all recovered. The Reed Commission had its proof.

Reed closed down Camp Lazear in mid-February and returned home to Washington, DC, to write up their report. "The Etiology of Yellow Fever" offered eleven conclusions. The first nine confirmed the transmission of yellow fever by mosquitoes, and not fomites, and explained the process of extrinsic incubation. The final two points set the course for further action: one stated that Reed and Carroll would continue to investigate the specific cause of yellow fever; the other, that yellow fever could be "most effectually controlled by measures directed to the destruction of mosquitoes and the protection of the sick against bites of these insects."[42] That task would go to Gorgas and his team.

## THEORY INTO PRACTICE

The day after Camp Lazear closed, Wood issued orders to begin yellow fever eradication in Havana, and as chief surgeon for the US Department of Havana, Gorgas led the charge. Given the new understanding of yellow fever transmission, the first step was to prevent mosquitoes from biting patients and redouble efforts to find yellow fever patients as soon as possible. Although Gorgas and Las Animas Hospital had such a good reputation that people generally reported their cases without the threat of penalties, the Americans now offered a substantial reward of fifty dollars for each case. Once patients were identified, they were swiftly isolated, screened in, and treated at home or in the hospital. Workers fumigated the patient's house and all contiguous buildings to kill any mosquitoes that might have had access to the sick.[43]

The next job was to get rid of mosquitoes altogether. Gorgas launched mosquito mitigation in the manner of a military campaign, whereby he and his workers killed mosquitoes as if people's lives depended on it. His department adopted Finlay's mosquito mitigation methods, and beginning in March 1901, teams fumigated every building in Havana, regardless of whether yellow fever had appeared in it. Sanitary workers used sulfur, camphor, or pyrethrum powder to knock out adult insects, then swept them up and burned them. To destroy mosquito eggs and larvae, sanitation workers would need to eliminate all exposed standing water in the city. With no dependable water source and few rivers, Cuban residents collected and stored rainwater in barrels or in cisterns below their homes, and this created ideal breeding grounds for *Stegomyia* that lived indoors and laid their eggs in still water. Gorgas's office therefore divided the city into twenty districts, deploying three hundred men in teams to inspect every building monthly for standing water where mosquitoes could breed. The US Department of Agriculture had shown the effectiveness of using oil to destroy mosquito larvae, so when sanitation teams could not eliminate a water source or screen or drain it, they oiled the surface.[44] Gorgas ultimately had fifty men charged with oiling cesspools and draining streams and pools throughout Havana, using the military's unique authority to execute such detailed and stringent measures.

With political and financial support from his superiors, Wood and Sternberg, Gorgas recruited and retained a dedicated group of colleagues who approached the job as a scientific and public health endeavor.[45] He hired Joseph Le Prince, an English engineer who had earned civil engineering and master's degrees from Columbia University, to improve and refine their mosquito control measures. Le Prince and his coworkers innovated as they gained experience and knowledge and by June, for example, were using ounces rather than pounds of pyrethrum per 1,000 cubic feet. Le Prince rose to become the general inspector of the Department of Sanitation and developed a lasting friendship with William and Marie.

Gorgas also recognized the importance of educating the community about mosquito control because he needed their cooperation if his department's invasive measures of home inspection and water source elimination were to succeed. Gorgas and

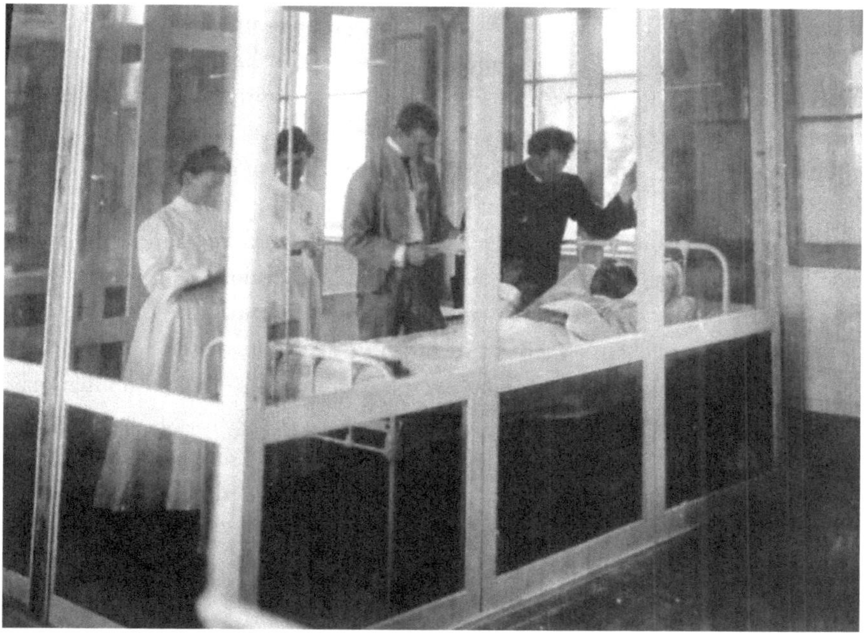

FIGURE 6.3. Photograph of a yellow fever patient screened to prevent transmission of disease by mosquitoes, archived in the Gorgas Papers at the Library of Congress. Library of Congress Prints and Photographs Division.

his staff therefore worked hard to educate people about the "wigglers"—larvae—in their water supplies. They showed housewives the larvae in their water barrels and in the cans of water they put beneath table legs to prevent ants from climbing up. Gorgas's energy and tact were critical to the campaign. Marie later wrote that her husband "became a familiar figure on the back streets of Havana—poking around tin cans and refuse, checking rain barrels, talking to housewives, delivering small spontaneous lectures, and making converts." She claimed that "whenever he rang a front-door bell, a beaming señora would greet him almost invariably with the same words: 'No hay mosquitos aquí, señor' [No mosquitoes here, sir]."[46] Gorgas and the Sanitary Department had broad enforcement powers, including possible fines and even jail time, but in contrast to the repressive Spanish colonial regime, they used these powers sparingly. American public health officials levied some $2,500 in fines for violations but ultimately collected only $50.[47]

Mosquito mitigation worked. Yellow fever deaths in Havana fell from 310 in 1900, to 17 in the first three months of 1901, and none in the next three months.

From May 7 to July 1, 1901, no yellow fever cases were recorded in the city at all.[48] As Gorgas began the work, he sent reports to Reed in Washington, who enthusiastically asked questions, gave advice, and celebrated the unfolding victory. As they began to see that they had found a means to control yellow fever, they engaged in a revelatory correspondence. "I begin to feel like rejoicing that I ever was born!" Reed wrote to Gorgas. "You are doing a splendid work for your corps and profession in Havana."[49] Gorgas responded, "Yours was the guiding hand in the whole matter," adding "I am very happy to shine in the more humble role of being the first to put your discovery to extensive, practical application."[50]

In the wake of the Army Medical Department's typhoid scandal of 1898, Reed felt that vanquishing yellow fever would serve as an antidote to their humiliation.[51] As he sought to take full credit, however, he disparaged Cubans, complaining that with "so many ignorant doctors" in Havana, it was impossible to report all yellow fever cases. "They will conceal their cases, do what you may; and these cases will be the foci for other cases."[52] Gorgas countered diplomatically, "I feel confident that there is very little concealment of cases; and I do not feel much anxiety on this score."[53] When Reed's fears proved to be unfounded, he admitted, "It shows that your acquaintance with the local conditions were [*sic*] much better than mine."[54] But he chided Gorgas for giving too much credit to Finlay for the mosquito theory. "I suppose that being back in Havana that you feel that your duty to 'honey up' that simpering old nabob."[55] Now Gorgas responded archly. "I do not 'honey up to the simpering old idiot' a bit. I think he is an old trump as modest as he is kindly & true." Gorgas judged Finlay's selection of the *Stegomyia* as the carrier of yellow fever "the best piece of logical reasoning that can be found in medicine anywhere." Then a salve to Reed: "Your name will be remembered in medicine with Jenner & Wills long after the old Dr. has been forgotten so do not begrudge the old man his little need of praise."[56] Reed apologized, but the first sallies in the contest for credit had been launched.[57]

## THE CONVERSION OF DR. GORGAS

Years later, after Gorgas's death, Jefferson Kean severely—and unfairly—criticized him for being slow to embrace the mosquito theory. But as early as December 13, 1900, Gorgas admitted to Henry Carter, who had become a close friend, "I was very averse to receiving the [mosquito] theory, but a few absolutely positive experiments outweigh any amount of negative evidence."[58] He was, however, reluctant to believe that mosquitoes were the *only* means of transmission, to the exclusion of fomites. The army's Typhoid Board had just shown that typhoid bacteria could be transmitted by houseflies carrying bacteria from latrines to food as well as through tainted water and food.[59] Thus, when Wood and Kean issued Circular No. 5 in April 1901, directing the discontinuance of disinfection for yellow fever, Gorgas did not stop disinfecting bedding and clothing for five more months.[60] A physician more than a scientist, and witness to so much pain and death from yellow fever, he hesitated to abandon all of the measures he had used for years against the disease.

Gorgas recognized his skepticism and in late 1901 explained the progression of his thinking to the editor of the *Philadelphia Medical Journal*, who had asked him for a paper on sanitation and yellow fever. A southern physician, Dr. John Purnell, of Vicksburg, Mississippi, had written to the journal arguing that while mosquitoes might transmit yellow fever, fomites did as well. Gorgas was sympathetic, writing, "My own personal experience with this disease had so impressed me with the belief that fomites were the principal, and practically the only, carrier of the disease that I had scant belief in the mosquito theory."[61] He then outlined the Reed experiments and noted that at their conclusion, "while I was convinced that yellow fever was conveyed by the Stegomyia mosquito, it was not proven that it was the only way." Only after yellow fever had disappeared entirely from Havana, he explained, was he willing to accept mosquitoes as the sole source of transmission and to stop disinfecting patient homes. Gorgas advised that if physicians were not entirely convinced, they should at least add "killing mosquitoes to their methods of disinfection."[62] He then invited Purnell and other southern health officers to Havana to see their work for themselves.

Once fully convinced of the mosquito theory, Gorgas was relieved. He wrote Reed on August 26 that he considered the yellow fever question "settled," and that "the discovery that it is the mosquito alone that conveys the disease will enable us to manage it."[63] Disinfecting homes of the sick was disruptive, unpopular, and damaged property; it thus discouraged reporting. Simply fumigating against mosquitoes, however, "damages nothing, only keeps them out of their room for an hour or two and kills the mosquitoes." As Gorgas told Reed, "Everything that minimizes the trouble and inconvenience to the people at large . . . is a great help in popularizing these measures, and in preventing opposition to their enforcement."[64]

No yellow fever appeared in Havana in August, and when a patient arrived in port already sick and died in September, Gorgas told his colleagues that it was likely the last case they would see.[65] Malaria deaths fell too, from 247 in the first six months of 1900 to 75 during the first six months of 1901.[66] "I hardly expected any such sweeping stamping out of the disease as we have apparently done so far this year," Gorgas told Carter.[67] But he remained cautious. Although researchers confirmed that yellow fever victims were not infectious after three days, Gorgas isolated his patients for five days. He also continued to screen the deceased, because "whether the mosquito will, or can, feed upon a dead body, I do not know."[68] Gorgas could, however, also make fun of skeptics. He liked to tell the story of a group of visitors touring the mosquito laboratory at Las Animas. While Gorgas was showing them mosquito eggs, larvae, and newly hatched adults, some netting slipped, allowing some mosquitoes to fly about the room. They had not fed on yellow fever patients so were not dangerous, but the men rushed for the door to flee the insects. Gorgas recounted, "Our visitors laughingly acknowledged that, at any rate, their unconscious selves had been convinced of the correctness of the theory of mosquito transmission."[69]

Newspapers reported the results in Havana with enthusiastic headlines: "American Success in Havana" (*Chicago Daily Tribune*); "Havana Purged of Fever" (*New York Times*); "Dr. Gorgas Says Mosquito Crusade Has Eradicated Disease in Havana" (*Washington Post*); and "Havana Is Now Healthy" (*Jacksonville Metropolis*).[70] In Tuscaloosa the Gorgas family eagerly read the news and contracted with a clipping service to keep track of stories about William.[71] Gorgas also sought to spread the word on how to fight yellow fever. Monthly reports were the lifeblood of army administration, and Gorgas began to wield these to great effect, ordering hundreds of extra copies of his monthly health reports and sending them to sanitarians, physicians, and others around the world.[72] *Public Health Reports* began to publish his monthly updates on the falling rates of disease in Havana, and *JAMA* and *The Lancet* followed his progress as well.[73] As early as March 1901, Gorgas noted that Jacksonville, Mobile, and New Orleans had higher death rates than Havana, and that while those cities had historically imposed quarantines against ships arriving from Havana, in the future, "Havana will have to guard against them."[74] The *Washington Post* disapproved of Gorgas's optimism, though, and suggested that he be more circumspect and "avoid that role of prophecy in which so many great and good men have come to lasting grief."[75] The newspaper had a point, because Gorgas and his colleagues soon came to grief.

## VACCINE?

Since Edward Jenner introduced smallpox vaccination in 1798, scientists had been seeking similar ways to induce immunity against other diseases. In recent decades Louis Pasteur and others had experimented with attenuated cholera, anthrax, and rabies pathogens to develop vaccines against those killers, with some success. Now Gorgas and his colleague Juan Guiteras proposed to do the same. Cubans acquired immunity through mild attacks of yellow fever during childhood, and Guiteras hypothesized that yellow fever germs weakened as they successively passed through mosquitoes and in such attenuated form could be used to make a vaccine. Gorgas therefore in February 1901 asked Sternberg for funds to set up a laboratory at Las Animas Hospital so Guiteras could conduct experiments, "to see if some general system of inoculation would not be feasible and justified."[76] Sternberg and Wood approved, so that summer, while the Sanitary Department was killing mosquitoes, Guiteras inoculated thirty-four American and Spanish volunteers using the Reed Commission protocol of informed consent. At first no yellow fever cases developed, and they blamed cool weather for hindering the extrinsic incubation of the virus in mosquitoes. But in August, when Guiteras inoculated sixteen more volunteers, one man allowed eleven mosquitoes to bite him and developed a well-marked, though not dangerous, case of yellow fever. However, when those same eleven mosquitoes bit seven other volunteers, tragedy ensued. Six became very sick and three of them died. Spaniards Antonio Carro and Cumperino Campa were inoculated on August 8 and 9, and both died within a week. The third death was Clara Maass, a nurse, age twenty-five, of East Orange, New Jersey. Maass had arrived at Las Animas in the fall of 1900 after serving in the army training camps and the Philippines during the war. She volunteered for the trials hoping to become immune so she could travel to other tropical posts and earn better pay. Over the summer she allowed herself to be bitten by infected mosquitoes five times, until on August 18 she finally fell ill. She developed a severe case of yellow fever, and on August 24, Gorgas had to inform her family of her death.[77]

It threatened to be a scandal. American newspapers cried, "Fatal Experiments," and Clara's mother told a reporter, "My daughter's death seems little short of murder."[78] The young volunteer's informed consent absolved the team in Havana of such charges, but Gorgas and Guiteras stopped the experiments, and Gorgas offered compensation for the deceased volunteers' families.[79] He told reporters, "I hold myself responsible for what occurred and I cannot sufficiently express my sorrow."[80] As Gorgas told Reed, "I had hoped that through the mosquito we had a means of giving mild cases that would protect, but these cases show that the severest form of yellow fever can be transmitted by one or two mosquito bites." The "death of these patients," he said, "makes all success taste of gall and wormwood, and casts a gloom over the Sanitary Department."[81] Mosquitoes were not invincible, though, and Gorgas's success in eradicating them and yellow fever from Havana outshone the dismal failure of the vaccine trials. Press criticism soon died down.

Reed, Carroll, and Gorgas presented papers on their work at the September 1901 American Public Health Association annual conference in Buffalo, New York.[82] Gorgas now set his sights on the American South, telling Carter, "My ambition is soaring. What I want to tackle now is New Orleans, after she has been well infected." After Havana, though, it would be "too easy a job."[83]

## "FILTERABLE VIRUS"

The final phase of the American yellow fever project involved Reed and Carroll's continuing efforts to find the pathogen. Scientists would not be able to actually see viruses until the development of powerful electron microscopes in the 1930s, but Carroll continued to examine blood samples from patients at Las Animas, looking for the actual physical pathogen that caused the disease. In one experiment he passed infected blood through a clay filter that could screen out larger bacterial pathogens and injected it into three volunteers. When they developed yellow fever, it showed that the infecting agent was a "filterable virus," meaning that it could pass through filters and was therefore smaller than bacteria. This demonstration foreshadowed the virology of the twentieth century.[84]

## THE CUBAN REPUBLIC

In addition to ridding Havana of yellow fever, the United States assisted Cuba in breaking free of Spanish domination, restoring the economy, and building up the urban infrastructure with sewerage systems, roads and bridges, a justice system, schools, and a robust network of hospitals to prepare the island for self-government. Most of these projects were paid for by $57 million in Cuban revenues from customs and internal revenue, with the United States paying only for the occupying troops.[85] Political reform was less successful. Secretary Root ordered a census of the island in anticipation of widespread voting, but conservative male citizens recommended suffrage only for literate men twenty-one and older who were native Cubans or Spaniards and had served in the Cuban Army, or men who owned at least $250 in property. This enfranchised only 105,000 of the 1.6 million Cuban population. The constitutional convention incorporated these measures in a new constitution for the Republic of Cuba to take effect on May 20, 1902.

Also, as Wood and the occupying American army were avowing their support for Cuban independence, Congress was retreating from those promises and passed the Platt Amendment to a military appropriations bill laying out several conditions before the United States relinquished control. One permitted the United States to maintain a naval station at Guantánamo Bay to support commerce and ensure that no other foreign power gained control over the island. Another required the government of Cuba to implement public sanitation plans, so that "a recurrence of epidemic and infectious diseases may be prevented," which meant not only in Cuba but in southern US ports.[86] Cubans angrily denounced the demands but yielded to the United States and incorporated the amendments into their constitution. The measures and associated corporate investments would bind Cuba to the United States for decades.[87]

Gorgas did not opine on these developments but did observe that massive government spending in Cuba had improved the social conditions, and that with no military to maintain, every Cuban peso collected in taxation was being spent "upon the people themselves." He felt convinced that this was possible only under the US military rule and "could not occur under a civil government."[88] With implicit support for Cuban independence but reservations about the future of democratic self-government on the island, he told Amelia, "The best government in the world is a one man despotic government—provided your despot is a good & able man," but added, "The trouble with despotisms is that you can never insure this."[89]

America thus left Cuba with a fragile economy dependent on sugar and tobacco, and a limited governing electorate of Spanish and Creole upper classes. These conditions would lead to a populist revolt only four years later and, under the Platt Amendment, cause the United States to reoccupy the island.[90] In the meantime, however, Cuban and American officials, including William and Marie, attended a ceremony on May 20, 1902, to lower the American flag and raise that of the Cuban Republic. Most of the Americans then left for home on the next steamer, but a handful, including the Gorgases, remained in Havana. William had orders from Leonard Wood to continue "investigations in regard to the relations between yellow fever and the mosquito."[91] Gorgas, however, was already thinking of new frontiers.

CHAPTER 7

# Will Panama Be Safe Enough to Build a Canal?

> I would rather die five or six years earlier in this struggle such as we would have in Panama, trying to accomplish some work that would benefit all mankind, . . . than live five years longer in the pleasant, but much narrower, field in which I am now living.
>
> —William Gorgas to John Ross, January 1904

As Gorgas and other public health officials had hoped, the Cuban work freed the southern United States from a primary source of yellow fever and the attending fear and disruption. To honor the Medical Department's work, Secretary of War Elihu Root recommended that Congress recognize both Reed and Gorgas, promoting Reed to full colonel and Gorgas to lieutenant colonel. The "brilliant character of the scientific achievement, its inestimable value to mankind, the saving of thousands of lives, and the deliverance of the Atlantic seacoast from constant apprehension," he wrote, "demand special recognition from the government of the United States." The Office of the Surgeon General (hereafter, OTSG) prepared dossiers on the two men, describing their accomplishments and including letters of endorsement from key individuals and organizations.[1]

Gorgas was already thinking about his next job and, as early as February 1902, had launched a campaign urging that a physician and sanitarian be named to the Panama Canal commission, preferably himself. A French effort to build the canal in the 1880s had been thwarted by yellow fever, which killed thousands of workers and engineers, and devastated French investors. Although the Panama campaign would be expensive, Gorgas told Surgeon General Sternberg, "the methods worked out at Havana could be so modified as to be applied successfully at the Isthmus."[2] He requested an assignment in Washington, DC, so that if and when the United

States gained access to Panama, he would be close by to advise the canal commission. The job of preventing this kind of disease toll greatly appealed to him, he told Amelia, "if they will give me the power and some extra pay."[3] This vision set William Gorgas on a path of controversy and strife as well as national and international success and acclaim.

## PROMOTION AND TRAGEDY

As they awaited their promotions, Gorgas and Reed pursued different paths. Gorgas set his sights on Panama, while Reed led the research effort to find the yellow fever germ and promote the mosquito theory in the scientific world. The theory was beginning to take hold.[4] When yellow fever broke out in Laredo, Texas, near Fort McIntosh, instead of moving the entire army command to escape infection, the post's medical officer was able to keep all five of his yellow fever patients from dying and contained the outbreak by imposing a quarantine and implementing antimosquito measures.[5] Other communities, north and south, began forming mosquito brigades to clean up their neighborhoods for comfort as much as for disease control. As one newspaper observed, the value of "real estate would undoubtedly go up in Jersey and the Long and Staten islands if the evil reputation of the mosquito were no longer a blight on suburban property."[6] In a step of great import, William Osler incorporated the new information in the fourth edition (1902) of his definitive medical textbook, *Principles and Practice of Medicine*, recommending Gorgas's four means of control—preventing mosquitoes from biting yellow fever patients, screening buildings, destroying adult mosquitoes, and eliminating mosquito breeding places near residential areas. Osler's textbook did not, however, adopt Gorgas's gentler regime for treating patients and continued to recommend mercury and strychnine.[7]

Throughout the spring of 1902, Jefferson Kean advocated for fellow Virginian and friend Walter Reed to succeed George Sternberg as surgeon general. In June, however, Secretary of War Root named Col. Robert M. O'Reilly instead, on the basis of seniority. Gorgas quickly wrote to O'Reilly urging that a medical officer be assigned to the Isthmian Canal project. "I would like to be that member," he told his new boss.[8] The new surgeon general made no commitment to Gorgas regarding Panama but did assign him to a post in Washington, DC.

The Gorgases left Havana in September 1902 with a glow. "No more interesting story in the history of medicine has ever been told," wrote the *Medical News* of Gorgas's accomplishments in Havana, "than the disappearance of yellow fever from that city."[9] The new president of Cuba, Tomás Estrada Palma, hosted a dinner in Gorgas's honor, causing the *New York Times* to observe that "no American official who has been on duty here under the government of occupation has gone away from Cuba with more good wishes from the Cubans than he. The people have for him a genuine feeling of gratitude."[10] Many Cubans may have recognized Gorgas's public health work, but they also appreciated his diplomacy in implementing the rigorous measures.

After Gorgas was settled in Washington, O'Reilly sent him to a medical congress in Cairo, Egypt, in December 1902, to give an account of the Medical Department's accomplishments in Havana. While in Egypt he could examine sanitary conditions at the Suez Canal and, on the way home, stop in Paris to consult with the French on the health measures during their failed canal project. William was reluctant to leave Washington before the Panama commission was appointed but persuaded Marie to go with him, and the couple departed New York on the *Futoria* of the Hamburg American Line on November 19, 1902. Before he sailed, Gorgas took the precaution of buying extra life insurance but assured his brother, Dick, that he did not "feel any symptoms of an early demise. On the contrary we are both in first rate trim."[11]

Not so, Walter Reed. In October he started to feel too fatigued to give his lectures, and by November he was in so much pain he went to bed. Suspecting that he had appendicitis, Reed consulted his colleague at the Army Medical School, Maj. William C. Borden, who immediately admitted him to the hospital at Washington Barracks. Upon operating, Borden found a burst appendix and necrotic tissue. Reed was critically ill. He lingered only a few more hours and died on November 23, 1902, at the age of fifty-one.[12] Borden, Kean, and others were bereft. Gorgas learned of Reed's death at sea, en route to Cairo, and observed to Amelia, "No single man in medicine in his generation has done work that will directly save as many human lives as Reed's discoveries in regard to yellow fever." Thinking of Reed's widow, Emilie, he added, "He leaves his wife and daughter with about $20,000 which with their pension will make them comfortable."[13] Not everyone agreed. According to Kean and Emilie, before Reed went into surgery, he said to Kean, "I am not afraid of the knife, but if any thing should happen I am leaving my wife & daughter so little, so little."[14] Kean took this comment to heart and looked after Reed's widow and his legacy for the rest of his life.

On his first trip overseas, while Marie was quite seaworthy, William found he was a terrible sailor and suffered from seasickness throughout the twelve-day voyage. This problem would plague him for life but not deter him from sailing the seas.[15] When they finally disembarked onto solid ground in Egypt, they toured the Suez Canal, which had been completed in 1869 and linked the Mediterranean and Red Seas. Gorgas found the desert landscape differed greatly from the "low

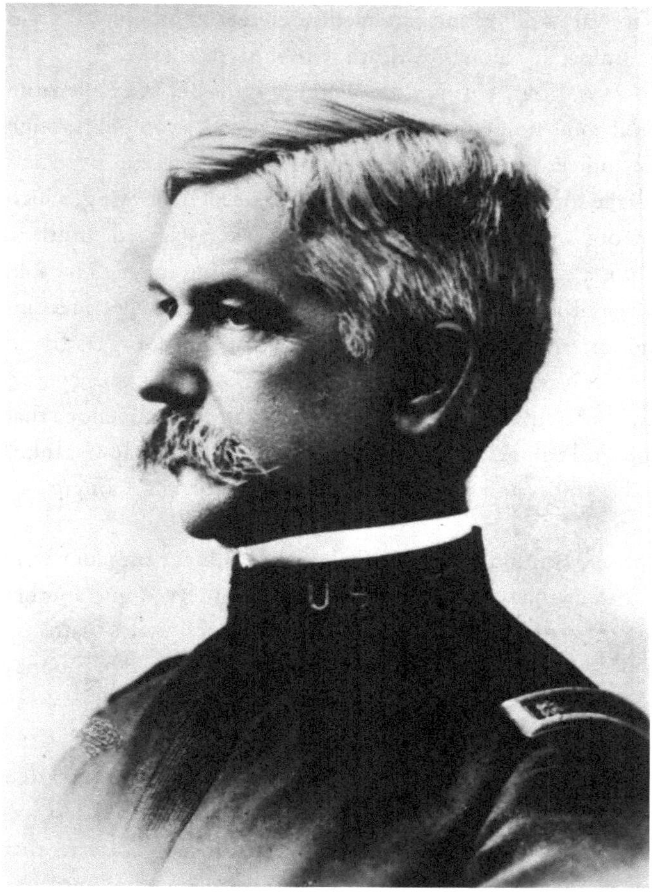

FIGURE 7.1. William C. Gorgas, n.d. National Library of Medicine.

swampy country, alternating with rugged mountains" landscape of the Isthmus he had read about, and he therefore pronounced it all "a very interesting trip, though I did not get much information that was useful to us at Panama."[16] William and Marie climbed the pyramids, visited museums, dined with health officials, and sent postcards home to their family.[17] Traveling through Italy, they visited the Coliseum in Rome. There, Gorgas turned morbid. He had just seen a painting portraying the lions and the Christians and now conjured up that image as he sat in that ancient arena. He imagined the terror of the thirty men, women, and children "drawn together in a little group away from the door from which they knew the lions were to come." He also considered what the gladiators would feel, both conqueror and conquered, as the victor "drove his sword through the heart of his helpless opponent."[18]

Given his proximity to war as a boy and as a medical officer in Siboney, Gorgas seemed to live more comfortably alongside death than most people.

As Gorgas sailed to Paris, Kean, who was now working in the OTSG, cabled him to cut short his trip and come home to help shepherd his promotion bill through Congress. All military officer promotions required congressional approval, and jumping ranks such as the surgeon general was proposing needed lobbying, which would be difficult if Gorgas was on a junket in Europe. Gorgas agreed. "Both in point of pay and honor, a colonelcy would be a very big thing for me," he told Amelia, adding that even if it did not pass, it was an honor to have been recommended.[19] The promotion bill had stalled after Reed's death, but Gorgas's friend John Ross, now at the US Naval Museum of Hygiene in Washington, urged Surgeon General O'Reilly to action. Since Reed had died, O'Reilly recommended that Gorgas be promoted to full colonel in Reed's place, an even larger jump in rank.[20] Secretary Root agreed, so Ross and Kean worked with members of Congress to carry the legislation.

The unorthodox promotion did not go unchallenged. Military surgeons were a small cadre and as they circulated through various posts observed one another carefully—if not jealously—following the progress of their colleagues' paths up the army ranks. Maj. Valery Havard, with whom Gorgas had worked at Siboney and Havana (and who had initially refused to evacuate Gorgas and Theo when they were sick with typhoid) objected to the legislation because it would promote Gorgas over thirty-five other medical officers, including himself. He argued that Gorgas had nothing to do with discovering mosquito transmission, and that it was merely "the accident of Major Gorgas being chief sanitary officer of Havana that gave him the opportunity."[21] Gorgas was hurt by Havard's opposition, telling Theo, "As we were personal friends, I am sorry that he has feeling in the matter. I do not think that he has grounds for any feeling."[22] While Havard and other officers had a legitimate grievance, Secretary Root countered that Gorgas's achievement was "a great object lesson to the world" on how to rid the tropics of mosquito-borne diseases. Gorgas may not have been the only medical officer capable of doing this work, Root stated, but "in all life the rewards are given to the men who are fortunate enough to get this opportunity."[23]

Despite the opposition, the promotion became law March 3, 1903, and the *Atlanta Constitution* announced, "Southern Man Goes up Higher: Services of Major William Crawford Gorgas Honored by Congress."[24] Gorgas was gratified. "It is the first time an Army medical officer has been directly recognized by Congress," he told Amelia. "It places me in a rank that would have taken me about 15 years to reach in the ordinary course of promotion and increased my pay $80 per month."[25]

Gorgas's promotion after Reed's death may also have sown the seeds of Jefferson Kean's jealousy. Congress did recognize Reed's work by naming the Army Medical Department's new, modern army hospital in Washington after him, and authorizing pensions of $100 a month for his and Jessie Lazear's widows.[26] But with Reed and Lazear dead, Carroll in poor health, and Aristides Agramonte in Havana, Gorgas was in a position to receive the lion's share of the recognition and rewards for the American success in Cuba. The *Washington Post* announced, for example, "Yellow Fever Stamped Out: Dr. Gorgas Says Mosquito Crusade Has Eradicated Disease in Havana."[27] In June 1903 the University of Pennsylvania awarded Gorgas an honorary doctor of science degree, as did his alma mater, the University of the South. He was becoming famous.

## HISTORY OF PANAMA

The Isthmus of Panama stood as the great bridge from the Old World to the New, the Atlantic to the Pacific, and from North to South America. In the late nineteenth century, as the United States sought dominance in the Western Hemisphere, many Americans considered the Isthmus of Panama vital to regional access and control. Several government commissions investigated the geographical and political options to gain access and influence there, and Gorgas now sought to leverage his promotion and new acclaim into a seat on the most recent Isthmian Canal Commission.

Since the first Spanish ship appeared on the coast of Panama in 1501, the narrow isthmus has had a dynamic history. By the 1520s the Spanish were transporting silver from the Inca Empire across the Isthmus by foot, donkey, and mule, to galleons headed for Spain.[28] These riches financed the expansion of the Spanish Empire, making Panama City one of the richest outposts of the New World. After Panama declared its independence from Spain in 1821 and joined Simon Bolivar's newly created Republic of Colombia, the region became a relative backwater until midcentury when Americans, spurred by the discovery of gold in California, began using the isthmus as a shortcut across the continent. The dangerous ocean voyage between New York and San Francisco around the horn of South America took four or five months, whereas a land crossing via Panama—only fifty miles and a few days on foot and by mule—cut the time to six weeks. In the 1850s, when the American-owned Panama Railroad Company built a rail line across the isthmus, the trip became faster and safer. The railroad was built at immense cost: 5,000 to 10,000 laborers died from disease and accidents during the five years of construction, but it became a commercial success. The first paying passengers made the four-hour crossing for twenty-five dollars, and between 1849 and 1859, roughly 20 percent of the people who traveled to California from the eastern United States did so by way of Panama. American and Panamanian investors got rich, and to protect those investments, the United States intervened militarily in the Colombian province of Panama thirteen times between 1856 and 1903.[29]

Despite the disease threat, the region seemed ideal for a canal, and in 1879 French diplomat and entrepreneur Ferdinand de Lesseps, architect of the triumphant Suez Canal, announced he would build a similar sea-level canal across Panama. During the 1880s, de Lesseps's company raised the funds and recruited thousands of Caribbean workers to dig a trench following the rail line, but as Gorgas had observed, Panama had a different environment than Egypt. Costs ballooned, mud and rockslides filled in new cuts, and yellow fever and malaria killed thousands of workers. De Lesseps gave up and in 1889 sold the operation to another French company, which kept on digging just enough to maintain the franchise rights.

Over the years the US government explored various routes across Central America, but the commissions had narrowed options down to Panama or Nicaragua. In the 1890s interest mounted in a shorter passage between the oceans, as US naval power expanded to compete with the British and German navies, and the country acquired new territories after the war with Spain. When it annexed Hawaii in 1898, the United States gained a port and naval base to protect Pacific trade.[30] In 1899 Congress created yet another Isthmian Canal Commission, chaired by Navy Admiral John G. Walker, to determine the most feasible and practical route to build a canal.

A new, powerful impetus toward building a canal came in September 1901, when Vice President Theodore Roosevelt assumed the presidency after the assassination of President William McKinley. Gorgas, though a Democrat, had always admired Roosevelt, perhaps drawn to his great energy and his vision of using government to harness modern science and technology to benefit society. TR now declared his support for a canal and pursued negotiations with Colombian and Nicaraguan officials and French investors in Panama for access to an appropriate strip of land. The beleaguered French, led by businessman Philippe Bunau-Varilla, lobbied the Americans to use the Panama route so that they could recoup their losses. Congress obligingly passed legislation in June 1902 authorizing the purchase of the French holdings. The United States then negotiated with Colombia to pay $10 million and $250,000 annually for a ninety-nine-year lease to a six-mile-wide canal zone. Gorgas approved. "My heart is so set upon the canal proposition," he told Amelia. "It seems my work will be much more useful there than anywhere else."[31]

## JOCKEYING FOR POSITION

Throughout 1903, during the negotiations for land, Gorgas and the Medical Department lobbied for a central role in the project. Secretary of War Taft, Surgeon

General O'Reilly, and. Leonard Wood all urged the president to name Gorgas to the commission. O'Reilly wrote that Gorgas was "in every way fitted to the chief sanitary Authority in the undertaking." He pointed out that as a southerner, Gorgas was not likely to become disabled by Panama's hot climate and that he was immune to yellow fever. Moreover, given his practical experience in mosquito mitigation, to select someone else would be to "experiment where it is possible to be certain."[32] Gorgas and his colleagues, however, heard nothing about a Panama commission assignment and were afraid that "in the press of business the matter might be overlooked when the president came to make the appointments."[33] The OTSG solicited support for his appointment from national medical organizations. The AMA, for example, created a special committee to make the case to President Roosevelt, and *JAMA* provided the drumbeat of support for modern sanitation in the canal project.[34] They had competition, however. Sensing glory, the Army Corps of Engineers, the Marine Hospital Service, and the Navy Bureau of Medicine were maneuvering to have their men assigned to the canal project.[35] In June 1903, however, Admiral Walker sent Gorgas an encouraging if noncommittal note suggesting that Gorgas would at least get a position on the staff. It said, "I am looking forward to seeing you assigned to duty in connection with sanitary measures on the Isthmus."[36]

As Gorgas became the standard-bearer for medical involvement, he gathered around him a circle of colleagues who saw digging the Panama Canal as the next "war" and wanted to be in on the action. These included two of Gorgas's closest friends, Henry Rose Carter and John Ross. Gorgas wanted Carter to manage the quarantine operations at Panama, with the enticement to the aging sanitarian that he "might have a little more opportunity for investigating some of the dark points in yellow fever."[37] Ross, he thought, should administer hospitals, because "no hospital that I have ever known anything about was run so entirely for the benefit and interests of the patients as Las Animas was under your jurisdiction."[38] Siboney veterans Louis La Garde or Theo Lyster could be his second in command. Gorgas also recruited C. L. (Charles Lincoln) Furbush, a medical officer who had worked with him in Cuba, and Joseph Le Prince, the English engineer who had intelligently and enthusiastically pursued mosquito mitigation in Havana.

While waiting on the Panama project, Gorgas used his time on temporary duty on Governors Island, New York, to publish several articles on mosquito mitigation and yellow fever eradication.[39] He and La Garde, who was following developments in Washington, also optimistically made plans. They calculated that to staff the hospitals and clinics they would need thirty or forty "medical men" of high ability from universities like Johns Hopkins or Harvard, and that with such talent, they could make great strides in tropical medicine. "When hereafter anyone undertakes to look up the literature of tropical diseases on the Isthmus," La Garde told Gorgas, "our experience may stand out as an intelligent guide instead of the mass of confusion which the present literature offers."[40]

Gorgas watched the events closely, but in August 1903, the Colombian legislature rejected the treaty, opposing an American presence in the region. President Roosevelt was furious, and O'Reilly told Gorgas the Panama matter was "apparently hopeless."[41] Gorgas was nevertheless able to advance the yellow fever project when he traveled to Paris in October 1903, for a public health conference to update international agreements regarding infectious diseases. There he was gratified when the conference adopted his recommendations on yellow fever with a strong resolution "stating that yellow fever is transmitted only by the mosquito and not at all by fomites and that only such quarantine measures are necessary as look to this method of conveyance."[42] This was, he told Marie, "more advanced ground than any of our associations in the United States have yet taken."[43]

The outlook on the Panama front also brightened when the French canal financier, Philippe Bunau-Varilla, quietly approached Panamanian businessmen who had long chafed under the Colombian rule and encouraged them to declare independence from Colombia and pursue the canal and its financial promise as a sovereign nation. When they sought reassurance from Roosevelt for such audacity, he quietly conveyed his support for a rebellion. Therefore, on November 3, Panamanian leaders declared their independence from Gran Colombia and simply arrested two Colombian generals and the governor of Panama at a luncheon in Panama City. American gunboats appeared in the Panama harbors to protect the rebels, but the only official death occurred when a hapless civilian was killed by a shell fired into Colón from a Colombian ship. The United States recognized the Republic of Panama on November 13.

Bunau-Varilla, now an agent of the new country, negotiated a fresh treaty whereby the United States would pay $10 million to Panama, and $250,000 annually, the same as the Colombia agreement, but expanded the strip of land for the canal zone from six to ten miles and changed the lease from ninety-nine years to "in perpetuity." The treaty also included language stating that the United States would protect Panama's independence but gave the Americans the rights, access, and power that "may be necessary and convenient for the construction, maintenance, operation, sanitation and protection of the said Canal." Of most import to Gorgas, Article VIII gave the US government virtually absolute power over the sanitation and public health of the Canal Zone. It stated that the cities of Panama on the Pacific coast and Colón on the Atlantic "shall comply in perpetuity with the sanitary ordinances whether of a preventive or curative character prescribed by the United States." If they failed to do so, the United States had the right and authority to enforce those ordinances.[44] Bunau-Varilla's treaty concessions shocked many Panamanians, but the revolutionaries could not go back to Colombia. As one historian put it, "humiliation was . . . preferable to hanging."[45] They signed on November 18, 1903.

As the Panama project approached viability, Gorgas was still unsure he would be included and in his frustration wrote an intemperate letter to the secretary of state via Surgeon General O'Reilly. They needed a sanitary man, he insisted, because "these gentlemen have not the remotest idea of what sanitation in the United States needs and none at all of the importance in the tropics."[46] He warned that a meager congressional appropriation of $105,000 for sanitation would be money wasted in Panama. "It was probably gotten up hastily by gentlemen not familiar with the needs of modern tropical sanitation," he wrote. "Estimating the cost of burying a dead man at $25, the $100,000 would pay the funeral expenses of only 4,000 men," the expected death toll from only one year.[47] Such an outburst—unusual for the equable Gorgas—did nothing to advance the Medical Department's cause, and O'Reilly was not pleased. "Here is your letter back," he replied. "You are wasting powder." Gorgas put the letter away, and a few weeks later the surgeon general gave him another writing assignment. He asked Gorgas for a short, practical treatise on how to get rid of yellow fever, keeping it simple and free from technical language. "Just tell what you did in Havana," said O'Reilly. Such an article would "be good for the country, honorable to you and credible to the Corps." He added, "Write it in English – not Spanish."[48] Now Gorgas tried to be more patient. He told John Ross that if he could not go to Panama, he enjoyed living in New York and could "browse around very contentedly in my present pastures." But, he added, that would mean that "one is not accomplishing very much for his fellow man."[49]

The US Senate finally approved the treaty drafted by Bunau-Varilla in February 1904, and Roosevelt appointed the Isthmian Canal Commission (hereafter, ICC) under supervision of Secretary of War William Howard Taft on March 8, 1904. Taft named Admiral Walker chairman and Gen. George Davis, the army member of the commission, governor of the American Zone in Panama, along with five civilian members, mostly engineers. Roosevelt and Taft did not appoint Gorgas or any other public health expert to the ICC. The sanitarians would have to be satisfied to be on the commission staff.

Four days after the commission was named, Gorgas finally received a telegram from Walker advising that they would sail for Panama on March 29 for a six-week inspection tour.[50] Things were looking up. If not yet formally appointed to the

Panama post, Gorgas was at least involved at this stage. Upon reading in the paper that Gorgas was going to Panama, New York physician Alexander Lambert, Theodore Roosevelt's personal doctor and hunting companion, invited Gorgas to dinner to discuss the project.[51] The two men met the next day, and after a productive—and, as it turned out, fateful—dinner conversation, Lambert followed up with a letter to Roosevelt supporting Gorgas's involvement.[52] But days later the medical officer received some horrible news.

## MARIE'S HEALTH

Marie had escaped death from yellow fever at Fort Brown in 1882, but she never again enjoyed robust health. William monitored her health closely and reported on her ups and downs in his letters home. Writing from Cuba in 1901, for instance, he told Amelia, "Marie is not in first rate health, but pretty well for her."[53] In New York, in June 1903, he wrote, "Marie has not been well for the past two weeks. A return of her old diarrhetic trouble. She looks a good deal pulled down."[54] Then in early 1904, just as they were awaiting word of his assignment to Panama, Marie found hard nodules on her left arm and a suspicious lump on her breast. The first thought would have been breast cancer—a horrible diagnosis in 1904. The couple turned to a trusted friend and one of the leading experts in the field, William Mecklenburg Polk, a gynecologist at Cornell Medical College. Polk was the former Confederate officer and man on horseback in a slouch hat at Brierfield whom Gorgas had so admired as a boy. Dr. Polk now recommended tissue biopsies, but with William set to sail to Panama, he and Marie decided to wait until he returned. They had been working for this Panama opportunity for a long time, and a visit to the surgeon could wait until he returned. Marie put on a brave face. While Gorgas was in Panama, she wrote to John Ross, who was with him, reporting that the lump was not growing or becoming more painful, so she was not worrying about "the tumor or whatever it is." She added, "I just don't believe it amounts to anything," and that she would be fine until "you unkind medicos worry me with possible operation, etc."[55]

## FIRST TRIP TO PANAMA, APRIL 1904

The first of dozens of voyages Gorgas would make to Panama set off on Easter Sunday, April 3, aboard the Panama Railroad Company's SS *Allianca.* The party included members of the Canal Commission, led by Walker; medical officers Gorgas, Ross, and La Garde; and army engineers Cassius Gillet and William Black, who had been working on the canal plans for a year. Despite smooth sailing, Gorgas was seasick until La Garde "dosed him." He nevertheless relished the adventure, noting he was "farther south than I have ever been before," and told his family, optimistically, if not naively, "The commissioners are a very nice set, and I am glad to have the opportunity of meeting them. They treat me quite as one of themselves."[56]

During their three weeks in Panama, while the engineers surveyed the physical landscape and inspected the mechanical infrastructure left by the French, Gorgas and his team inspected the hospitals and clinics left behind by the French and assessed health conditions to determine what kinds of resources they would need to keep canal workers healthy. About 40,000 people resided in the newly acquired territory and that number would grow to 100,000, with 50,000 to 60,000 laborers and their families living along the canal route in more than a dozen villages. They surveyed Panama City, on the Pacific side of the isthmus, and the city of Colón on the Caribbean or Atlantic side, and the towns in between. Unlike in Havana, they would fight mosquitoes in the city and the countryside because, in addition to yellow fever, Gorgas intended to control malaria, which no one had ever tried to do in such a large population. His team therefore took blood samples from Panamanians and West Indians who had worked for the French to check for malarial parasites and examined children for enlarged spleens that indicated malaria infection. From their initial investigations, they estimated that between 50 and 80 percent of the people in the Canal Zone were infected with the parasites, and while many of them did not experience symptoms, mosquitoes could easily spread the disease to others. The party stayed in Colón during their visit, and Gorgas was amused when they were invited to dinner in Panama City, on the other side of the isthmus. "It is somewhat startling," he wrote, "to contemplate traveling from the Atlantic to the Pacific for a dinner engagement, but at Panama this is not unusual."[57]

Returning to New York on April 27, Gorgas began to work up detailed plans for the public health side of the enterprise, putting together a $1 million budget proposal for sanitation in Panama, similar to the one he had executed in Havana.[58] To tackle the enormous task, he laid out the requirements for hospitals and medical system staff, and the labor and supplies such as screening, lumber, and insecticides required to screen and fumigate homes and barracks, drain swamps, eliminate mosquito propagation areas, and inspect the results. He proposed providing each town along the canal route with clean water, good sewerage and sanitation, and a system of hospitals. The team would develop a health record for each inhabitant in the zone and administer a daily dose of quinine to those with malaria. By thus treating those infected with disease, they could "gradually eliminate the human being as a source of infection within a year."[59] Gorgas also made the bold if not rash promise to the ICC and the press that he would clean up Panama and make it habitable in one year, by July 1905.[60]

The United States gained control of the Panama Canal Zone on May 4, 1904, and Gorgas sought to generate support for his sanitation program by publishing articles on the health challenges of Panama in the journal *Engineering Record*, and an opinion journal, the *Review of Reviews*. He acknowledged that building the canal would inaugurate what is "probably the largest, most difficult and most important engineering work ever begun by man" but insisted that Panama was not a death trap, and that it would not be "fatal to live there." The Canal Zone, he explained, was "a compact little territory of 500 square miles," and with proper government authority and sanitary measures, he was confident he could quickly control mosquito-transmitted disease.[61] "We anticipate no trouble on that score," he told a reporter. "That problem was solved in Havana, and the same principles will be applied to the Isthmus of Panama."[62]

As Gorgas and his colleagues developed their plan for Panama, he and Marie scheduled her biopsies before William's next trip to the isthmus. Although surgery was much safer than just decades before, any procedure was risky in an era before antibiotics. John Ross was so worried that he sent self-addressed postcards to William so he could mail him daily updates on Marie's surgery and recovery.[63] Dr. Polk biopsied Marie's left breast and arm on May 17, 1904, and diagnosed the growths as cancer. In 1904 that was considered a death sentence.

## TO PANAMA, JUNE 1904

As Marie recovered from the biopsies, Gorgas finally received a one-sentence letter from Admiral Walker: "My Dear Doctor. I saw the Secretary of War to-day and in my presence he directed General Chaffee to order you to report for duty, etc., so that I reckon the matter will now go through without hitch."[64] The next day the War Department formally relieved Gorgas from his duties in New York and ordered him to report to the ICC, along with the associates he had recommended.[65]

But now, at the last minute, a dispute threatened Gorgas's assignment, when Surgeon General O'Reilly angrily objected to Secretary Taft's proposed $2,500 annual salary for Gorgas. It was more than he had earned as an army colonel, but only one-third of that for chief engineers on the project, aggravating a sensitive political rivalry. O'Reilly thought it unfair to Gorgas personally, and "injurious to the medical profession whose representative he is." Gorgas, he wrote, "was the only man in America who had a record of successful achievement in tropical sanitation on the great scale and under conditions much resembling those on the isthmus." Such a low salary would depress compensation to the physicians and sanitarians working under him, and O'Reilly was "unwilling to assist in a policy which must result in a poor sanitary service." If the commission did not pay Gorgas $10,000 annually, it would be "resented by the entire medical profession of the country."[66] Gorgas was afraid that O'Reilly was so angry that he would withdraw his appointment entirely. He cautioned his boss that "there were plenty of men ready to take our places and all that would be accomplished would be the loss of the most important sanitary work ever undertaken by our corps."[67] He hoped things would blow over and that O'Reilly would calm down. They did and O'Reilly agreed to send Gorgas to Panama at the lower salary.

As the Panama Canal commission departed from New York Harbor on June 21, 1904, William left Marie with in-home nursing care and once again boarded the *Allianca*.[68] He was joined by Le Prince, as chief sanitary inspector in charge of mosquito mitigation; Henry Carter, to command the marine sanitation and quarantine operations; John Ross, in charge of the twenty-five hospitals along the canal route; and Louis La Garde, to run the six-hundred-bed general hospital in Panama City. Ten other medical officers, including Theo Lyster, were on board, as well as an apothecary and three female nurses. Mary Eugenie Hibbard, a nurse who had served with Gorgas in Cuba and was immune to yellow fever due to an attack there, would serve as chief nurse for the hospital system.[69] Gorgas also found positions for one of La Garde's nephews and Alexander Lambert's uncle.[70]

Once they were en route to Panama, Gorgas wrote to thank O'Reilly for his support on the salary matter but agreed that the low salary indicated "that the Commission does not appreciate the whole importance of the sanitary work at Panama."[71] He was unfortunately correct. Before they departed, Gorgas told the press he had recommended three hundred physicians to care for the fifty thousand men working on the canal.[72] But concerned about costs and skeptical about the need to control mosquitoes, instead of the $1 million Gorgas had requested, Walker authorized only a staff of seven physicians and $50,000 for sanitary and hospital supplies. Gorgas was nevertheless upbeat. As one reporter noted, Gorgas had "no doubt that Americans will be as successful in Panama as they were in Cuba, and by the same means."[73] But Gorgas and his colleagues got off to a rocky—and deadly—start, and the next year would severely test Gorgas, both personally and professionally.

# PART III

# NATIONAL TO INTERNATIONAL RENOWN, 1904–1914

## CHAPTER 8

# Dark Days at Home and in Panama

I am so thankful . . . to know that you are still living,
and that we are to meet again in this world.

—William Gorgas to Marie, February 1905

"We were just three old codgers," remembered Henry Carter about those first days in Panama. He, Gorgas, and Joseph Le Prince were hardly old, though; Carter was only fifty-two, Gorgas fifty, and Le Prince, born in 1875, not even thirty. But arriving in Panama in the extreme heat of the tropics tested their health and vigor. "It rained four times a day," Carter remembered, and "when it stopped raining and the sun came out it was like opening the door of a furnace."[1] The men moved into the second floor of an old French building in Ancón, over the chapel where the yellow fever funerals had been held.[2] They shared a room and one dresser. "Gorgas had the top drawer, I had the middle, Le Prince the bottom," Carter wrote. "If any guests came, they put their things on the floor!" They used Carter's trunk as a washstand, slept on cots, and hung their clothes on nails on the wall. They protected themselves from insects and dust with flowered curtains purchased from a Chinese shopkeeper in Panama City. They had no lamps, and Carter was the only one who thought to bring candles, so they shared them among fifteen officers. The ration was one-fourth of a candle per night. "No man dared to go to bed without killing all the mosquitoes in his net, and there had to be quick work before the candles flickered out." The Americans soon bought all the wire netting they could find in Panama and screened off a portion of the upstairs porch that they called "the cage." There they would sit after dinner, safe from the mosquitoes, "talking shop and enjoying the soft, cooling breezes and a lovely view."[3] William Gorgas spent many Panama evenings like this, smoking a cigar, reviewing the day's work, and philosophizing about life and death. Over the course of his time in Panama, his hair, while still somewhat dark in Cuba, turned completely white.

## JUNE TO DECEMBER 1904, MONTHS OF FRUSTRATION

Having cleaned up Havana, Americans faced a more daunting challenge in Panama. The American Zone comprised five hundred square miles of jungle and swamp bracketed by two cities, Colón and Panama City. Marie would later draw a vivid portrait of the isthmus. The vegetation "was an impenetrable mass of palm trees, banana plants, mangroves, creepers of all kinds, bamboo, cotton woods," she remembered. Animal life was "a never-ending panorama" of monkeys, parrots, and parakeets. "Birds of the most variegated plumage filled the trees; wild turkeys, wild boars, and wild hogs swarmed the tall grass, and poisonous snakes, great lizards, tarantulas, and all manner of reptile and insect life covered the oozy ground." The general impression, she wrote, was "one of dank terror."[4]

William was less gloomy about the landscape and enjoyed tromping through the jungle. He was more concerned with the potential death toll from yellow fever and other diseases than tarantulas, calculating that during the French construction years in the 1880s, one-third of the workers were sick every year and at least twenty thousand died, most of them from mosquito-borne disease.[5] Despite the horrific death toll, the French had dug a lot of dirt, completing one-fourth to one-third of the digging required, and left behind steam shovels, trains, and more than 1,500 structures, including hospitals in Panama City and Colón, all of which the Americans acquired. These hospitals had seen a lot of death, but Gorgas and his colleagues believed that new scientific knowledge would enable them to succeed where the French had failed. Political opposition, however, would prove more daunting than the mosquitoes and would sorely test the sanitarians.

Aside from his outburst the year before, Gorgas had developed a finely tuned political sense. He knew when to speak up and when to lie low, how to marshal support from key groups and individuals, and how to avoid grandstanders and grandstanding. He took care to educate the public, the press, elected officials, and local communities to better understand and support his work. He also chose his colleagues well and in Panama graduated from the team leader he had been in Havana to a manager of men. The "old codgers" were soon joined by several talented young physicians eager for adventure, including Lloyd Noland, assistant surgeon; Edward P. Beverly, assistant physician; and A. I. Kendall, chief of laboratories. Several of them stayed on in Panama for many years. Noland later wrote that Gorgas's "choice of men and the attitude of his corps, their loyalty and their steady and unlimited devotion to him and his ideals were determining factors in his success on the isthmus." Noland observed that few people complained about overtime, due in part to Gorgas's leadership. "Men did for love of him and bore for the love of him what they have never done or borne for pay or the ordinary obligation of official duty." The early years in Panama were difficult, said Noland, but "formative not only for our organization but for our chief as well. I saw him grow."[6] In Panama, Gorgas had an open-door policy and remained accessible to his staff, a practice he would maintain as surgeon general.[7]

When the Americans arrived in the Canal Zone, many of its forty thousand residents were Afro-Caribbeans from Barbados and Jamaica who had worked on the canal during the French era. Twenty thousand lived in Panama City, ten thousand in Colón, and another ten thousand in twenty small towns along the canal route between the cities. Gorgas's team found no yellow fever in those communities when they first arrived but knew that it was a "strangers' disease" and that the arrival of thousands of new workers would spark an epidemic. In addition, with more than half of the Panama residents harboring malarial parasites, mosquitoes could quickly transmit that disease to newcomers. Gorgas estimated that, as the canal project ramped up, by the end of 1905 he would need to protect fifteen thousand workers from yellow fever, malaria, leprosy, plague, and other tropical diseases that simmered in the region.[8] He also understood, as Marie recalled, "that all the blame for the outbreak of disease would be charged to his negligence."[9]

His team therefore needed to get to work immediately. The sanitation program was critical for the project because "if we lost from yellow fever fifteen hundred or sixteen hundred Americans every year," Congress would halt it.[10] The ICC, however, stymied them from the start. Adm. John Walker was so concerned about costs and so hostile to the mosquito theory of disease transmission that he questioned Gorgas's plan. The commission also decided to manage the project from Washington, so to Gorgas's great frustration, he did not have direct access to the chairman but had to work through various ICC bureaus to secure supplies and personnel. Chief engineer John Wallace prioritized construction orders over medical and sanitary ones, so Gorgas's team had trouble getting the staff and materiel they needed requisitioned through the ICC bureaucracy. Even getting General Davis, governor of the Canal Zone and the only ICC member residing in Panama, to sign official documents was impossible until Gorgas and Carter assured him that if any problems ensued, it would be their fault and not his.[11] In the book Gorgas later wrote about the Panama project, *Sanitation in Panama,* he deemed these factors initially "fatal" to the health and safety of the zone, because the ensuing delays cost scores of lives. Nevertheless, he wrote, "we all commenced work with a great deal of enthusiasm, determined to do the best we could under the circumstances."[12]

The first job was to keep yellow fever from arriving in Panama from elsewhere. Henry Carter and his PHS staff therefore established quarantine stations at Panama and Colón, where they fumigated ships and required isolation for all passengers who had not been exposed to yellow fever or were suspected of harboring an infectious illness.[13] Not everyone appreciated the importance of these measures. Governor Davis broke quarantine by leaving his ship against regulations, and when Gorgas challenged him, the governor tried to "set him right," telling him, "On the mosquito you are simply wild. All who agree with you are wild. Get the idea out of your head." Everyone, Davis asserted, knew that filth caused yellow fever.[14] Gorgas explained that his job was to "carry out the quarantine laws of the Panama Republic," so when the governor refused to obey those laws, "My plain duty, it seems to me, is to report the matter to the proper Panaman [*sic*] official."[15] He added that if Panamanian President Amador had broken the regulations, he would have reported him as well. The matter was dropped, but it did not endear Gorgas to his superiors.

With a quarantine in place, the next job was to attack the mosquitoes. The Department of Sanitation's first municipal inspection found *Stegomyia* larvae in almost every house in Panama City. Dozens of structures stood in disrepair and unscreened against mosquitoes. Some were so decrepit that one hospital building they fumigated for mosquitoes produced twenty bushels of dead bats as well. While Gorgas and his colleagues felt that they were preparing for war with a deadly enemy and needed an army of inspectors and a mountain of supplies, the ICC held sedate meetings in Washington, repeatedly refusing or ignoring his procurement requests or referring them to subcommittees for consideration.[16] Whereas Leonard Wood had supported Gorgas's work in Cuba, Davis insisted that Gorgas clean up Panama and Colón instead of chasing insects. For example, when Gorgas requisitioned tons of newspaper for sealing buildings before fumigation, commissioners denied the order, believing it was "too much reading material for his department."[17] The ICC also rejected his requests for ambulances and laboratory equipment, and when he asked for one hundred trained female nurses, the commission approved forty. Since there was no yellow fever in Panama when the Americans arrived, and Panamanians were immune, members of the commission did not understand Gorgas's urgency to get his supplies and hospitals in order. "He knew that yellow fever was coming—that with the arrival of this great body of non-immunes it was inevitable," Marie wrote, "but he was almost powerless to prevent it." Still, he told her, "We've got to work and show them."[18]

The commission agreed to modest repairs to the Miraflores hospital, a cluster of old French buildings that could accommodate 160 patient beds, but allotted only $1,600, or $10 per bed. They allowed $800 for a hospital roof, but no funding to repair the floors, so the order to carpenters was to "leave no hole through which a man's foot would pass." Soon the hospital was full of sick and injured workers except for two empty beds. That was a success, Gorgas later explained, because "two more sick men than beds is a failure."[19] Le Prince recalled those early months in Panama as "excruciating," because they were "fighting a war without ammunition."[20]

The first case of yellow fever showed up in a few short weeks, when Charles Cunningham, a Scotsman who had come to Panama to work on the police force, developed a high fever. The hospital was not ready for patients, so Gorgas isolated Cunningham in a house, and Le Prince rushed to kill all the mosquitoes where the Scotsman had been living. Gorgas and his nurses treated Cunningham with all of their skill, but he died on July 14.[21]

By late July, Gorgas was so frustrated that he sent a nine-page letter to Admiral Walker explaining that he had promised to eliminate yellow fever and reduce malaria from the Canal Zone by July 1905 under the assumption that he could get organized quickly and put his plans in operation. Having to go through so many agencies, however, to get screens for the hospital wards, shovels, fumigating supplies, and the staff to do the work was putting him months behind. He understood that the supply and engineering departments were large and preoccupied with ramping up to dig the canal, but his department had to be in place before the digging began if workers were to be protected. Asking Governor Davis for every dollar he needed on a daily basis, he explained, was a waste of everyone's time. Gorgas therefore sought a free hand in ordering supplies and construction materials until the other departments were organized. The sense of a ticking bomb comes through in Gorgas's tortured explanation of the bureaucratic snarl he faced. "Years from now the chief of [the Supply Bureau] would have gotten thoroughly organized, and my requisitions would be filled very promptly. But that will be too late for me. My work will have been either a success or a failure by that time."[22]

The ICC met the letter with silence, and when Gorgas was in Washington a few weeks later to plead his case, he learned that the commissioners viewed it as a power grab. Walker told him that the mosquito theory was "balderdash" and that Gorgas just needed to clean up the zone.[23] Not grasping the mosquito theory, the ICC members thought him and his team prone to fanciful or impracticable ideas. "They thought us visionary and more or less lost confidence in us," Gorgas wrote. And he knew that if the Panama project failed, his reputation would be ruined.[24]

## CANCER

As William contended with the ICC bureaucracy and fought the first cases of yellow fever, Marie recuperated from her surgery in New York.[25] Devastated by her grim prognosis, Gorgas told his sister Ria that he was considering leaving Panama. He would be willing to "stick it out" with the ICC, "but with the possibility of Marie's having only a year or two of life, I do not want her to lightly bury herself down here." He was heading home on leave, and while there, planned to "have some earnest talks and if Marie agrees I will ask to be relieved from this duty."[26] But before he returned, there was more bad news. Dr. Polk found another lump on Marie and operated immediately, on September 21, 1904. This time Polk removed her left breast and the lymph nodes in her left armpit and performed a lumpectomy on her right breast. Gorgas quickly got an extended leave and went to New York, where Marie was still in the hospital, suffering from the ether used for the operation.[27] There they began to explore their options.

In the early twentieth century, cancer stood eighth in the cause of death for Americans.[28] Breast cancer was the most common form for women and was often not detected until tumors became hardened, visible, and or even ulcerated.[29] With little understanding of the cause of cancer or how to treat it, physicians could only report on their clinical experiences in medical journals and conferences. They debated whether cancer was a disease that spread locally or systemically, and by the time Marie was diagnosed, the prevailing view was that early local detection and surgical removal could prevent metastasis and save lives or at least ease the pain of the tumor and help patients die more comfortably.[30] William Osler described the various ways breast cancer could spread throughout the body. "An early diagnosis of the condition and an early recognition of its helplessness may lessen the terrible ordeal of the poor victim and mitigate not only her sufferings, but those of the near relatives." Hardly reassuring, he recommended a liberal use of "morphine, enough morphine! Given freely and without fear in doses sufficient to keep the patient comfortable, affords the only possible relief."[31]

Surgeons also debated breast cancer surgery techniques, and William Halsted at Johns Hopkins University was the leading authority in the United States. Trained in Europe, Halsted learned more gentle approaches to surgery and took advantage of improved anesthesia and antisepsis to carefully dissect the breast and surrounding tissue to find and eliminate signs of cancer.[32] He used rubber gloves to prevent surgeons and surgical nurses from spreading infection, but he also began to employ increasingly radical surgery to attack tumors, excising not only the cancer tumor and the breast but also the surrounding fatty tissue, lymph nodes in the armpit, and even pectoral muscles under the breast.[33] Many surgeons adopted the "Halsted Method" or modified it in accordance with their skill and experience.[34] This form of radical mastectomy prevailed in the United States until World War II.

Surgeons also discussed whether to remove a woman's ovaries along with a

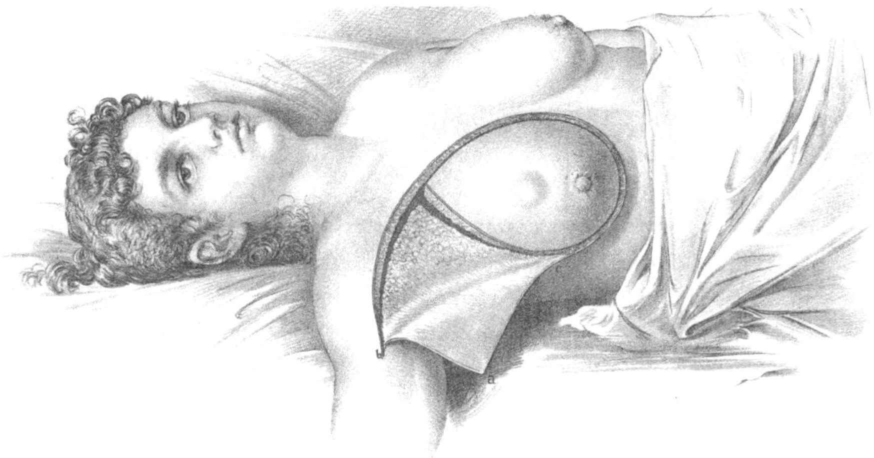

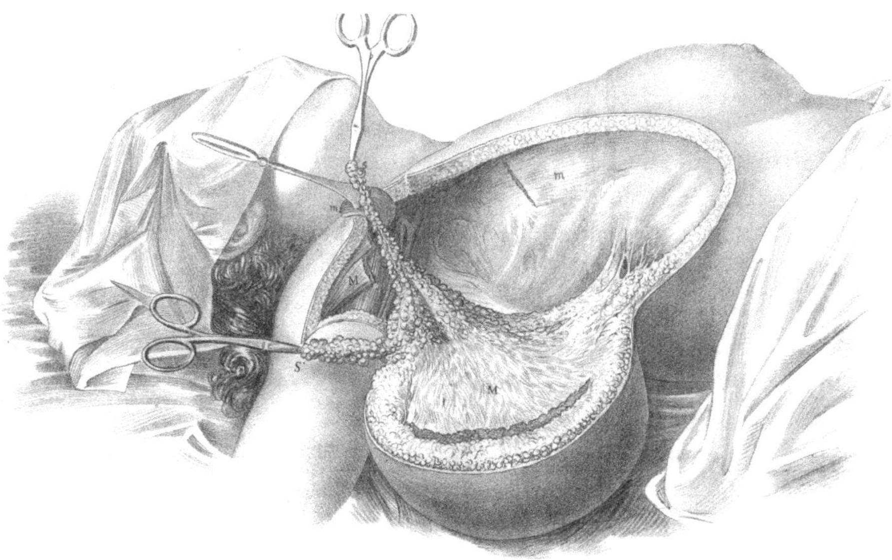

FIGURE 8.1. Plates X and XI from Halsted's landmark 1894 paper showing his incision and dissection for the radical mastectomy. W. S. Halsted, "The Results of Operations for the Cure of Cancer of the Breast Performed at the Johns Hopkins Hospital from June 1889, to January 1894," *Annals of Surgery* 20 (November 1894): 497–555.

mastectomy. Hormones were not yet well understood, but some physicians reasoned that the ovaries and the breasts were connected in women's physiologies, so that disease in one organ could travel to the other. Abdominal surgery was dangerous, though, because a tear in the bowel could cause a fatal infection. One physician described the procedure in detail but admitted, "I have not had the courage or the faith to do it myself."[35]

Radiation therapy was in its infancy in 1904. Only ten years earlier, German scientist Wilhelm Röntgen had discovered that certain rays could penetrate solid substances, terming them "X-rays." Almost immediately, physicians and scientists were experimenting with X-rays on myriad diseases and conditions, including ulcers, psoriasis, tuberculosis, goiters, and cancers.[36] One physician concluded that "like strychnine and arsenic, the x-rays are safe and useful when properly prescribed and administered; but like them, too, they are capable of doing terrible damage."[37] The Gorgases also explored therapies using an ultraviolet light treatment, something called the Coley fluid, and a bacterial vaccine developed by a New York physician.[38] These were all radical, dangerous procedures in a time before antibiotics or safe blood transfusion.

With such a bleak medical landscape before them, William proposed to Marie that he resign his army commission so they could live her last years together. She refused, insisting that he stay on the Panama project. So when she was strong enough to travel in the fall of 1904, with Aileen in boarding school, they packed up their things in New York and went together to Panama.[39] While Marie recuperated during the late fall, William cared for thirteen new yellow fever patients in Ancón Hospital, three of whom died.[40] A visit from Aileen and a school friend provided some cheer during Christmas, but John Ross had to resign and go home on account of persistent malaria.[41] Before Ross left, however, he and Theo removed another cancerous lymph node from Marie, using cocaine as anesthesia. Gorgas noted in his journal, "Marie quite sick afterwards."[42]

The Gorgases now had a fortuitous encounter. Dr. William Keen, a surgeon at the Women's Medical College and Jefferson Medical College in Philadelphia and on the AMA committee overseeing the Panama project, came to the isthmus in late December. A generation older than the Gorgases, Keen had served as a surgeon in the US Army during the Civil War. He visited the Gorgases over the holidays with his two daughters, and the families became lifelong friends.[43] Keen examined Marie and proposed two major surgeries at his hospital in Philadelphia—one to clean the lymph nodes on her left side and remove her ovaries, and the other, a mastectomy on the right side, all followed by X-ray therapy.[44] He explained that removing the ovaries was, basically, worth a try. "Of course, the majority of cases are not influenced for the better, but there is a reasonable number who are cured, or in a few other cases, if not cured, are benefitted."[45]

These were drastic measures, and William and Marie were not sure she would survive, but Marie decided to go forward. "Though I can see she dreads it greatly she has made up her mind to have it done," he recorded in his journal.[46] She still insisted that he stay with the Panama project and not come to Philadelphia for the surgery. Gorgas was torn. With a growing number of yellow fever cases and increasing panic among the Americans on the isthmus, "I do not think that I ought to leave, or rather Marie does not think that I ought to," he told Dick. "I would throw up the whole job if it were not that she urges me to hold on. So I will not leave with her." But, he added, "it is a lonely condition for her." William called upon friends and family for support, arranging for a close colleague C. L. Furbush to meet Marie's ship in New York and asking Dick to visit her every weekend. Overly optimistic, however, he predicted that "in two or three weeks I will have yellow fever here under control & when Dr. Keen fixes the date for the second operation I will come on to be with Marie."[47] A few days later, Marie departed for Philadelphia.

William and Marie's correspondence as they worked together through the calamity of her breast cancer and his struggles with the ICC reveals a marriage of partnership and mutual respect. At each step in the unfolding crises, they took time to consult with each other, weigh the enormity of what each was facing, and then make decisions as a couple. Sharing their life together as long as they could was paramount, but Marie also knew firsthand the terror of yellow fever and the importance of William's quest to fight it, both for him and for the nation. If given a chance, she too would join in that endeavor.

## RED TAPE AND YELLOW FEVER

Shortly after Marie left, the USS *Boston* arrived in the port of Colón with six cases of yellow fever on board, two of them Japanese mess stewards. One of them was too ill to move and died on the ship. The ship's medical officer, Dr. O. Rholhase, also died at Gorgas's hospital after telling Carter through his high fever, "I ought to have known, I ought to have known."[48] Searching for the source of the outbreak, a sanitation team found a dishpan in the ship's kitchen swimming with *Stegomyia* larvae. "You can imagine the stir and excitement there is everywhere," William told Marie in his journal. "Carter and La Garde will not let any of their family leave the hospital grounds and none of our non-immunes go downtown at any time."[49]

Gorgas tried to remain upbeat and reported to Surgeon General O'Reilly that the quarantine system was working well in Colón and Panama. They had three hundred men doing mosquito work along the strip and in a dozen dispensaries in the towns to treat malaria. "We have accomplished everything which could have been accomplished with what has been allowed by the commission." But, he admitted, his problems obtaining staff and supplies were threatening his goal to free the zone from malaria and yellow fever in six months. It might take two or three years.[50] Meanwhile, panic widened in Panama. Yellow fever diagnoses mounted, with nineteen cases and three deaths in January; fourteen cases with nine deaths in February; and eleven cases with three deaths in March. Fearful Americans were leaving in droves, some even choosing to ride in steerage on the first ship they could find. "Anything to get away from Panama," Gorgas told Dick. "Grim care sits behind my saddle and has hugged me tight down here."[51]

Facing a professional crisis, Gorgas also feared he would lose his wife, who was preparing for her operations with William Keen. The surgeon had laid out his views on breast cancer in an 1894 article, recommending early amputation of the breast "while it is a local tumor and not waiting until it is a giant trouble." Keen recommended that women find a good surgeon and then leave it up to him whether to remove only the tumor or the breast, or also clean out the armpit. He explained, "You may do the best operation in the world according to the best rules, and yet if you leave these infected glands you leave a fire burning that will burn down the house." But he was almost cavalier about the chest muscles, stating "You need not be very particular about the pectoral muscle itself. If it be infected, the whole of the muscle should be sacrificed."[52]

Marie's first surgery was on February 2, and Keen wrote to Gorgas immediately afterward, describing the procedure. He first attended to the left chest, where he "cleaned out the armpit" and removed three hard nodules on her arm over the bicep. He then moved to the abdominal area and removed both ovaries "without any trouble at all." Finding the appendix greatly enlarged, he removed it as well, and pathology reports from tissue samples confirmed cancer, including an "early cancerous invasion of the skin."[53] Marie was under ether for the operation, but after the first twenty-four hours, Keen declined to give her morphine, because if the abdominal surgery had sparked an infection, increased pain would alert him so he could go in and cut out the infected tissue. On the fourth Marie was well enough to cable William that she was doing well and still did not want him to come to Philadelphia. Gorgas was relieved and gratified. Marie had written to him before the surgery, and while the letters have not survived, he replied to them in his journal. "They are lovely sweet letters," he said, "just as if they came to me from Heaven, where you might have been now. If you had gone, they would always have been a comfort and solace to me. But I am so thankful, as I read them, to know that you are still living, and that we are to meet again in this world." When Furbush sent a cable saying that Marie was doing well, he wrote, "What a load is off me! And I am so relieved to know that Charlie is with you. With such good news, I feel like a different man tonight."[54]

Keen gave Marie twelve days to recover and then removed her right breast, including the pectoral muscle, and excised lymph glands in the armpit. This time Marie had "very much less suffering," because unlike after the abdominal surgery, Keen gave her opium for pain. He reported to Gorgas that within days she was able to "do up even her back hair, the supreme test of the usefulness of a woman's arm."[55] No cancer was found on the right side, but Keen believed that "widespread cystic degeneration" of the right breast confirmed his decision to remove the entire breast, as he had seen similar cystic breasts become cancerous.[56] Keen recommended that Marie have X-ray treatment in the area of the left breast, armpit, and left upper arm. He closed saying, "Mrs. Gorgas has been a delightful and most appreciative patient."[57] William and Marie were grateful to Keen for the rest of their lives.[58]

## THE OTHER DR. REED

The canal project meanwhile hung in the balance. Theodore Roosevelt was so frustrated by the panic and the work standstill that Secretary Taft sent physician Charles A. L. Reed, a personal friend and former AMA president, to investigate. Before his arrival, Gorgas provided Reed with a memo outlining the problems caused by the ICC's failure to act on his requests and suggesting changes.[59] He conceded that an "ounce of quinine" was a small matter compared to a steam dredge, but he needed to cut the red tape and be assigned staff in the supply and disbursing departments dedicated to supporting the Sanitation Department. He also recommended that "the Chief Sanitary Officer report directly to the supreme authority."[60]

Reed was in Panama for fifteen days in February, staying in the medical staff compound, touring the zone, and discussing the various problems with Gorgas, Carter, La Garde, and Le Prince. After returning home, he wrote his report in two weeks, submitted it to Taft, and unwisely sent a copy to the *Journal of the American Medical Association*, which published it immediately. It was a bombshell. After lavishly praising Gorgas's program, Reed issued a scathing indictment of the commission's management, writing that they were "ignorant of [Gorgas's] purpose." One can imagine Gorgas cringing as he read that Reed was "impressed with the efficiency and zeal of the sanitary staff; with the fact that very much has been accomplished in the way of sanitation under exceedingly adverse circumstances." Reed continued, "Colonel Gorgas and Major La Garde are both officers of high-grade and extensive experience and are gentlemen of recognized integrity." Unfortunately, they were buried under seven layers of command beneath Secretary Taft.[61]

Reed recited a litany of commission misdeeds, such as buying cheap X-ray supplies that were incompatible with the equipment in Ancón Hospital, questioning requests for screening and fumigating supplies, and authorizing only forty female nurses when Gorgas asked for one hundred. Reed saved his sharpest barbs for Commissioner Carl E. Grunsky, a civil engineer, who oversaw Gorgas's requisition requests. The ICC, he wrote, "especially Mr. Grunsky," repeatedly denied requests for carpenters, mosquito teams, and men to dig ditches and drain swamps. "The responsibility for the present existence of yellow fever on the Isthmus," Reed charged, "can be placed nowhere else than on the ICC, more especially on Mr. Grunsky." President Roosevelt, he concluded, should ask the whole commission to resign.[62]

Alarmed that the report made him seem insubordinate and resentful, Gorgas sent a copy to Marie. "You see the report has a bitter, personal tone toward Mr. Grunsky and the commission. I do not feel that way at all." Many people, he told her, "apparently think I am on the inside. . . . But you and I know that I'm not." He was sorry that the report was published and feared that it was "more likely to injure me, than anyone else." He admitted, though, that he was "glad of the opportunity of getting the facts as they are, before the secretary."[63] In the OTSG, Kean told Gorgas that "our breath was taken away" by the report. "It is certainly a hot number, but we fear its publication by him at so early a date was somewhat ill-advised."[64] Years later Marie's assessment was more positive. "Never has ridicule served a better public purpose than this pamphlet of Dr. Reed."[65]

Secretary Taft, unfortunately, was not convinced. He believed that Gorgas had "no executive ability at all," and told Roosevelt that the sanitarian wanted an "entirely free hand in the matter of ordering construction supplies and the employment of subordinates."[66] Alarmed, Gorgas immediately dictated a letter to Taft seeking to quash any idea that he was power grabbing or asking the commission to place a million dollars at his disposal. "Nothing that I have ever said or written can fairly be construed into any such proposition," he told Taft. "This would be entirely illegal, and if it were legal, I would not wish to have any such unnecessary responsibility." But he did need more control over his program and proposed submitting to the ICC periodic estimates for expenditures, which, once approved, would then give him free access to the funds to purchase supplies and hire people as needed. Therefore, he told Taft, he needed direct access to the "supreme authority" of the project.[67]

Gorgas sent copies of the letter to O'Reilly and to Roosevelt's physician friend Alexander Lambert, who was on a hunting trip with the president in Colorado, explaining, "All that I want to do is to disabuse the Secretary's [Taft's] mind as to the idea that I had made any such childish or puerile proposition as the commission have evidently represented to him that I have."[68] Lambert showed Gorgas's letter to Roosevelt and reported that it "removed the false impression Reed had given about you both in the mind of the president and the Secretary of War. The president expressed himself as pleased to read it and get the right ideas in his mind." Roosevelt, in fact, had already decided to replace the commission and sent Gorgas's letter to Theodore Shonts, his next choice for ICC chairman. Lambert told Gorgas that if he would "talk frankly and bluntly to Com. Shonts you will get what you want."[69] He then reported that the hunting was good, and the president got a big bear and two bobcats.

As Gorgas was trying to save his career, Marie underwent six weeks of X-ray treatment during March and April in New York, and William's sister Ria, a trained nurse, went up from Tuscaloosa to be with her. Although Marie was out of immediate danger, Gorgas was still torn between his duty to his work and that to his wife. He was loath to leave Panama without conquering yellow fever, lest he appear to be fleeing, and he confided to Dick that he had to stay, "unless I wanted to separate from the work with a certain amount of reflection on my motives." If Marie had wanted him with her, he would have gone, but, he said, "She cabled me not to come so here I am. Marie is certainly grit from the top of her head to the soles of her feet. I pray the dear girl will be rewarded for her courage and determination." But it was a dark time. Alone in his house above the old yellow fever wards, Gorgas ruminated about yellow fever victims past and present. "It is a melancholy pleasure to sit on the gallery, smoke, listen to the sighing of the royal palms and think of the ghosts that people this old building." His wards were not fifty yards away, and he told Dick, "I have two or three poor fellows getting ready for the great journey. All foreigners at present. A French Catholic priest and two Italian boys."[70] Gorgas especially worried about the "poor little priest" who was delirious and twitching, "a very bad symptom in yellow fever."[71] Ancón Hospital records, however, show that all three survived.[72]

Gorgas escaped the tension, both personal and professional, visiting with his colleagues, and riding horses around the countryside. He wrote frequently to Marie and tried to keep her spirits up. "You have done nobly and all that you could, to get well. And I believe you will."[73] Mary Price, a neighbor in Ancón, started seeing William walk by their house every evening toward sunset. When she asked him about it, he explained that he and Marie "had formed a pact, when separated, to commune in spirit at the same hour & together see the sun go down." Mary Price never forgot it and told Marie the story years later.[74] As William wrote in the journal one night, "Good night. It is 9 o'clock. I will think of you at 930. I've had the little parlor clock repaired, and time myself by that."[75]

In the wake of the Reed report, Kean and Gorgas had a tense exchange of letters in which Kean said the surgeon general encouraged Gorgas to "rattle around and make demands," and urged him to "replace indolent, inefficient, and unenergetic men of your personnel by men of known energy and activity."[76] When Gorgas did not reply, Kean reiterated a few weeks later that he and O'Reilly would assist him in any way, but with regard to Gorgas's staff, "We all hope that you will not let your kindness of heart lead you to holding on to men that are not perfectly satisfactory." They wanted Gorgas to replace several men, including Carter and La Garde, adding that while the surgeon general had strongly defended Gorgas, "he thinks and I do too that you are inclined to be softhearted with your assistants." O'Reilly added, "So fire the bunch and make us happy."[77] The correspondence troubled Gorgas, and he sent it to Marie. "You can see from Kean's letter, that the Surgeon General wants me to stir around and demand things, but I think I better keep quiet until I can see which way things are going."[78]

Gorgas took a few days to calm down and then fired back a response, complaining that Kean and the surgeon general were "very bloody minded to be so eager to get off the heads of La Garde and Spratling." He did not appreciate their judgments of him, either. "You and Gen. O'Reilly sit up in Washington criticizing my soft heart, meaning my soft <u>head</u> without knowing a damn thing about it (pardon the expression)." He added, "If you cast reflections upon the consistency of my cardiac organ, you might at any rate give me credit for good judgment and diplomacy in my year down here and balance my mushy heart by saying something about good firm cerebral tissue." Regarding Panama politics, "We are in the worst political kettle down here you ever struck," and while he was grateful for the surgeon general's support, "I flatter myself that I know Latin American municipal sanitation about as well as anyone can." He concluded, "I have made many sacrifices in the last four months (you can probably imagine what they were) to stay here. Every inclination was to ask to be relieved, and it was always not entirely clear in which direction duty pointed, but as things have turned out I am glad I stayed." In fact, "I feel pretty cocky" about the situation down here, and O'Reilly should not worry because "I believe yellow fever has been eradicated, and I believe that malaria has been controlled."[79]

Gorgas's clerk, Harry Bovay, long remembered that day and that letter. In the yellow fever panic he had decided to leave Panama and was in the office writing his resignation letter when Gorgas came in and asked him to take dictation. As Gorgas outlined everything he was contending with, Bovay later remembered, "He used the word 'Damn' in that letter and it was the only time in my whole ten years with him that I heard him use an ill word." The young clerk was moved. "The load he was carrying and the inspiration coming from his wonderful soul in the dictation of that letter caused me to tear up my resignation."[80]

Despite Gorgas's confidence, yellow fever continued to spread through the vulnerable workforce. After no cases from March 23 to April 17, nineteen cases suddenly flared among the clerks in the administration building, four of them fatal, including an American architect named Johnson, who died on April 30. Le Prince recalled that the young man had ridiculed the sanitary crew for their insistence on screening doors and windows but then got yellow fever himself.[81] Johnson's death hit Gorgas hard. In a long letter to the architect's fiancé, he said that he knew Johnson from playing cards and riding horseback on the isthmus, and that the architect was universally liked in Panama "on account of his laughing and merry disposition and great kindness of character." Gorgas told her that when Johnson fell ill, the young man was not alarmed, because he "thought that it would be of great benefit to have it and get through it, and that he hoped soon to be an immune." Johnson had her photograph by his hospital bed and spoke of their approaching marriage. Gorgas consoled her that he died "without any evidence of pain, simply becoming more and more heavy and comatose, and finally life ceased with a single convulsion."[82] The next day Gorgas ordered the administration building closed and fumigated repeatedly.[83] And, despite the fact that they had worked so closely together in recent years, Gorgas finally agreed to replace La Garde as head of Ancón Hospital with a "younger and more active man."[84]

## A NEW COMMISSION

When Roosevelt returned from his hunting trip, he dismissed the entire seven-man commission in May 1905 and appointed a three-man body which he hoped could act more expeditiously. It was a strong group. Theodore P. Shonts, a railroad man, would be chairman; Charles E. Magoon, one of the most respected men in diplomacy and government, governor of the zone; and John Stevens, another railroad man, chief engineer. Significantly, they would live in Panama, not supervise from Washington. As the senior military official in Panama, Gorgas asked to be in charge during the transfer of power, and Taft agreed, making him acting governor from May 9 to May 25.[85] But just as it seemed Gorgas was in the clear, the epidemic worsened, and he came to the brink of losing his position. Thirty-three more people contracted yellow fever in May, and eight died. Cases reached a peak of sixty-two with nineteen deaths in June, causing another exodus of Americans from the Canal Zone. From April to June, five hundred American employees—three-fourths of the total—had fled, including the project's chief engineer, John Wallace, and his wife. Some observers worried that people fleeing Panama might bring yellow fever to the United States, and newspapers ran ominous cartoons of Yellow Jack challenging Uncle Sam.[86]

Shonts and Stevens arrived in Panama at the end of July. Stevens immediately saw that the Department of Sanitation was the only one that was properly organized, and that Gorgas had "an utter lack of cooperation on the part of his immediate superiors."[87] He also quickly determined that in order to recruit clerical and skilled laborers to the Canal Zone, the workforce needed better living and working conditions, so on August 25 he halted all digging on the canal until proper quarters could be constructed and health conditions brought under control along the lines proposed by Gorgas.

Shonts was less impressed by Gorgas's work and asked Taft and Roosevelt to replace him with Dr. Hamilton Wright, a civilian who did not believe that mosquitoes transmitted yellow fever. Roosevelt was inclined to go along with his new commission head but decided to confer first with his two closest medical advisors, William Welch at Johns Hopkins and Alexander Lambert.[88] Welch explained to him that mosquitoes did indeed transmit yellow fever and assured him that Gorgas was the best person to rid Panama of the pests and the disease. When Lambert visited Roosevelt at his home on Oyster Bay to discuss the matter, the president complained that Panama was still filthy, smelled bad, and just needed to be cleaned up. Lambert listened and then reiterated the scientific argument for mosquito mitigation and told him that the whole canal project rested on his decision regarding Gorgas. "If you choose the old way, you will fail as the French failed," he warned him, but "if you back Gorgas and his ideas and clean up the mosquitoes you will make it possible to have that canal." Now Roosevelt listened. "I never appreciated before how essential it was but I do now and 'by George' I'll back Gorgas and we will do it," he told Lambert.[89]

Roosevelt finally directed Shonts to give Gorgas the political support and resources he needed, and the new chairman accordingly made the Department of Sanitation an independent bureau with Gorgas reporting directly to him. After that, according to Marie, "the support which Mr. Roosevelt had promised Dr. Lambert that night at Oyster Bay he never failed to give."[90] Jefferson Kean thought he and O'Reilly should get credit for saving Gorgas, because he had struggled during the early months in Panama, and "several times but for the valiant backing of the Surgeon General would have lost his job."[91] Gorgas, however, felt obliged to Stevens. The new chief engineer had expressed confidence in his department from the start, and Gorgas once told him, "I knew very well that you were the only one of the chief officials who believed in the sanitary work we were doing, and who was not taking active measures to oppose us."[92]

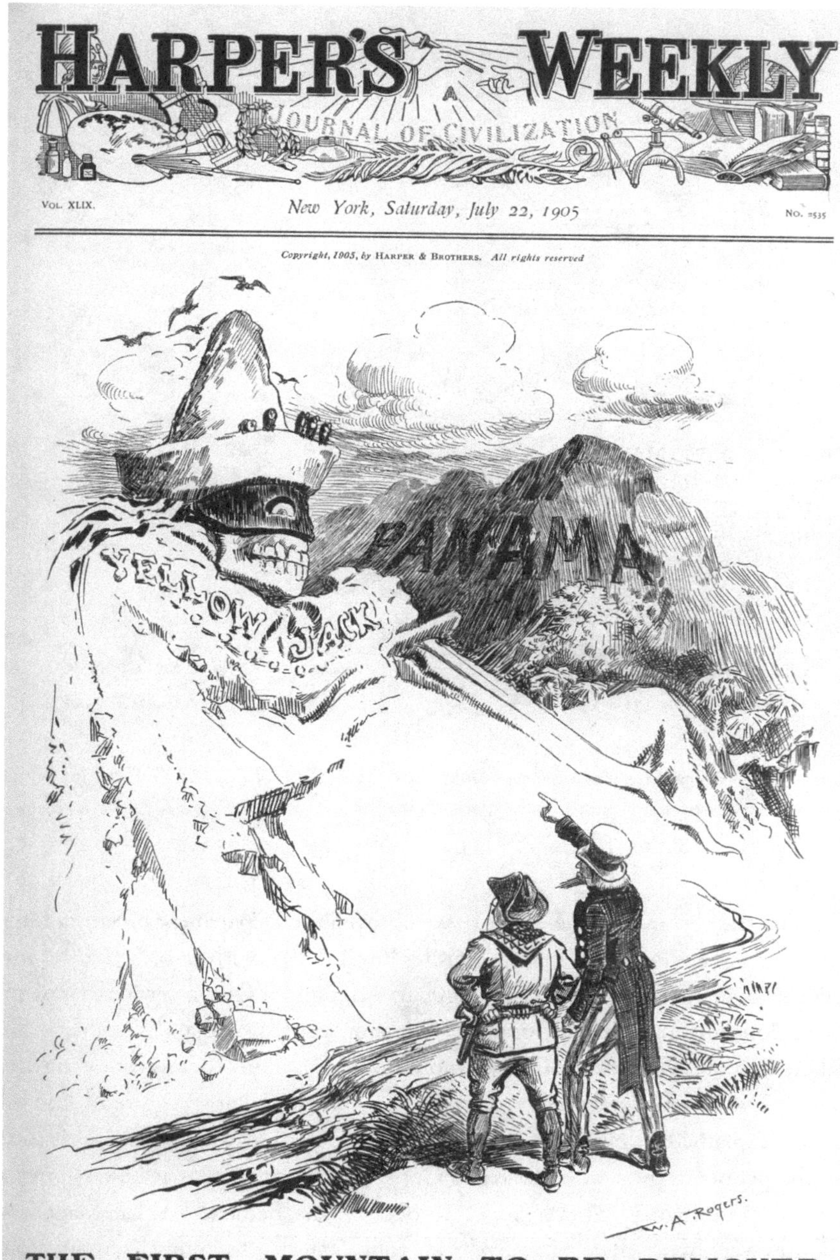


FIGURE 8.2. "The First Mountain to Be Removed," cartoon. *Harper's Weekly*, July 22, 1905. Courtesy of the University of Alabama Libraries Special Collections.

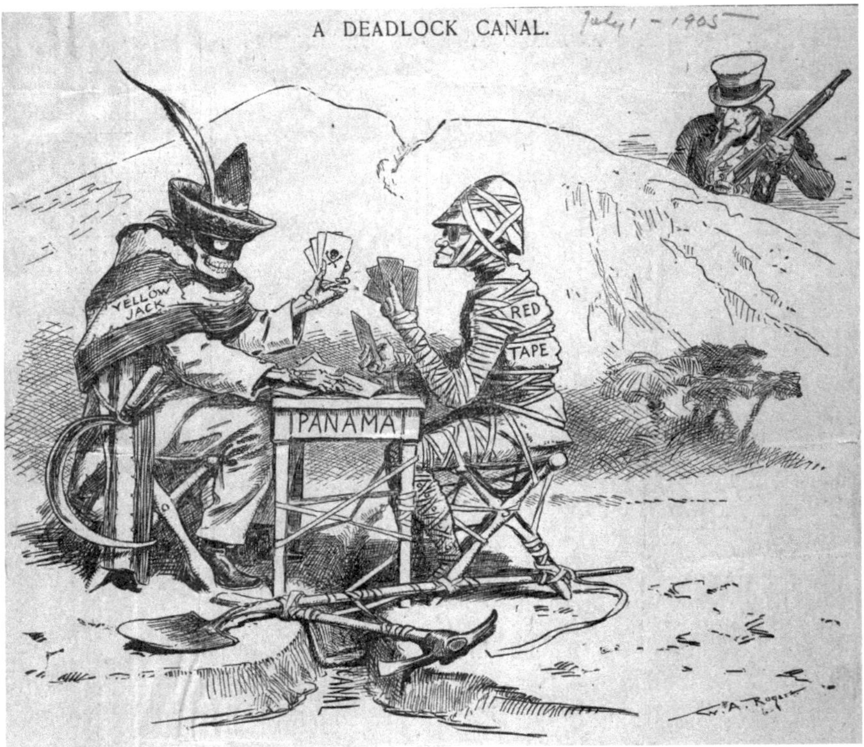


FIGURE 8.3. "A Deadlock Canal," *Piqua Daily Call*, Piqua, Ohio, July 1, 1905. Courtesy of the University of Alabama Libraries Special Collections.

Under the new management, the ICC approved the Department of Sanitation's budget of $656,444 for the year beginning July 1, 1905, with salary increases for senior staff, including a jump from $3,000 to $10,000 for Gorgas, twice that of an army colonel or a member of Congress.[93] Magoon assured Gorgas, "Money, means and men, to the extent of the Commission's ability to supply them, are at your disposal. We've relied upon you to ascertain and determine what is required." And by "we," he explained, "I mean the President, the Secretary of War, the Commission, and the people of the United States."[94] Gorgas told John Ross that he was promised "far more than I had ever hoped to obtain," and he believed that Magoon's promises were "more than skin deep."[95] He told Kean that he appreciated Surgeon General O'Reilly's faith in him but added, "Of course, I know that yellow fever and Gorgas cannot exist at the same place."[96]

# CHAPTER 9

# Halcyon Days for Panama Public Health

> These two years of 1905 and 1906 seem the halcyon days for the Sanitary Department. It was really during this period that our work was accomplished. By the fall of 1907, about all of our sanitary work had been completed.
>
> —William C. Gorgas, *Sanitation in Panama*

WITH WILLIAM'S POSITION NOW MORE secure and Marie's surgery complete, they moved their household to Panama to live their last months or years together. They had no idea or even hope that Marie would survive for long. But Gorgas's salary was now ample enough to hire staff to help her manage the household, and everyone was relieved they were together. Amelia told Marie, "I feel so happy that you can be with Willie during this trying yellow fever strain." She knew that Marie would excel as "the first lady in the Canal."[1] Many Americans believed that the Panama waterway would increase the United States' dominance in the region and even the world. William and Marie would be agents of that process and help advance American civilization in the Canal Zone. They carried with them their belief in the power of public health, modern medicine, science, and technology to improve people's lives, as well as the values of white supremacy and social stratification that were powerful sinews in the body politic. As historian Marixa Lasso has put it, "Between 1904 and 1907, Panamanian municipalities became American municipalities."[2] Sanitation was the tip of the spear in this process.

## ERADICATING *STEGOMYIA*

By mid-1905, with the ICC's support and resources, the Department of Sanitation could finally fight disease on all fronts. Now, compared to his original total budget of $50,000, Gorgas spent $90,000 on screening alone, and another $50,000 to renovate Ancón Hospital.[3] His yellow-fever-fighting weapons included city ordinances, hundreds of tons of insecticides, miles of lumber and copper screening, and several thousand workers. To ferret out all cases of yellow fever, as in Havana, the department offered a $50 reward to anyone who reported a case, and then isolated the patient at home or in hospital and fumigated their room or house. Workers also killed as many adult *Stegomyia* as possible and destroyed their larvae and breeding areas.[4]

*Stegomyia* are domestic creatures. They like to live in inhabited houses, do not stray far from home, and prefer to lay their eggs in clean, still water. Like the Cubans, Panamanians depended on rain for their water supply, storing it in cisterns and barrels inside and outside their homes, which provided ideal breeding areas. Gorgas issued a decree to help change old habits: "Breeding of mosquito larvae (wigglers) is prohibited within the limits of the city of Panama and the occupants of premises will be held accountable for violation of this regulation."[5] But many Panamanians, largely immune, did not share the Americans' sense of urgency in mosquito eradication, so offenders could be fined five dollars in gold. With this authority sanitation crews entered homes throughout the zone to mosquito-proof water containers, covered barrels with wire gauze, replaced water scoops with spigots, and oiled pools of water where mosquitoes might lay their eggs.

In a key part of the program, sanitation officials followed up with weekly inspections to ensure that the mosquito populations remained in check. Inspectors soon found violations in Gorgas's hospitals, where nurses set bed legs in tins of water to prevent ants from climbing up and annoying patients, and in Ancón's gardens, where workers put pans around fruit and vegetable plants to prevent the leaf-cutting ants from devouring them. The cans, swimming with mosquito larvae, had to be banned.

Sanitation engineers meanwhile, headed by Joseph Le Prince, studied the enemy.[6] They soon discovered that *Stegomyia* constituted 90 percent of the Panama mosquito population, compared to only about 5 percent of the mosquitoes in Havana. To get rid of them, the department ended up fumigating houses in Panama City three times to destroy several generations of mosquitoes, using 120 tons of pyrethrum and 300 tons of sulfur. Gorgas revealed that it required "all of the insect powder that could be found in the market of the United States."[7]

They developed a variety of traps and investigated *Stegomyia*'s reproductive processes, feeding habits, and flight range to better destroy them. Gorgas's department also employed mosquito catchers to track down and catch individual insects with test tubes and kill them with chloroform. Gorgas spoke of their work with some humor. He asked a scientific congress in Lisbon in 1906, to sympathize with the

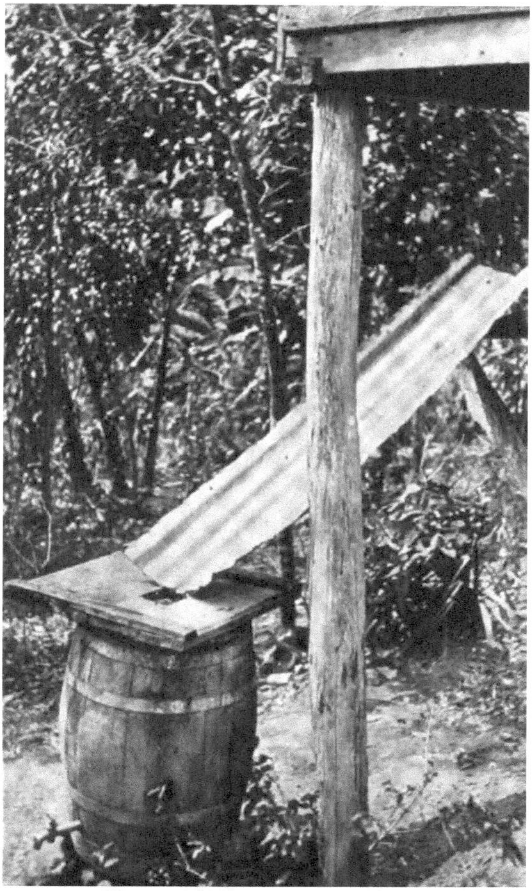

FIGURE 9.1. Covering water sources to prevent mosquito propagation. Joseph Le Prince et al, *Mosquito Control in Panama*, 90.

FIGURE 9.2. (*below*) Plates of water to prevent leaf-cutter ant infestations in gardens provided perfect habitat for mosquito breeding. Joseph Le Prince et al, *Mosquito Control in Panama*, 18.

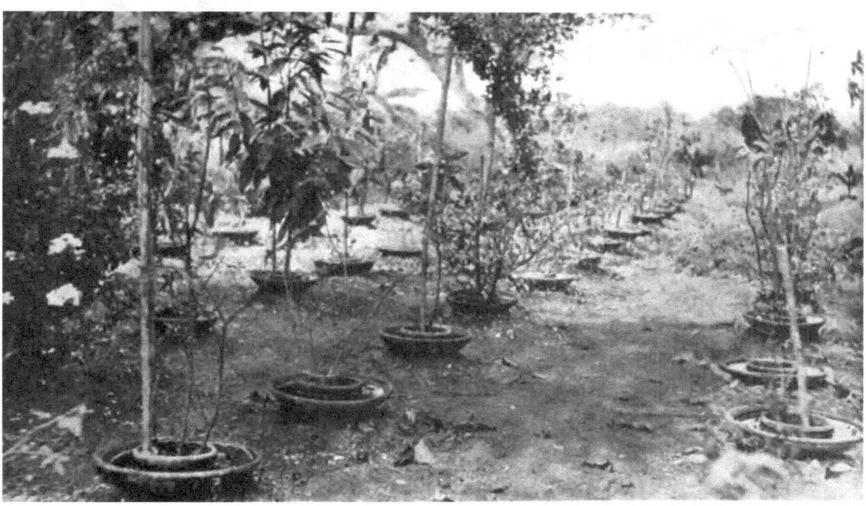

"unfortunate yellow fever parasite," who lived comfortably in the female *Stegomyia* mosquito, but if he wanted to continue his species, he must leave her and "seek the body of his deadliest enemy—man."[8]

Mosquito mitigation was one of the hallmarks of the Panama Canal construction era for locals and visitors alike. Laura Carter remembered that when her family first arrived in Panama in December 1904, her father, Henry Carter, said not to worry about boa constrictors or tigers in the house, but if they saw or heard a mosquito, "you must stop everything else and look for that mosquito until you find it, no matter how long it takes." During their days in Panama, they never left water in glasses or a screen door or window open or did anything that would "aid and abet our worst enemy—the mosquito."[9] Mary Chatfield, a stenographer from New York who landed a job with the ICC, told her family, "I am frequently ordered out of my room in the early dawn so that the sanitary department can fill it with burning sulfur."[10] Some of the locals protested. Miss Fania de Obarrio asked Le Prince to change his team's fumigation schedule, because her family was going to have their annual feast, and such an interruption would be "a calamity."

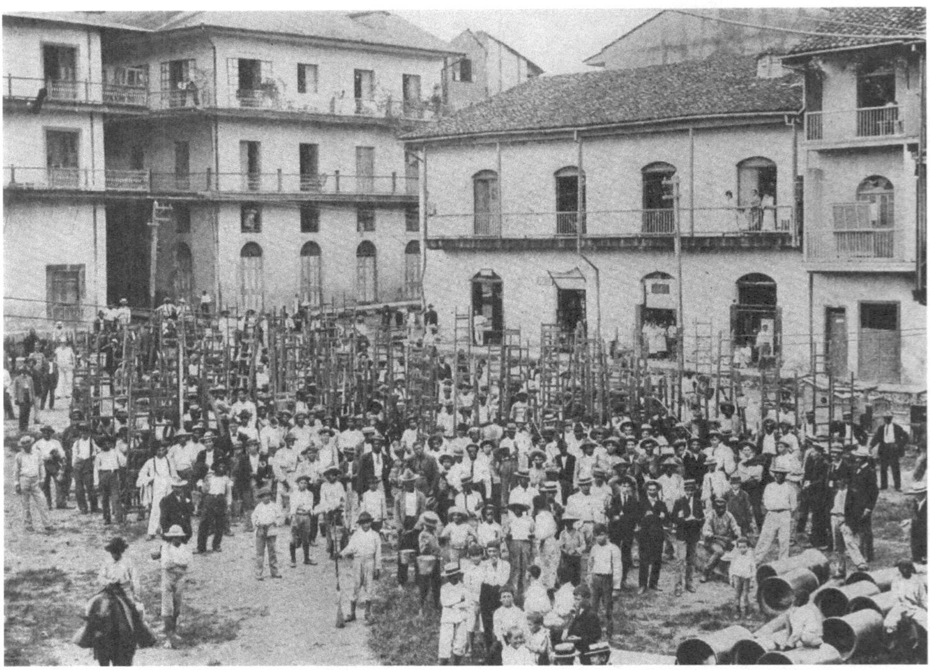

FIGURE 9.3. Fumigation brigades against yellow fever mosquitoes in Panama, 1905. New York Public Library Digital Collections.

He apparently did not comply, because the next day she asked Gorgas to tell Le Prince that their house was in excellent sanitary order and their rain barrels had been removed. She hoped that Gorgas would stamp out yellow fever, but "our dear Lord will certainly bless you and bless your work if you are kind enough to give us all a good long rest from fumigation."[11]

Other Department of Sanitation methods were equally invasive—such as drawing blood samples to test for malaria parasites, and demanding changes in latrine construction and cooking and washing practices.[12] As in Cuba, Gorgas pursued a diplomatic approach of education, incentives, and penalties, or, as one visitor put it, a "tactful policy," to enforce sanitation regulations.[13] Gorgas's gentle manner also seemed to endear him to the locals. His Spanish name may have been reassuring, and while he was nowhere near as adept as Marie at the language, he could say a few words of Spanish such as "buenos días" and "gracias." Whereas the first ICC chairman, George Davis, did not visit the nation's first elected president, Dr. Manuel Amador, or attend Panamanian ceremonies until Washington directed him to, William and Marie became friends with local physicians, including Amador, who was also a physician, and his wife.[14] So comfortable was the friendship that when Mrs. Amador expressed skepticism about Gorgas's ability to rid Panama of yellow fever, they made a wager: she would embroider a dozen handkerchiefs with his initials if he succeeded. What Gorgas wagered is unknown, but within a year Mrs. Amador presented him with the beautifully embroidered handkerchiefs.[15] Gorgas also required his staff to be considerate. When the OTSG told him he needed stronger assistants in Panama, he replied hotly, "I do not want a man who will *make* anybody clean up his back yard; I want him to *persuade* him to clean up his backyard; that is the key to my business."[16] One Panamanian official was amazed when some friends, "boiling over with wrath," went to Gorgas to complain about fumigation, but once he made them see the benefits of yellow fever eradication, "all came away reconciled." He remarked, "If Colonel Gorgas were not here, it would have taken a regiment of Marines and bloodshed to have carried out your fumigation."[17]

Disease mitigation required broad compliance and effective communication, but Gorgas recognized that operating under martial law also facilitated his efforts. In a 1906 article, he compared the situation in Panama to that of Holland residents living under the protection of dikes. "Eternal vigilance here is the price of freedom from epidemics," he explained. Panamanians had to learn to live under sanitary laws, and the locals (whom Gorgas called "natives") were rapidly learning to report yellow fever cases of their own accord. Gorgas explained, "Sanitary law operates harshly upon the native," because his department cleared people's houses of grass and bamboo, eliminated pools of water, and changed refuse disposal. When

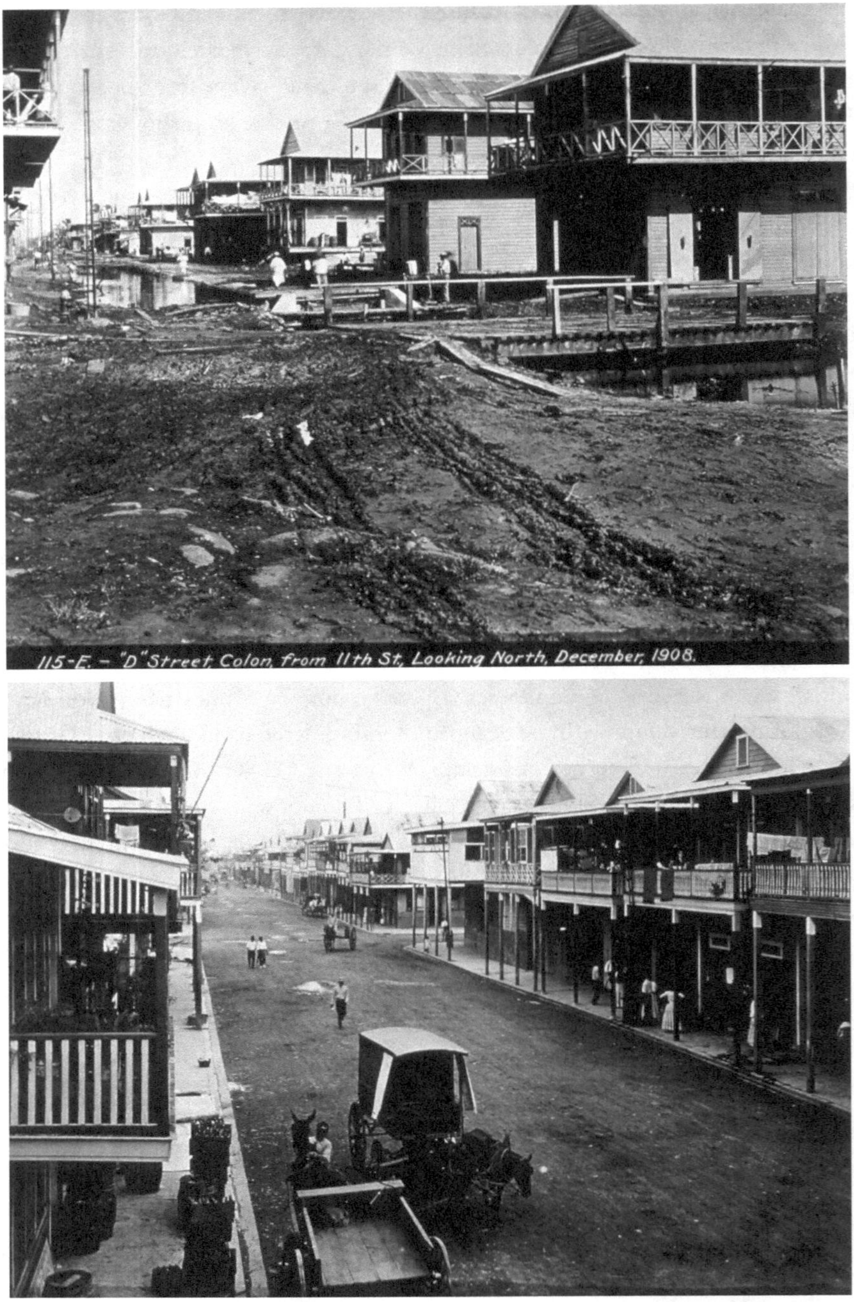
115-E. – "D" Street, Colon, from 11th St, Looking North, December, 1908.

FIGURE 9.4. Street in Colón before and after American sanitation efforts. National Library of Medicine.

some people resisted, "a fine for the first offense and imprisonment for the second are making them active cooperators with the system."[18] But Gorgas insisted upon leniency for those who ultimately complied. In August 1905, for example, his department issued 156 warnings but collected only twenty-six fines. The Panama Canal Treaty obligated the United States to install sewage and water systems in the zone, and once these projects were completed, first in Panama City and Colón, and then in smaller towns, many *Stegomyia* breeding places disappeared and waterborne diseases diminished.

During the epidemic Gorgas visited the yellow fever wards once or twice a day, "principally in order that I might keep in the closest possible touch with the yellow fever situation," he told Amelia, "and secondly because I like the work." The work, however, at times made him pensive, and one fall evening, sitting on his veranda, he reflected. "The moonlight and the royal palms and the great Pacific are outside as quiet as the grave, and in the shadows of my room I can hear the rustle of the ghosts, of the dozens of gallant French engineers who gave their lives in this gallant fight down here." He mused in a letter to his mother, "More men have died of yellow fever in this building than in any other building now standing," and pondered the greed of the bankers and financiers that sent men to their deaths. "What bitterness they must have felt when they saw the useless sacrifices they were making and when they saw how they were being betrayed by the shameless money sharks at home."[19]

But yellow fever was coming to heel. Gorgas and his team watched cases decrease steadily from a high of sixty-two cases and nineteen deaths in June 1905, to forty-two cases with thirteen deaths in July; and twenty-seven cases with nine deaths in August.[20] That month he noted in his journal, "Still chief sanitation officer of Commission."[21] In September there were seven cases and four deaths, October had four cases and two deaths, and finally in November, there were no cases or deaths.[22] Conditions, in fact, improved so much that Secretary of War Taft came down in November to inspect the project. After months of frustration, the secretary was now pleased. He told reporters that he found employee morale greatly improved, and the sanitary conditions excellent, and "believed that by continuing the present methods yellow fever could be controlled, or at least its ravages considerably diminished."[23] The ICC annual report recorded 450 vacant hospital beds and that mosquitoes were so scarce that people slept without mosquito netting. Panama was no longer a death trap or a "White Man's Grave," as the British called their tropical colonies. Back in New York for his home visit over the holidays, Gorgas bragged to reporters that the Panama mortality rates were so low, it would be like digging a canal between New York and Philadelphia.[24] He was content. Yellow fever was well in hand, and his job, for the moment, secure. On the personal front, Marie's health seemed to be improving, and all of his siblings were home in Tuscaloosa for the holidays for the first time in many years.

## THE MEDICAL SYSTEM

Now Gorgas turned to modernizing Panama's extensive medical system. While his immediate goal was eradicating yellow fever and taming malaria, his larger mission was "to improve the general health conditions of the force, so that the canal might be built in this tropical jungle with as little loss of life as might be."[25] The US army traditionally calculated the "non-effective rate" of a given unit or camp as the number of soldiers per thousand who were unavailable for duty, such as men under medical care, on leave, or in detention.[26] Hospitalizations caused people to miss work and consume medical resources, so the medical officer's job was to keep the non-effective rate as low as possible. In Panama, Gorgas's soldiers were the canal workers, and he wanted to keep as many workers well and on the job as possible.[27]

The Americans inherited a medical system that included two large, well-equipped hospitals in Ancón and Colón, a convalescent home on Tobago Island in the bay outside Panama City, medium-sized hospitals of twenty to one hundred beds in each of the twenty sanitation districts, and numerous smaller dispensaries in villages scattered across the zone. Each district also had its own cemetery.[28] The ICC established separate sanitariums for the insane, people with tuberculosis, and victims of Hansen's disease (leprosy). The centerpiece of the operation was Ancón Hospital, which the French had built on a beautiful tract of land on the northeastern slopes of Ancón Hill, which received refreshing ocean breezes and had spectacular views of Panama City. Gorgas judged the hospital to be better situated and equipped than any in the United States at the time. The five-hundred-bed compound had ninety-six structures with pavilion-style wards standing on cement pillars to keep them off the jungle floor, and only twenty-four beds each to promote air circulation and afford ample floor space for patients. Other buildings included quarters for nurses, a chapel, and storerooms, and the Mount Hope Cemetery located on a nearby hillside.[29] Some buildings had long porches and covered walkways between them to protect staff and patients from the tropical downpours, and orange and lime trees, and bananas and coconut palms graced the campus throughout. The Americans added libraries, an X-ray building, and two large recreation rooms. Like other army hospitals, Ancón functioned like a plantation, producing its own food in gardens, an orchard, a dairy of fifty-four cows, and a poultry yard of two thousand hens.[30] When Gorgas's team took over on May 4, 1904, they inherited eighty patients. They admitted their first patients on July 15, and by the end of 1905 had treated more than 1,100 sick and injured.[31]

Ancón soon drew patients from beyond Panama and became the largest hospital in Latin America. Theo Lyster established an ear, nose, and throat department, which attracted patients from afar. The smaller medical centers were able to do emergency surgery, but Gorgas preferred to have more serious cases treated in either of the two major hospitals. His department converted a baggage car into an ambulance on rails to transport the seriously sick and injured. It was properly screened, with canvas benches and cots, and, according to Gorgas, "manned by a trained white male nurse and a negro assistant." The trains ran between Colón and Ancón at 10:00 a.m. and 2:00 p.m., and the forty-seven-mile trip took about two hours, passing by more than twenty stations along the way.[32]

Gorgas and the new ICC intended medical care to be accessible and affordable—public health in the true sense. They put physicians on salary to discourage them from seeking paying patients and made them responsible for everyone in their hospital district, not just canal employees. ICC employees received free medical care, and family members of skilled workers paid $1 a day for ward treatment or $1.50 for a private room. Family members of laborers who earned less than $50 a month paid 30 cents a day. The Panamanian government paid 75 cents a day for nonemployees and their families, and other patients paid $2 a day.[33]

Gorgas wanted his physicians to be "accurately informed" as to what sicknesses were occurring in their district, so they could alert their colleagues of outbreaks and quickly take precautions to control them.[34] The department's medical duties included surveillance and recording of disease incidence, investigating the causes of outbreaks, enforcing sanitation and preventive measures, and researching new ways to treat and control illnesses.[35] Screens on mess tents and latrines made them flyproof to prevent typhoid, and the new water and sewer systems removed many disease pathogens. In 1908 sanitation teams trapped and poisoned eleven thousand rats to control bubonic plague and destroyed 973 dogs with strychnine to control rabies.[36] Medical staff vaccinated all new canal employees against smallpox, and when a child from Cartagena arrived with smallpox in 1907, health officials were able to find everyone who had been in contact with her and confined the spread to thirty-three cases with only one death, an excellent record for such a deadly disease.[37] These programs were so effective that Gorgas grew accustomed to stating in his monthly reports: "There were no reported cases of yellow fever, plague, smallpox, or typhoid."

With time Gorgas adjusted his staff. Except for his close colleagues Carter and Ross, he learned to prefer young men who could "get out on the line and do professional service." He told Kean, "I do not want any more men that I cannot order around anywhere."[38] Seeking to demonstrate the power of modern medicine and the excellence of the Medical Corps, Gorgas recruited some of the best health

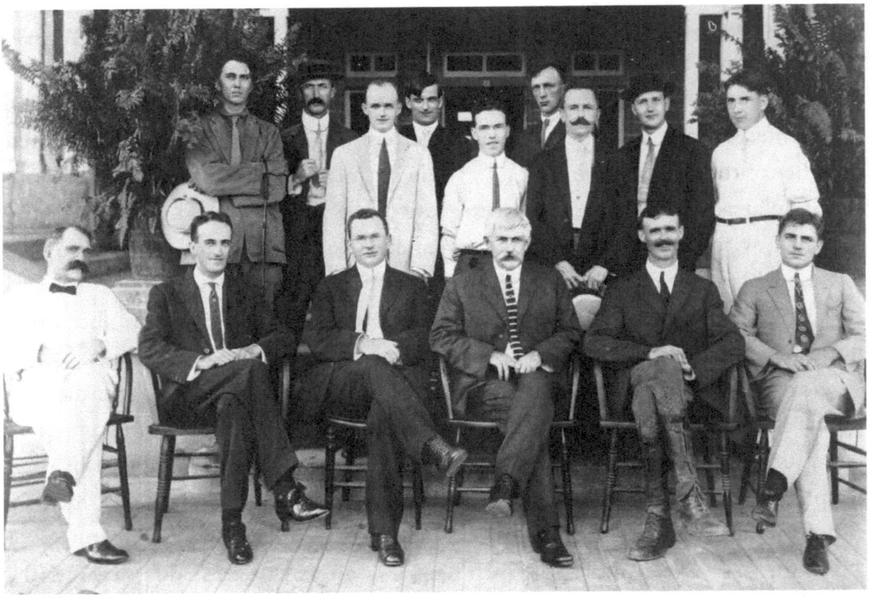

FIGURE 9.5. Ancon Hospital medical staff, 1906. In the first row, Samuel Darling, second from left, Gorgas center, and Joseph Le Prince, second from right. National Archives and Records Administration.

professionals in the country, insisting on the highest standards of education and experience. William Welch sent two or three newly graduated physicians from Johns Hopkins medical school every year, and *JAMA* announced opportunities for surgeons, physicians, pharmacists, and trained nurses, so that Gorgas received more applications than he could accept. At its peak, Gorgas proudly reported, the Department of Sanitation had 102 of "the very best class of physicians and surgeons," and 130 trained nurses from the "best training schools in the United States."[39]

Gorgas was always on the lookout for talented physicians. When he and Marie were in New York looking for a family doctor, Gorgas read some papers by W. E. Deeks about cardiac problems and nutrition. When they met with him, however, instead of discussing their own health problems, Gorgas asked Deeks to come work in Ancón Hospital, which he did.[40] Another recruit was John H. Purnell, the Mississippi doctor who had been skeptical of the mosquito theory. He joined Gorgas's team in 1905 as a health officer, and when he died of kidney disease in 1908, Gorgas spoke admiringly of his "ability and tact" in working with the public.[41] It took two years for Gorgas to persuade C. L. Furbush, with whom he had worked in Cuba and who had helped Marie during her cancer ordeal, to come to

Panama. In June 1904 Gorgas recruited him to be the health officer of Panama City, explaining, "your executive ability and knowledge of the Spanish character would be invaluable to me."[42] When Furbush declined, Gorgas tried again in 1905. Few men understood the mosquito work, he wrote, so he would "raise heaven and earth" to get him to come.[43] Furbush eventually agreed and worked closely with Gorgas until the latter retired in 1918.

Although the Army Medical Department did not fully embrace female nursing until World War I and from 1901 to 1917 employed only about a hundred nurses annually, as he had in Cuba, Gorgas employed female nurses from the start. He and his chief nurse, Eugenie Hibbard, adopted a paternalistic management style, not uncommon in American hospitals at the time, of requiring nurses to be single and to live in dormitories on the hospital grounds. With Gorgas's support Hibbard also carefully guarded her profession. Upon arrival in 1904, she and her staff, proud of their scientific training, were aghast at some of the practices of the Sisters of Charity nurses who had remained in the isthmus after the French occupation. The nuns did not understand the danger of mosquitoes, or the importance of netting over patient beds, and would feed very ill patients against doctors' orders. The women at first agreed to let the American nurses take over patient care, with the sisters in charge of ward administration, but the sisters guarded the bed linen so carefully that the Americans could not change the patient beds as often as they deemed necessary. After this and other failed efforts at compromise, the Sisters of Charity returned to France.[44]

Gorgas often got high marks for his treatment of patients and staff. One nurse remembered a morning Gorgas and Carter were making the rounds when a very sick yellow fever patient said that he would like some German pancakes. This surprised Gorgas, who advised against feeding very sick patients, but he turned to the nurse and asked her to get pancakes for the man. When the patient showed improvement the next morning, Gorgas ordered German pancakes for him every day until he left the ward. Another nurse remembered a Sunday when a female patient "who was the head of a notorious bad house" was ready to leave the hospital. Gorgas was there that morning, and "with true southern courtesy he led her down the steps and handed her into the waiting cab—as if she had been a princess."[45] Another employee said that as a boss Gorgas also "had the happy faculty of saying 'No' with better grace and without hurting than any big man I have ever known."[46] Gorgas could be stern with his staff, however. While the army provided uniforms to male doctors and orderlies, it required nurses to buy their own uniforms. In 1907 Gorgas increased the requirement to include caps and rubber-soled shoes, and the nurses protested the added costs. When he did not relent but just gave them more time to transition to new attire, some of the disaffected nurses returned home.[47] On another occasion Gorgas told a nurse who had malaria and would not take her quinine, "Well, my dear young lady, here we all have to take quinine and if you continue to refuse it, the best thing for you will be to go home as soon as you are well enough." He added, "I will see about your transportation." And home she went.[48]

Romance presented another management challenge for Gorgas. When a Medical Corps colleague recommended that he hire a nurse he and his wife had met in the Philippines, he explained, "She is a young, pretty, refined and well educated woman and I know you will like her, if you ever see her."[49] Gorgas responded, "I have no objection to her being refined and well educated, but I am now rather sore on young and pretty female nurses." He had already lost two nurses because they married doctors, and now those two men "do not pay as much attention to doctoring as they ought to."[50]

## PANAMA DOMESTICITY

The Canal Zone became so safe that President Roosevelt and his wife, Edith, came down in November 1906, during the rainy season so Roosevelt could see the zone at its worst.[51] Arriving on the USS *Louisiana,* the couple were met by a crowd of thousands in Colón and then took the train across the isthmus to Panama City. They stayed at the ICC's Tivoli Hotel, a section of which had been screened, at Gorgas's insistence, just in time for their arrival.[52] While Edith settled in at the hotel, Roosevelt jumped into Gorgas's carriage and asked to inspect Ancón Hospital. They visited the wards, met with doctors, nurses, and patients, and the president was favorably impressed. Over the next three days Gorgas accompanied the presidential party as they inspected construction sites. "We had a very strenuous time with the President," he reported to the former Governor Davis (with whom he was still friendly). "For the three days he was here we had the heaviest rainfall I have seen. . . . He went everywhere," Gorgas marveled. "You can imagine what we all looked like after a day in Culebra mud."[53] The visit to Colón Hospital brought disaster, however, when Roosevelt found unsanitary conditions in a toilet room that an inspector had not reported. He reprimanded Gorgas on the spot and followed up with a letter of presidential instructions to correct the problem.[54] Gorgas was devastated. "President Roosevelt has criticized my work," he told Marie. "No doubt I shall at once be relieved." More levelheaded, Marie thought the president had overreacted to one oversight despite the overall progress. Sure enough, before he departed, Roosevelt asked the Gorgases to walk with him to his steamer. Their final conversation left Gorgas in such high spirits, he whispered to Marie, "I don't think we'll pack our trunks just yet!"[55]

Roosevelt returned home with high praise for Gorgas and other officials. In a special address to Congress, he equated them with military heroes entitled to the same credit as men of a victorious army. The conquest of yellow fever, he said, would "stand as among the very greatest conquests, whether of peace or of war, which have ever been won by any of the peoples of mankind."[56] The speech thrilled Gorgas: "I do not think that an army medical officer ever had such recognition in a Presidential message. It probably marks the acme of my career."[57] During his visit Roosevelt had approved a plan to streamline the ICC management, and when Gorgas wrote to tell him of the success of the new plan, Roosevelt responded with a personal letter to Gorgas. "If ever there was a man who won his position strictly on his merits, you are the one," he wrote. "I am glad to hear how well you think the new organization is doing."[58] The Gorgases treasured the letter, and decades later when Aileen donated her parents' papers to the University of Alabama, she gave them a transcribed copy, noting, "I kept the original of this letter."[59]

While in Panama, Roosevelt recognized women's work and their struggles in the zone. "Mighty few things that are worth doing are easy," he said, and "sometimes it is rough on the men and just a little rougher on the women." TR was impressed that the wives who joined their husbands "turned in to make the best of everything and to help the men to do their work well."[60] Former Panama governor Davis, an army officer, had not wanted ICC employees to bring their wives, believing women did not belong on the frontier, in military camps, or in an alien environment like the tropics. But army families like the Gorgases had long been living on the frontier, and Davis soon found that it was difficult to keep men on the project without women. Turnover was so high among the foremen, subordinate engineers, and skilled craftsmen that it was impossible to organize an efficient workforce, and in 1905 a group of West Indian workers called a sit-down strike, protesting, "No women, no work."[61] Bosses and workers, white and Black men alike all wanted their families with them. Davis relented and allowed women and children in the zone.

As army officers and civilian engineers brought their wives to Panama, Marie remembered, "We each had our little tropical home," and she filled their house with flowers.[62] Describing her veranda, she wrote, "Overhead butterfly orchids and the Semana Santas interlaced their long shoots heavy with yellow and purple blooms. Here and there were tubs of the Holy Ghost orchids, long tree ferns, vari-colored foliage and jungle plants in abundance—yet not interfering at all with the spacious and restful air of the porch."[63] Marie much preferred the atmosphere in Panama to that of the frontier forts of the 1880s and 1890s, and as the community grew, she noted "a colony of charming and interesting men and women found themselves in intimate association."[64] Panama also introduced the Americans to bananas, mangos, pineapple, and coconuts, and wives quickly worked to acquire fresh milk and a more varied diet than the "old codgers" had enjoyed.

When Marie arrived in 1905, William asked Ancón Hospital's mother superior to recommend a maid to work for them, someone who had been "reared in a good family" and spoke Spanish. She suggested Tranquilina Gustamante, a Panamanian, who would work for the Gorgases throughout their ten years in Panama. During Marie's annual visits to the United States, Tranquilina managed the household. William wrote in his journal during one such trip that Marie "arranged everything, and told me just what I was to do, and I have done as she told me. Her little maid, Tranquilina, looks after my clothes and rooms."[65]

While many of the women in the zone were there as wives, others came for employment or adventure. At first the ICC stated that it was "not the policy of the Commission to hire women," but by 1908 some two hundred American women were on the ICC personnel rolls. Most were nurses and teachers—117 female nurses and twenty-five women schoolteachers—along with clerks, dietitians, timekeepers, telegraphers, postal clerks, and storekeepers. Eighteen women worked for the Panama Railroad. By 1911 the ratio of white women to white men was 1:3, up from 1:6 in 1906. The ICC and Gorgas at first prohibited female employees from going into Panama City and required some unmarried female employees to stay in their rooms from 9:30 p.m. to 6:30 am. Whether these rules were to protect the women from danger or prevent them from engaging in bad behavior—or both—was not clear.[66]

Progressive reformer Gertrude Beeks visited Panama in June 1907 to assess the social conditions. While generally positive about the project, she called for improvements in working and living conditions for laborers, and more family-oriented communities, better schools, and activities for women and children. She also recommended women's clubs to bring together the women of the Canal Zone, and soon the Federation of Women's Clubs had groups in at least nine towns.[67] In addition to social events, these clubs offered lectures and classes, and club members helped the churches, schools, hospitals, prisons, and asylums. As the wife of the senior officer, Marie organized Spanish classes for members, and a horticulture committee to help families beautify their gardens.[68]

The ICC encouraged clubs by directing that all churches in the zone include space for club or lodge meetings. The Red Cross and YMCA had organizations in towns across the isthmus, as did the Masons, the Elks, the Knights of Columbus, army and navy unions, and numerous college alumni fraternities. Gorgas was much in demand in these clubs. Over the years he was president of the Tivoli Club, and of the Canal Zone Humane Society, and presided at the opening exercises in the new YCMA clubhouse in Corozal.[69] (To run his meetings, he used a gavel made out of wood from the Gorgas home in Brierfield, which had been torn down.[70]) When the American nurses of Ancón Hospital established their own church, St. Luke's Episcopal, the Gorgases joined. William was the first leader of the congregation, and Marie played the organ.[71] In a gesture emblematic of Gorgas's paternalism and racism, he asked the church to offer services for Black workers, but at a different time of day than the service for white parishioners.[72]

## JIM CROW IN PANAMA

The Panama Canal was constructed during the apex of white supremacy in the United States, where *Plessy vs. Ferguson* in 1896 had made racial segregation the law of the land. Southern states and towns had erected a complex system of Jim Crow laws to keep African Americans in economic, social, and political subjugation. Theodore Roosevelt and Secretary of War Taft, Republicans from the party of Lincoln, also allowed segregation to take firm hold in Panama. While Roosevelt viewed the waterway as vital to US dominance in the region, he also saw his wider foreign policy as extending American civilization to "barbarous peoples," which he generally defined as nonwhites. "Barbarism has, and can have, no place in a civilized world," he proclaimed in 1901. "It is our duty toward the people living in barbarism to see that they are freed from their chains, and we can free them only by destroying barbarism itself."[73]

Construction of the canal was part of this effort but required a huge labor force. ICC labor contractors therefore had to recruit foreign workers, promising wages of ten cents an hour and free medical assistance and living quarters.[74] ICC leaders considered recruiting Chinese workers, but labor unions objected to the competition and cited the Chinese Exclusion Act laws. Managers therefore turned to English-speaking Black men from the British colonies of Jamaica and Barbados.[75] Consequently, from 1904 to 1914, more than 150,000 people migrated to the five-hundred-square-mile Canal Zone, two-thirds of them from the West Indies.[76] At its peak in 1910, the ICC employed 50,800 people, and the Canal Zone census reported people from more than a hundred countries, every state in the Union, and the territories of Alaska and Hawaii.[77] William and Marie thus occupied a lofty position in Panama's stratified and diverse society whereby American whites, most of them Protestant, sat uneasily at the top of a Latin and Catholic world where light-skinned Panamanians ran the country of Afro-Caribbeans and other immigrants, with Indians and mixed-race groups below them.

White supremacy permeated every aspect of life and work in the Canal Zone, creating a society that would be familiar to a son of Alabama. The ICC payment system reinforced racial stratification by paying white employees in gold coin, and

Black employees in silver. The origin of the system is unclear, but during construction of the Panama railroad in the 1850s, skilled workers were paid in gold, and unskilled in silver, a division that fell generally but not completely along lines of race. Gorgas explained to his family that "Negro employees are usually referred to as silver men, from the fact that when they first went down they were paid in Panaman silver currency."[78] But in 1907, at the insistence of American unions of skilled workers, mostly white men, the ICC hardened the lines, restricting the "gold rolls" to American citizens and Panamanian whites, "except where American or Panamanian labor or service of the character required is not available."[79] One historian called this demotion of Black skilled workers and railroad engineers "one of the most vicious episodes in canal history, remembered and resented deeply by West Indians for years afterward."[80]

By 1907 the ICC had organized everything according to gold and silver rolls, creating a system even more rigidly stratified than the Jim Crow South.[81] All employees, regardless of race, received pay while in the hospital if they were injured on the job, but gold employees got six weeks of vacation, better housing, food, and recreation facilities, and were eligible for paid sick leave for up to thirty days, benefits that silver workers, who outnumbered gold workers four or five to one, did not enjoy. Schools were free but segregated; the ICC hired white American women to teach in the twelve schools for white children, and West Indian men for the fifteen schools for Black children.[82] Social and educational events were also segregated by race and often by sex, reflecting white patriarchy. The *Canal Record* reported on bowling and baseball contests open to the "white public," and when Gorgas spoke at the Gorgona Club, it was advertised as open to "all white men."[83]

Chief engineer John Stevens was contemptuous of his Black workers, who toiled in the heat, humidity, and constant threat of industrial accidents, complaining to the ICC that "their disposition to labor seems to be as frail as their bodily strength."[84] Gorgas was equally contemptuous, telling Amelia that most of their Jamaican workers were "not by any means as good as our negroes. You can hardly believe it. But you do not know what shiftlessness is till you see Jamaican negroes pretend to work."[85] Gorgas did have a couple of African American physicians in Colón who were paid $50 a month in gold (compared to $150 to $250 for white physicians) and assigned to care for Black patients in segregated hospital wards and clinics.[86]

Within this racially segregated system, the ICC Department of Sanitation was nevertheless based on a public health model that sought to ensure the greatest health for the greatest number and was thus the most progressive part of Panama society. The free health care all workers received under the ICC was better medicine than many had ever seen. One West Indian, H. Pilgrim Wilkins, later told Marie, "Gorgas's sanitary achievements and health reforms knew no race, no color, no creed," and that we "of mixed blood of the British West Indies" are grateful for the sanitation.[87] Other visitors admired this approach. One reporter noted, "With a wisdom which far outruns that of the people of the United States, our government has decided that the health of the army . . . is as important as the security of property."[88]

As Gorgas was taming disease in Panama, Jefferson Kean was getting restless. In 1907 he complained that despite his success for the OTSG in getting Congress to improve the status of the Medical Department, he had little to show for it. He reminded Gorgas that he had "put in some good licks" for him, so Gorgas should return the favor. In fact, Kean wanted to succeed him as chief of sanitation in Panama, and he "would like you to back me for that position."[89] Kean may have had reason to think that Gorgas's position in Panama would soon be open, because about this time, Surgeon General O'Reilly asked Gorgas if he wanted to succeed him as surgeon general. Gorgas, however, recorded in his journal, "I would prefer to stay in Panama for the present and told him so."[90] This decision to turn down the highest prize in the Medical Corps puzzled the ambitious Kean. Gorgas's ambition, however, lay in fighting mosquitoes and disease.

# CHAPTER 10

# Fighting Mosquitoes and George Goethals

I have had considerable trouble down here in managing my affairs for the past year.

—William Gorgas to Jefferson Kean, July 1908

As late as 1906, the ICC and Congress had not yet decided whether to dig a sea-level canal that cut completely through the mountain range or to construct a waterway with a system of locks and dams that could carry ships over the mountains. Gorgas thought that a sea-level system would be better for commerce and sanitation, moving people and goods more quickly across the isthmus, but he told Amelia that "the beautiful Lake that would be formed among the mountains by the lock plan has a wonderful fascination for me."[1] In June 1906 President Roosevelt signed a law authorizing a canal with three locks on the Atlantic side, three on the Pacific side, and a lake in the middle created by damming the Chagres River at Gatun. With this finally determined, chief engineer John Stevens got the Panama Canal project on track, literally, by making the railroad the backbone of the project. He devised a system whereby steam shovels emptied their spoil onto special railcars that then transported the dirt and dumped it at Gatun to build the dam that would create Gatun Lake. The dam would then generate power which would—voila!—run the railroad and locks.

In late January 1907, however, ICC chairman Shonts resigned to take a job running the New York City transportation system, and just days later, seemingly out of the blue, Stevens resigned as well. Roosevelt offered to abolish the ICC and put him in sole charge of the project, but the chief engineer told the president he could not continue. In a breathtakingly impolitic letter to Roosevelt, Stevens said that despite the "honor" or "glory" of the work, it did not appeal. The canal was "only a big ditch." He would rather be a railroad engineer, a position more attractive to him than even the "Presidency of the United States." Nor could patriotism compensate for the sacrifice of time with his family and low government salary.[2] Outraged and amazed by Stevens's dismissal of honor, duty, and patriotism, Roosevelt wired him, "Your letter received and resignation accepted."[3]

Now Roosevelt turned to the army, whose officers, he figured, could not quit on him. Secretary of War Taft recommended Lt. Col. George Washington Goethals, a West Point graduate, army engineer of excellent reputation, and an expert in locks and dams. Taft knew and liked Goethals and had been urging Roosevelt to send him down to work as Stevens's "understudy." The ICC had not been receptive to the idea, but now that Stevens had resigned, Taft brought Goethals's name forward.[4] Frustrated with the inefficiency and continuous turmoil surrounding the canal project, Roosevelt decided to combine the positions of ICC chairman and chief engineer into one office and centralize authority and accountability in Goethals, beginning April 1, 1907. The president also appointed a new ICC under Goethals's leadership. This time Roosevelt did appoint Gorgas to the commission, but ironically, now that he finally became a commissioner, the ICC's power was diminished. Under the new system, power was concentrated in George Goethals's hands, which he wielded, according to Gorgas, "without gloves."[5]

## ARRIVAL OF GOETHALS, 1907

George Goethals was all business when he came to Panama. He stayed with William and Marie in Ancón when he first arrived, but the Gorgas charm was lost on the engineer. They kindled no friendship. The new chief soon took residence in Stevens's former quarters at Culebra, amidst the digging and the blasting in the middle of the zone, away from the more social environment of Ancón, where Gorgas and the medical staff lived. Goethals eschewed distractions. He had an immense job and reported directly to President Roosevelt, who was determined that "his" canal should be built. Goethals had to manage scores of engineers and accountants and oversee forty thousand workers from various countries as they struggled against the pitiless climate, merciless terrain, and fearsome earthquakes of the isthmus.[6] He had to work with Panamanian officials and corporations such as the United Fruit Company and the Panama Railroad Company, which owned much of Panama. University engineering schools clamored for a piece of the action, and workers, skilled and unskilled, made demands. All of this was done in full view of the national press and various congressional committees, delegations of which periodically descended on Panama to inspect the expenditure of taxpayer dollars. Goethals faced a raft of weighty issues in addition to those of health and sanitation:

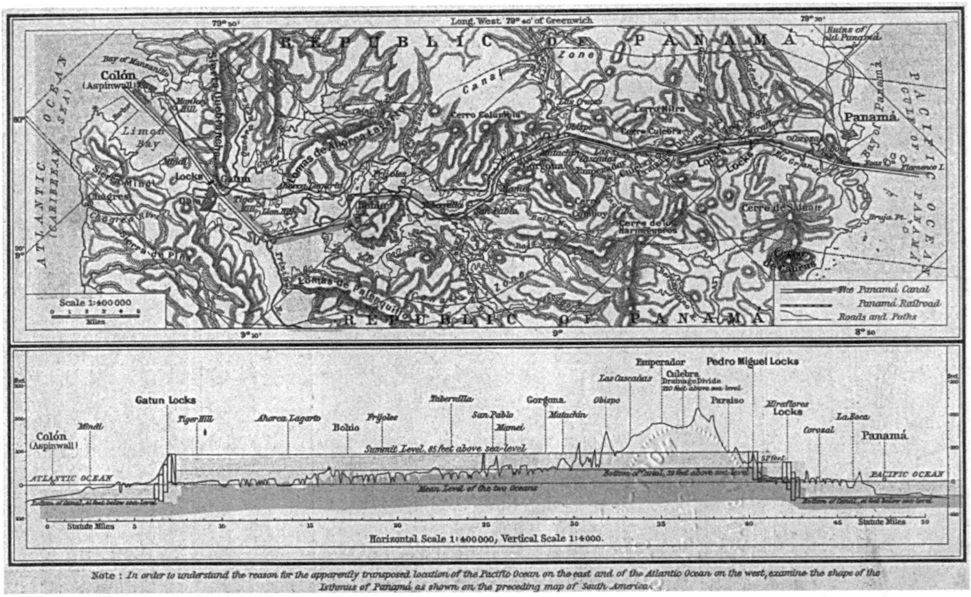


FIGURE 10.1. Section view and plan of the American scheme for a lock canal with a summit elevation of eight-five feet above sea level, prepared in June 1906. William R. Shepherd, *Historical Atlas*, New York: Henry Holt, 1911, 216.

how to compensate landowners whose property was flooded by the canal; how to cope with landslide upon landslide, which impeded progress; whether the canal should be fortified by military guard; and who should pay tolls for transiting the canal and how much should they pay. And he was under orders to deliver the canal on budget and on time.

When Goethals, the third chief engineer in as many years, received a cool reception upon arriving in Panama, he attributed it to resentment that the army was taking over the project. He therefore never donned his uniform or practiced martial ceremonies. He did, however, impose almost military discipline on the employees, adhering to a strict chain of command with himself as the ultimate authority.[7] The nicest thing Marie wrote about Goethals was that his appointment was "a fortunate one," because it was "based upon the assumption that the Canal needed a persistent driver; one who was possessed, above all, of administrative ability, a talent for handling large masses of men, and even a certain remorselessness of spirit in accomplishing his ends."[8] In an early example of his exercise of power, when steam-shovel men struck for higher pay within weeks of his arrival, Goethals, backed by Taft and Roosevelt, replaced them with strikebreakers at just slightly higher pay. One of

Goethals's managers, Robert E. Wood, found Goethals "stern and unbending—you might say a typical Prussian." Others referred to Goethals as a czar or despot, and Goethals himself said that TR's executive order of January 8, 1908, which concentrated power in him, "permitted the subordination of everything" and placed him at the head of "an autocratic form of government for the Canal Zone."[9]

Goethals therefore quickly assumed command and divided the canal project into three sections, each headed by a military engineer: William L. Sibert, engineer for the locks and dams, headed up the Atlantic division; David Dubose Gaillard had the central section at the Culebra Cut, blasting through the mountains; and Harry H. Rousseau oversaw the Pacific side of the canal digging. Rousseau was a naval officer, and Sibert and Gaillard had been roommates at West Point. William and Marie became especially close to the Gaillards and the Siberts. Gaillard was from South Carolina, and Sibert was a fellow Alabamian who attended the University of Alabama. His wife had even contracted yellow fever in Brownsville at the same time as William and Marie.[10] The engineers and Gorgas soon began commiserating about their new chief. Some people saw a regional divide within the canal upper management; historian David McCullough wrote that Goethals had a "keen dislike" for Sibert, Gaillard, and Gorgas, all three sons of the Old South, and they in turn resented a northerner coming down and taking credit for their accomplishments.[11]

While Goethals wielded the power, William Gorgas was still most closely associated with the canal. As a full colonel with three years' experience in the Canal Zone and an international reputation, Colonel Gorgas was superior in rank to Lieutenant Colonel Goethals and held respect across the isthmus. For example, when a traveler at the Tivoli Hotel restaurant asked if the water was safe, the waiter cheerfully replied, "Sir, the water is certified by Dr. Gorgas!"[12] Thus, while Gorgas wanted a free hand to continue to implement sanitary policy as he saw fit, Goethals saw Gorgas as his chief rival, and this set the stage for a contest between the two men that McCullough described as "intense almost from the outset."[13]

Goethals began to speak critically of Gorgas and his department, disparaging the sanitation work and mosquito chasing, saying that Gorgas and his team had merely followed methods worked out by Walter Reed, Ronald Ross, and others. Gorgas ignored such talk, but Marie heard it all and seethed. Her biography of William depicts Goethals as a tyrant who resented that Gorgas's department was "so much of an independent organization."[14] The Canal Zone was the "little province that Colonel Goethals ruled," she wrote, as he "flew about" in his little yellow motorcar that people facetiously called "the yellow peril" or stood at the center of things, "surveying the scene and issuing instructions, with an inevitable air of boss-ship." Comparing Goethals to her husband, Marie observed that one was "unyielding as a bar of iron, while the other was resilient to every human being; one was not particularly sympathetic or tolerant of any point of view except his own, while the other was open-minded." Whereas Goethals controlled by command, Gorgas did so by persuasion, good humor, and "never-dying patience." One was a man of few words, wrote Marie, while her husband, was a man "to whom human association was the greatest joy in life."[15] And to whom, she might have added, fighting mosquitoes was an urgent calling.

## BATTLING MALARIA AND *ANOPHELES*

With *Stegomyia (Aedes aegypti)* vanquished, the *Anopheles* mosquito, which transmitted malaria, now presented the greatest menace to the construction project. Gorgas had told a medical conference in 1906 that malaria was the most important disease in the tropics, because "the amount of incapacity caused by malaria is very much greater than that due to all other diseases combined." He knew because he had suffered the disease himself. "The mental depression caused by this general sickness can hardly be appreciated by any one who did not see it," he observed.[16]

Although yellow fever and malaria were both transmitted by mosquitoes, the diseases were quite different. Yellow fever was an acute, short-term disease caused by a virus that struck in epidemic episodes and was often fatal. Malaria was rarely fatal in adults but could kill children who did not yet have fully developed immune systems. Most commonly, malaria made people feverish and weak and generated high hospitalization rates as a chronic, long-term illness. Between January 1905 and September 1910, one-half of the patients admitted to Ancón Hospital, 41,000 out of 83,000, had malaria.[17] Malaria is caused by *Plasmodium* parasites that reproduce in the mosquito gut and are then transmitted to humans by the bites of female mosquitoes. The parasites take up residence in the human bloodstream and feed upon and destroy red blood cells, causing a cycle of fevers and chills every two days. The damage can clog arteries in the brain and kidneys, and often enlarges the spleen. By 1904 medical scientists had identified four different malaria *Plasmodium* parasites. The most common and malignant variety in Panama was the *Plasmodium falciparum*.

Whereas yellow fever patients were contagious for only the first three days of the illness, and survivors acquired lifetime immunity, malaria victims could recover but continued to harbor *Plasmodia* in their blood and could experience multiple episodes of active disease. They could also serve as a reservoir of pathogens for mosquitoes to transmit to other people. The mosquitoes that carried *Plasmodium* were different, too. Yellow fever's *Aedes aegypti* were urban and domestic creatures, confining themselves to inhabited areas, whereas malarial *Anopheles* were country cousins, preferring swamps and forests, making them much more difficult to find and destroy. While fumigation, screening, and draining of water sources worked well against yellow fever's *Aedes aegypti* that lived in and near people's homes, the swamp-dwelling *Anopheles* required additional measures. Marie aptly characterized the challenge: "Making war on the yellow-fever insect is like making war on the family cat, while a campaign directed against the malarial parasite is like fighting all the beasts of the jungle."[18]

Although some of Gorgas's Medical Corps colleagues would later say that he was a poor manager and not much of a scientist, the work done in Panama during the years 1904 to 1914 belies the charge. Gorgas presided over pathbreaking investigations in entomology, bacteriology, epidemiology, and sanitary engineering. He hired excellent scientists, got funding for them, gave them free rein, and celebrated

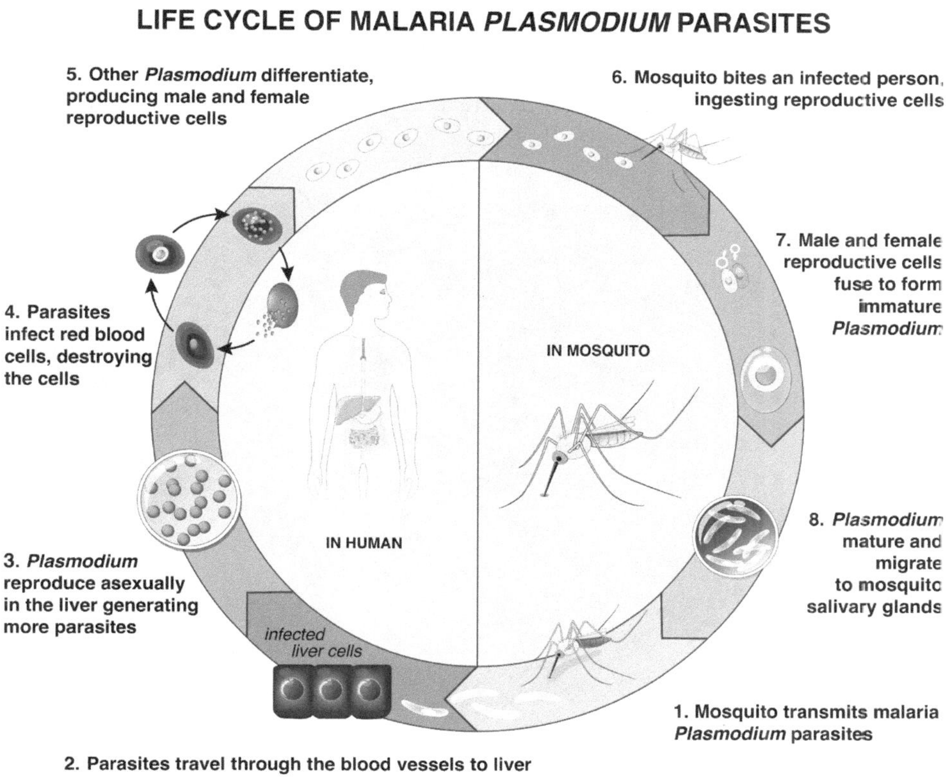


FIGURE 10.2. The life cycle of the malaria parasite. DesignUA/adobe.stock.com.

their successes. Some of the most important work was done by Joseph Le Prince in the field, and Samuel Darling in the laboratory, laying foundations for disease control and tropical medicine for generations to come.[19]

Gorgas and his colleagues set out to learn as much as they could about the enemy and what they believed to be 600 to 700 species of mosquitoes (today that figure is more than 3,500).[20] They wanted to know where they lived, what they ate, and most importantly, if they carried disease. Gorgas became so familiar with mosquitoes that at times he spoke of them affectionately. The *Culex solicitans* looked much like the *Stegomyia*, with its striped legs but did not carry yellow fever and was strong and bold, and could fly "twenty miles in one night before a favoring breeze." The *Stegomyia* had white bands on the body and leg joints and was "one of the feeblest species in its ability for flight and it is at once blown away and destroyed when it gets into a breeze," he explained in *Sanitation in Panama*. "It therefore seldom wanders from the house in which it is bred."[21] The long hind legs of the fearsome malarial mosquito, the *Anopheles*, "give her when at rest the appearance of standing on her head," but she was not very strong, so "two hundred yards is, in general, a good long flight for her." Regarding the mosquito larva, Gorgas said the *Culex* was sluggish and paid little attention to predators, but "the *Anopheles*

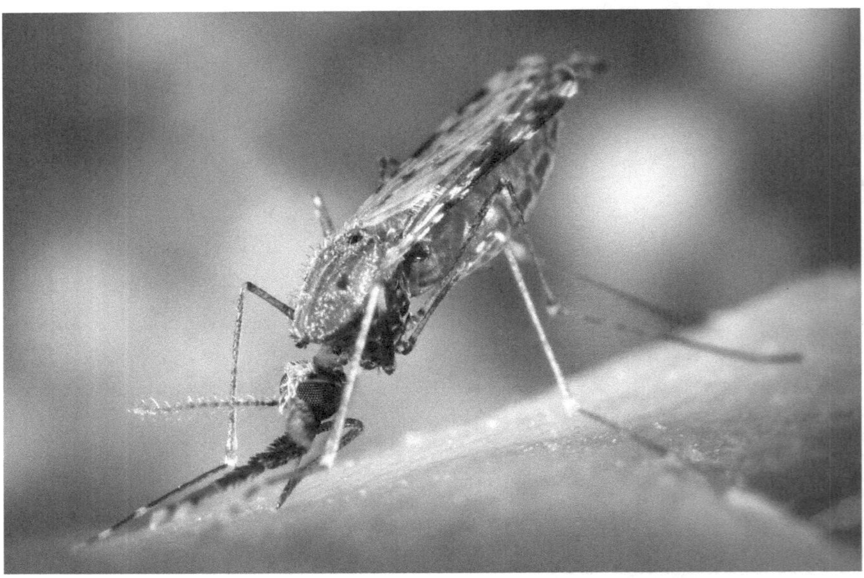

FIGURE 10.3. Female *Anopheles*, the malaria mosquito. Public Health Image Library, Centers for Disease Control.

larva is most noticeable from its superior intelligence. It will dive and seek shelter in the grass at any sound or shadow thrown upon the water."[22] Gorgas did not kill every mosquito he saw. When a visitor saw a mosquito land on Gorgas's hand, she was surprised that he let it sit undisturbed. Seeing that it was a male, he explained, "There's no harm in that fellow."[23]

The malaria campaign in Panama had three approaches: destroy the parasites in the victim's body; exterminate adult mosquitoes and their larvae; and reduce or destroy any habitat congenial to *Anopheles*. Unlike with yellow fever, physicians had medicine to treat malaria. Quinine, made from bark of the cinchona tree, could kill or at least reduce the *Plasmodium* in the blood, thereby serving as both a therapeutic and preventive drug.[24] Medical personnel confirmed malaria diagnoses with blood samples to identify the parasite, screened patients to prevent mosquitoes from spreading the infection, and then injected the patient with large doses of quinine, switching to an oral version as the patient recovered.[25] While the drug did not cure malaria, it helped people regain enough strength to return to work. Researchers found that three grains of quinine (about 0.1 gram) could suppress *Plasmodium* levels in the blood enough to keep a person relatively well and reduce the chance of transmission to the noninfected. Gorgas wrote, "No drug ever discovered has been as useful to mankind as quinin [*sic*]." Quinine's bitter taste, however, made it unpopular, so it was often mixed with tonic to mask the taste. Gorgas's department carried out a vigorous education campaign on the importance of quinine and dispensed it preventatively to Canal Zone employees, putting out quinine tonic and tablets at all eating houses, messes, and the Tivoli Hotel. During 1910 the Department of Sanitation dispensed more than a ton—2,526 pounds—of quinine. "No attempt was ever made to force anyone to take this prophylactic quinine, but explanation and persuasion were used to their fullest extent," wrote Gorgas.[26] But diplomacy was not enough. Whereas in 1906 forty thousand workers consumed forty thousand doses of quinine daily, three years later the department distributed only twenty thousand daily doses to forty-five thousand employees.[27] Gorgas learned that some workers tossed the tablets out windows. At one mess an old pet turkey gobbled them up until he developed "quinin[e] amblyopia," or blindness, and had to be confined until he recovered.[28] Although Ronald Ross recognized in 1910 that the quinine had deleterious side effects such as tinnitus, and Ancón Laboratory scientists investigated the problem, Gorgas did not mention this in his *Sanitation in Panama*.[29] He was trying to get people to take quinine, not scare them off.

Gorgas's deputy, Joseph Le Prince, focused on destroying adult mosquitoes and their habitat, and became a world expert on mosquito control. People long assumed

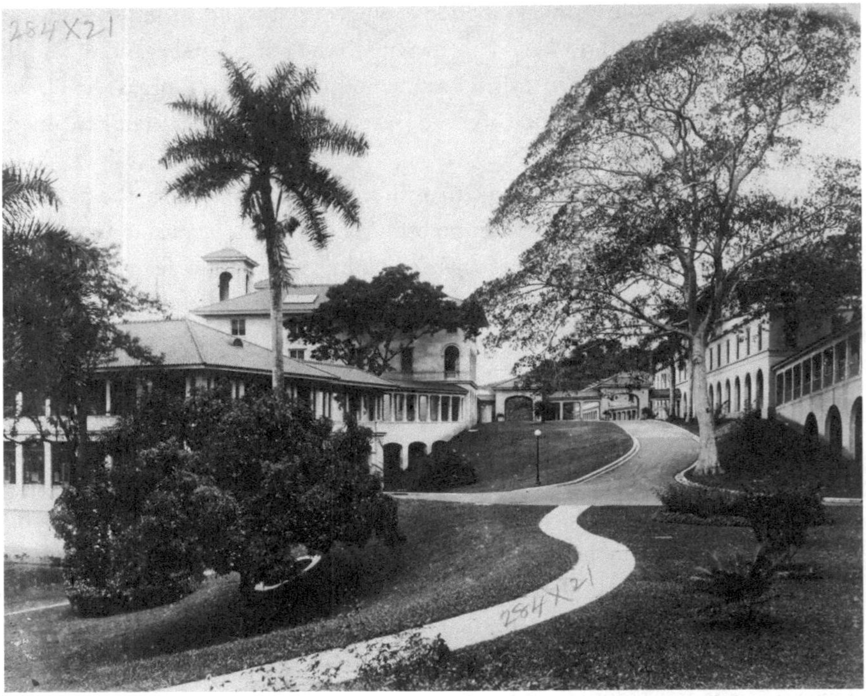


FIGURE 10.4. Mowed lawns and screened buildings of the Ancón Hospital complex. Samuel Taylor Darling Memorial Library Archives, US Army Medical Center of Excellence, Simson Library Digital Collections.

that wind could simply blow mosquitoes into a building, but when Le Prince tested this notion by placing traps in vacant, open houses, he caught no mosquitoes. Through trial and error, he learned that mosquitoes are attracted to human odors. Theorizing that mosquitoes followed the scent of human perspiration, he paid "very patient negroes," to act as bait for mosquitoes. The men lay on cots in an Ancón Hospital ward with pillboxes and a clock. "Each time a mosquito bit them, or tried to, it was captured and placed in a pillbox and the date and hour written on the box," explained Le Prince.[30] *Anopheles*, they learned, attacked inside buildings during all hours of the day, and "at night they became too numerous to make the work pleasant."[31] When they took the experiment outside the hospital walls, however, the mosquitoes "absolutely refused to follow a man out into the bright rays of the sun." Gorgas and Le Prince thereby discovered a powerful, plentiful, and cheap ally—sunlight. In another ingenious study, Le Prince and

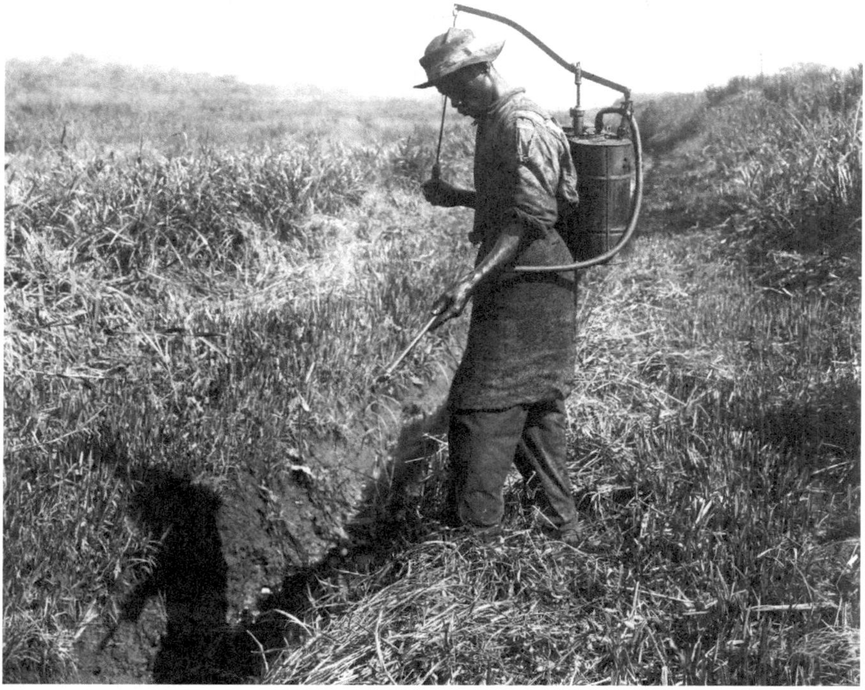

FIGURE 10.5. Miraflores, the Panama Canal Zone: A Department of Sanitation worker sprays larvicide into a ditch as part of a mosquito control program, 1910. National Archives and Records Administration.

his crew dusted mosquitoes with blue dye and then released them, setting traps to see how far the mosquitoes could travel. Upon finding that *Anopheles* would typically not fly more than two hundred yards in the open because they avoided the sun, researchers concluded that workers needed only to cut grass and drain standing water for two hundred yards around inhabited areas to effectively reduce malaria.[32]

The mosquito work was prodigious. As he had done in Havana, Gorgas divided the Canal Zone into districts—here twenty-five—each with a mosquito expert, an engineer, carpenters for screen maintenance, one or two quinine dispensers, and an inspector who supervised twenty to thirty men cutting brush and keeping drainage ditches clear. To reduce mosquito breeding areas and habitat, crews worked continually to eliminate standing water, attacking the jungle with drainage canals, and cutting grass and foliage to reduce or eliminate dwelling areas and rest spots for the *Anopheles.* Where water could not be drained, they used oil or larvicides.[33] Le Prince and crew also identified and bred mosquito-eating spiders and ants to increase predation and cleared bodies of water of vegetation and algae to allow fish to better see and eat larvae. In another ploy workers set out basins of fresh water to lure mosquitoes to lay their eggs in these attractive locations, and then emptied the containers periodically to destroy the larvae. If malaria cases increased, the inspectors had to find the offending mosquitoes and destroy them. In 1908 alone, for example, the "*Anopheles* brigade" for Panama City cut two and a half million square feet of weeds and grass, oiled 5,182 pools, and fumigated more than five million cubic feet of homes and buildings.[34] Gorgas calculated that his team ultimately constructed six million feet of open ditches, one and a half million feet of concrete-lined ditches, and one million feet of subsoil tiled ditches, all to carry away standing water.[35]

Gorgas's system became a model that he promoted, and it was adopted around the world. In 1913 he observed that all of the brush cutting "looked very much like vandalism on our part to see all the beautiful plants, rose bushes, flowers, etc., which had been for so many years carefully nurtured and cared for by our French predecessors, ruthlessly destroyed."[36] Such a remark seems to anticipate more recent assessments of the social and environmental costs of the canal construction. The engineering work and the formation of Lake Gatun destroyed many villages, displaced thousands of people, and irreversibly changed the landscape, allowing the introduction of invasive species, and, ironically, creating more mosquito habitat across the isthmus.[37] Mosquito eradication based on Gorgas's methods also altered the landscape and has had similar ecological and social consequences in other parts of the world that continue to be studied by scientists and policy makers.[38]

Fighting mosquitoes and disease also advanced in the laboratory under the direction of Samuel T. Darling, one of the scientists William Welch recommended to Gorgas. He had graduated at the top of his class at the College of Physicians and Surgeons Medical School in Baltimore in 1903 and in 1905 traveled down to Panama to build a state-of-the-art laboratory at the Ancón Hospital. In addition to conducting thousands of blood, urine, stool, and sputum tests for the physicians treating patients, his laboratory helped Gorgas's team better understand the tropical diseases they faced, publishing more than a hundred clinical and scientific papers. Darling investigated a broad range of diseases including rabies, leprosy, filariasis, tuberculosis, plague, typhus, pellagra, beriberi, smallpox, scurvy, and hookworm, and established the journal *Proceedings of the Canal Zone Medical Association*, which became one of the leading publications of tropical medicine in the twentieth century.[39]

Darling's work, like that of Le Prince, provided a scientific foundation for Gorgas's antimalarial program and produced groundbreaking research on *Anopheles*. Darling, for example, weighed mosquitoes before and after biting to determine how much blood they consumed and examined their stomach contents to learn how many *Plasmodium* were required to transmit disease. With his findings Darling recommended that instead of discharging malaria patients when their symptoms abated, they be kept in the hospital and given quinine until parasites were undetectable in their bloodstream and thereby prevent transmission.[40] Darling's team also determined that there were eleven species of *Anopheles* mosquitoes in the Canal Zone and that the most common species, *A. albinimanus*, was the most frequent perpetrator of malaria.

All of this scientific research and the mowing, screening, oiling, and mosquito chasing paid off. Hospitalization rates for malaria plummeted from a high of more than 10 percent of the workforce in July 1906 to only 0.5 percent during July 1913.[41] But Gorgas's goal for malaria in Panama was zero cases. He even drew a cartoon to that effect—the only such creative work found among his papers.

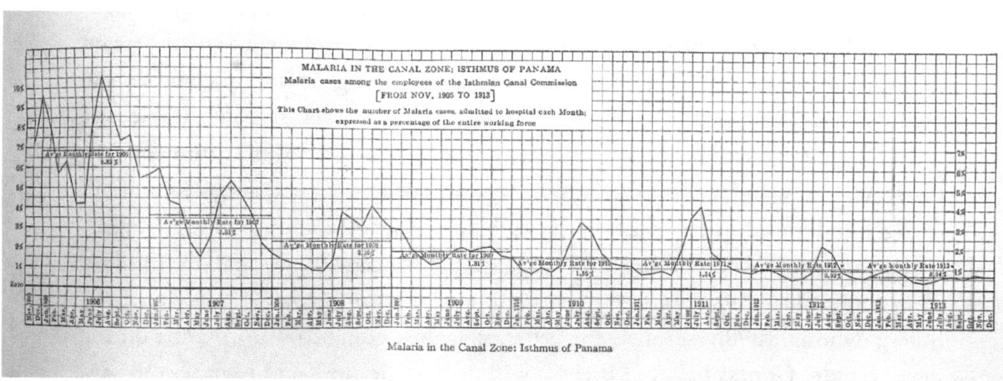


FIGURE 10.6. Chart showing the reduction in the number of ICC employees admitted to the hospital for malaria every month as a percentage of the workforce. The average monthly rate fell from 6.83 in 1906 to 0.54 in 1913, with a high of 10.5 percent in July 1906 and a low of 0.25 in May 1913. Le Prince, *Mosquito Control in Panama*, 226.

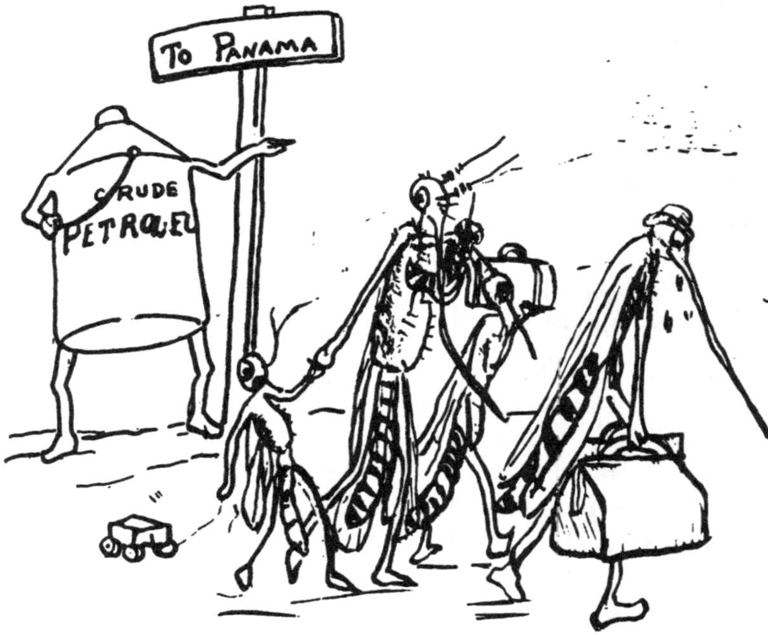


FIGURE 10.7. Cartoon by William Gorgas. Mary C. Gillett, *The Army Medical Department, 1865–1917*, 269.

## GOETHALS VS. GORGAS

By 1907 Gorgas seemed well on his way to eliminating all mosquitoes and associated diseases from the Canal Zone. That year a correspondent signed "Steam Shovel Man" told the *Canal Record* that since all buildings at the Culebra Cut site had mosquito netting, the mosquitoes were gone, and it was so comfortable that he was going to have his family join him as soon as possible.[42] With comments like these, it is no wonder that Goethals, intent on getting the canal completed under budget and ahead of schedule, began to balk at spending more money on mosquito mitigation, and this predictably aggravated the classic tension in the military between medical officers and the line command. Like Surgeon Gen. George Sternberg, who in 1898 cautioned the generals against going to war in Cuba during fever season, Gorgas believed they should devote the time and resources to save lives and keep workers healthy and on the job. Like the generals of 1898, however, Goethals wanted speed and economy in the execution of his project. Gorgas neither judged nor interfered with the engineering side of canal construction—his writings have few references to the engineering work—but rather observed with detached interest the huge steam shovels and thousands of workers digging the great ditch and building the locks and the huge Gatun Dam. The medical officer did, however, have a clear sense of his duty to control disease and care for the sick and injured in the Canal Zone and steadfastly resisted efforts from above and below to interfere with his work.

This contest was fought out over the next seven years as Goethals sought to undermine Gorgas and his program. He was reluctant to attack Gorgas directly, because the medical officer was popular and outranked him, so instead he challenged Gorgas's budget expenditures, blocked staff hires and raises, refused permission for him to travel, criticized the costs of hospital care, and used the Department of Sanitation as a dumping ground for problem employees. And, most troubling to Gorgas, Goethals transferred the responsibility for mosquito mitigation from sanitation and public health operations to the engineering and quartermaster's departments, threatening Gorgas's mission to *eradicate*, not just reduce, disease in the tropics.

The men clashed on personnel matters. When Gorgas gathered his friends and colleagues to work in Panama and wanted to pay them well, Goethals pushed back and challenged a raise for Le Prince and disapproved the salary Gorgas proposed for Furbush. Gorgas in turn resisted. "After thinking about the matter, I think that it would be wiser for me to let my recommendations with regard to promotions stand than to withdraw them."[43] When Gorgas offered Kean the command of Ancón Hospital, they discovered that the ICC chief had already promised the post to another medical officer.[44] Gorgas also resented Goethals's repeated criticism of his medical officers, complaining to the OTSG, "Who could imagine that a person of Goethals' position would persecute able and efficient men merely because he did not like their personality?"[45] When Goethals wanted to replace some of the sanitation inspectors, Gorgas cautioned that this must be done gradually, because it took time to train people in "anti-anopheles work," and that an inspector should, "above all, be a man of tact in enforcing the sanitary ordinances."[46] Goethals did meet some roadblocks. In January 1909, soon after George H. Torney became the new army surgeon general, Goethals went to him to recommend that a PHS officer replace Gorgas. Torney instead alerted Gorgas and told him to hold his ground for himself and for the Medical Department.[47]

Another way Goethals stifled Gorgas was to deny travel requests. In 1908, for example, he turned down his request to investigate a yellow fever outbreak in Costa Rica, and when the British Medical Association invited Gorgas to a meeting in England, Goethals denied leave as well, causing Gorgas to quip that he was happy to know that his "services are so valuable they cannot be spared."[48] Gorgas once explained to Goethals that "writing articles and delivering addresses is laborious and hard work for me, and I do not like it," but he needed to write and to travel because "it is most important for our work at large to give as wide publicity as possible to what is being done in the Isthmus."[49] Goethals was not convinced, but he could not object when Secretary of War Root appointed Gorgas to attend the Pan-American Scientific Congress in Santiago, Chile, in December 1908.[50] William and Marie traveled to the conference, where he spoke on his yellow fever and malaria work and met leaders in South American medicine. Before the trip, Gorgas met with Roosevelt at the White House (while TR was being shaved) to discuss the conference. When Roosevelt invited him to dinner the next evening, Gorgas responded that he already had plans but could break them. Roosevelt laughed, "I would not for the world interfere with your plans!" Gorgas's friends were appalled that he turned down a presidential invitation.[51] Roosevelt appreciated his guileless medical officer, though, and kept his word to support Gorgas and his work. During one round of Goethals's budget cuts, "the President kicked," Gorgas told the OTSG, and wired Goethals, "Hands off Sanitary Department."[52]

The tension in Panama was not confined to the men. Goethals's wife, Effie, complemented her husband's efforts by challenging Marie's status as first lady of the Canal Zone. Effie Rodman Goethals did not like living in Panama, but she was not about to be upstaged by Marie.[53] Mrs. Gorgas was president of the Panama Women's Club, but when Effie Goethals suggested to the other members that her husband could do more to help their husbands' careers than Gorgas could, they elected her president of the club and demoted Marie to chair of the Ancón Women's Club.[54] Such competition reached the national press in late 1909. The *Washington Star* blared, "Officers' Wives Are Waging War," and reported that while Mrs. Gorgas has been "the central and controlling figure of all social functions," there was now a "fight for social supremacy between the wives of two distinguished army officers." Another paper wrote that relations had become so bitter between the two women that rumors were circulating that the president would transfer the Gorgases from Panama.[55] *The World* asked, "Who Is Social Queen at the Isthmus?" and described a "long feud between two ambitious and beautiful women." The paper reported that Marie "sweetly smiled, concealed what ever discomfiture existed, and continued to remain First Lady of the Land because of her husband's senior rank."[56] But she was troubled enough to send newspaper clippings of the story to a friend, who wondered why someone would "purposely endeavor so to wound another's feelings."[57]

## GRASS AND POWER

The most bitter struggle between Gorgas and Goethals was over the mundane matter of cutting the grass. Gorgas believed that malaria rates were the best measure of his success in Panama and, as a medical officer, sought to keep his sick rate, or "non-effective" rate, as low as possible. He therefore kept a close watch on the mosquito work. Goethals, however, thought the grass-cutting budget was extravagant and believed that the Quartermaster's Department could do it more cheaply.[58] In a brilliant power grab, he proposed to shift the grass-cutting, ditch-digging, and screen-repair work from the Department of Sanitation to other ICC departments. Gorgas resisted the suggestion for several months, fearing that "sanitary grass cutting would suffer."[59] In July 1908, however, he agreed to the transfer of duties for a six-month trial, whereby the Division of Engineers would do the swamp drainage and the Quartermaster's Department cut the grass and collect the garbage under Department of Sanitation recommendation. If after six months operations were "not working satisfactorily," he proposed, "we return to the present plan."[60] When the transfer of duties was made effective September 1, the ICC predicted that "economy would result, friction be removed, and responsibility definitely fixed."[61] Gorgas and Goethals, however, had different ideas of what grass cutting was about: Goethals's quartermaster's crews mowed the lawns for aesthetic purposes, while Gorgas's sanitation employees cut grass as if people's lives depended on it.

Trouble began almost immediately. In November, Gorgas sent a twelve-page letter to the chief quartermaster, C. L. Devol, detailing the slow responses or simple disregard for requests for grass cutting, drainage work, and screen repairs. Devol's crews cut some grass too short and too often like lawns, he complained, while letting other areas grow tall, creating mosquito habitats.[62] Furthermore, canal digging continually changed the topography of the land, creating new mosquito breeding grounds across the isthmus, but quartermaster personnel neglected these and failed to clear out vegetation and pools of water near the workers' camps, leaving breeding places within one hundred feet of laborers' barracks. This lack of vigilance "affects our malarial sick rate very seriously," Gorgas warned, and the ICC would not save money if workers' malaria rates went up, because the cost of caring for those malaria cases would be "quite a considerable sum."[63]

Gorgas was frustrated. He told Torney, "I hoped my yielding would tend to smooth matters over between us but this has not been the case and I now have a much poorer machine to work with and my relations with Goethals are not better than they were before."[64] Everyone watched the test of wills, and Sibert later remarked that he had admired Gorgas's "polished pertinacity." When facing an impediment to his purpose, "he would start on another tack and always reached his goal without losing his temper."[65] But the grass-cutting affair hurt Gorgas's ability to control malaria. In 1910 the Canal Zone hospital system tallied 20,356 admissions, and 9,122, almost half, were for malaria.[66] "I had hoped to get rid of malaria all together on the zone, as was done with yellow fever and as was done with malaria in Havana," Gorgas told Kean, "but with a chairman such as Goethals, so antagonistic to sanitation, and not wishing success for the Sanitary Department, that is out of the question."[67]

Grass cutting remained a sore point. When in 1911 Gorgas sent the quartermaster a list of malaria rates in the various districts and asked that the grass cutting and ditch clearing be returned to his department, Goethals appointed a special committee to investigate. After a six-month study, the committee rejected Gorgas's request and instead recommended nineteen administrative measures to ensure the quartermaster's responsiveness to his department. This did little to satisfy anyone.[68] Screening became another point of contention, as Gorgas wanted to screen in all ICC quarters, including buildings for silver workers, whereas Goethals and the Quartermaster Department opposed the plan as too expensive. The result was a two-tiered system of screened buildings for white ICC employees and unscreened for the West African workers—and, to Gorgas's dismay, higher malaria rates.[69]

The contest between Gorgas and Goethals was intractable. Gorgas was so focused on his war against mosquitoes that he failed to credit the numerous other claims and exigencies on Goethals and the canal project. For his part, wrote historian Mary Gillett, Goethals continued to "belittle the chief sanitary officer and his department" throughout the construction period.[70] Journalist Arthur Bullard trenchantly described the situation in his 1914 book on the canal. Any visitor, he wrote, could soon see the war between Gorgas and Goethals. The greatest difference was in temperament. Goethals, he observed, "the practical, scrupulous administrator, makes a fetish of economy," while Gorgas was "imaginative and enthusiastic... [and] would like to kill every mosquito on the Isthmus and then begin on the rest of the world." Whereas Goethals was, "in a way, paterfamilias of the community, so Colonel Gorgas is the family physician. Goethals is farther aloof and authoritative. Gorgas is genial and sympathetic." Bullard agreed that the medical and sanitation operations were run with "less strict economy" than other departments, so it was therefore probably good that a "strong and rather hostile hand" kept the department in check.[71]

## FEELING THE YEARS

In 1908 Gorgas told Marie's surgeon, William Keen, that her health was "excellent, very much better than it has been for a good many years."[72] But William was feeling his age. Theo began treating him for a problem with his left eye in 1909 and told him not to read more than an hour a day.[73] The problem became serious enough that he had to wear dark glasses for a year. "I am still taking all sorts of care of myself," he wrote to Mamie. "Do not smoke, drink, and I'm looking after my diet, and am in the outdoors more than I used to be."[74] The problem persisted and in 1911 he told Jessie that "my left eye is useless but the right seems to be all right. I imagine that we were given double organs just for this very purpose, to compensate us in case we lose one."[75] Prone to such philosophizing, especially around his birthday, Gorgas told Amelia on his fifty-fifth that although he felt his decline, he was content. "I think that I have done a man's share of work in this life and look forward with pleasure to a period of rest."[76] But that would not come for a while.

# CHAPTER 11

# Making the Tropics "Safe for the White Man"

Our sanitary work at Panama will be remembered as
the event which demonstrated to the white man that he
could live in perfectly good health in the tropics.

—William Gorgas at Johns Hopkins University, June 1912

In mid-1910, the ICC members assembled on the steps of an administration building for their annual portrait. Most of them were in their tropical whites, but William Sibert and Gorgas were clad in dark suits and bow ties. The men were largely expressionless, except Gorgas, who stood a bit to the side, holding his Panama hat and smiling amiably for the camera. This pleasant photograph hid the tensions percolating among the men working for George Goethals, a man who found ways big and small to dominate his staff and dictate policy and practice in every aspect of Canal Zone construction and life. He often took credit for the accomplishments of his engineers and continued to challenge Gorgas and his public health and sanitation program. But Gorgas refused to be run off. Although he received several job offers, he would not leave the greatest engineering project in history before it was completed and became the only senior official to see the Panama Canal construction from beginning to end. Gorgas's mission to vanquish mosquitoes and disease was not only for the glory for the Medical Corps and his profession but toward a larger purpose: Goethals might be the master of the Panama Canal, but Gorgas would be the man who made the entire tropical world safe for white civilization.

## WHITE SUPREMACY AND MEDICINE

Theodore Roosevelt and other American imperialists sought to project the United States onto the world stage and compete with world powers in Europe and Asia

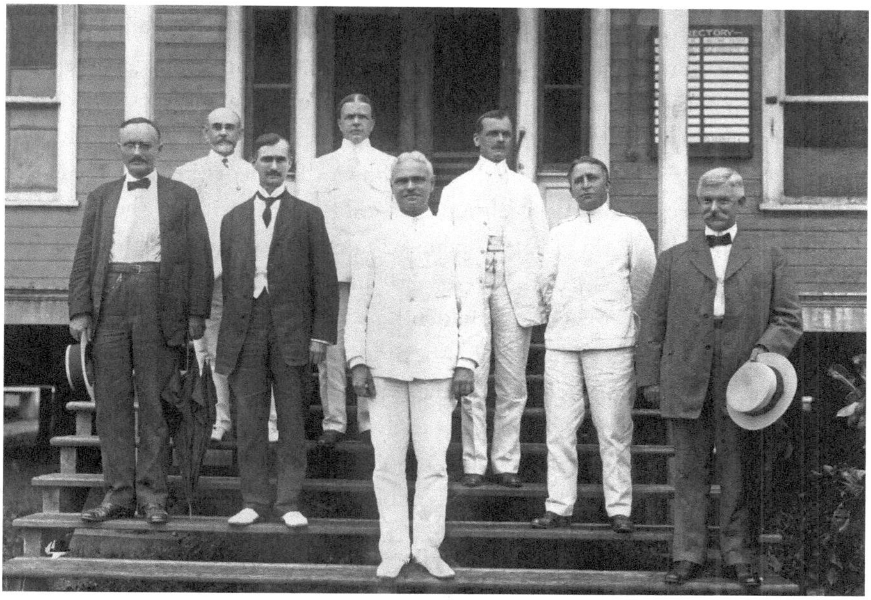

FIGURE 11.1. The Isthmian Canal Commission, 1909–1914. From left, William Sibert, Joseph Bucklin Bishop, Maurice Thatcher, Harry Rousseau, George Goethals, David Gaillard, Harry Hodges, and William Gorgas. Office of History, US Army Corps of Engineers, David Gaillard Collection.

for raw materials, consumer markets, and maritime coaling stations. Gorgas was leery of such overseas ventures, believing they shifted the national focus from domestic problems and economic reform.[1] But he shared with Roosevelt and their contemporaries an interest in extending American and European culture, science, and technology to the less developed, "barbarian" tropics. These new lands hosted pathogens and parasites alien to Europeans, some of which were deadly to native-born and newcomer alike, but others to which indigenous people had developed immunity. For centuries colonists had to simply endure these new environments, but now modern medicine began to tame the deadly diseases that killed would-be imperialists.[2] Men like Gorgas, Walter Reed, Ronald Ross, and George Sternberg were unlocking the mysteries of deadly disease to make the tropics hospitable to European civilization.

When in 1909 the AMA recognized Gorgas's work by electing him president, he used his inaugural speech to lay out the role of public health in advancing "civilization" and white supremacy. Leaving no doubt as to his purpose, he entitled the speech in Atlantic City, New Jersey, "The Conquest of the Tropics for the

White Race." Gorgas focused on malaria and described in detail his department's malaria mitigation methods—mosquito destruction, swamp drainage, brush cutting, screening, the dispensing of quinine pills, and continual inspection and oversight—which enabled him to cut the malaria rate by three quarters. Such advances in tropical sanitation, Gorgas stated, "have shown that the white man can live in the tropics and enjoy as good health as he would have if living in the temperate zone." And, he added, it was not "difficult or expensive to achieve this." The consequences for such disease control were vast: "I dare to predict that after the lapse of a period, let us say, equal to that which now separates the year 1909 from the Norman conquest of England [1066], localities in the tropics will be the centers of as powerful and as cultured a white civilization as any that will then exist in the temperate zones."[3] It might take centuries, but science and public health would ultimately enable "white civilization" to dominate the earth.

The speech was reported by numerous publications, including the *New England Journal of Medicine*, the *Chicago Medical Recorder*, the *Tampa Morning Tribune*, *JAMA*, and *The Lancet.* "Life in the tropics for the Anglo-Saxon will be more healthful than in the temperate zones," announced the *New York Times,* predicting that within two or three centuries the tropics would once again become centers of human civilization and production.[4] Even a children's magazine noted that "white civilization shall some day flourish on the banks of the Niger, the Congo, and the Amazon."[5] Gorgas was not alone; other Americans were trying to make the Philippines habitable for white occupiers, as were the British and other European powers in tropical colonies in the Caribbean, Africa, India, and Southeast Asia. Many, like Gorgas, argued that modern medicine would help people in the countries they occupied, but the primary impetus was to protect the health of the colonizers.[6] White supremacy was not, of course, merely a rhetorical concept. Jim Crow was alive and well and brutally enforced in the United States, where in 1909 alone, sixty-nine African Americans were lynched, including seven men in Gorgas's home state of Alabama.[7]

In Panama the ICC's racially prescribed "gold rolls" and "silver rolls" governed all economic and social organization, and segregated medical clinics and medical personnel's racial prejudices resulted in inferior care and higher sick and death rates for Black workers. Whereas Black people outnumbered whites by more than three to one in the Canal Zone, they had a 20 percent higher death rate, 11.40 per 1,000 compared to 9.03 per 1,000 for whites.[8] Many of those workers died unnamed, invisible to the racialized power structure. Gorgas's annual sanitary reports often included the names, ages, dates, and causes of death for white Americans but provided no such information on Black laborers. A vignette from Ancón

Hospital in 1909 illustrates such racism. The hospital had about five hundred patient beds segregated by disease, age, race, and sex: about three hundred beds for Black male patients; eighty for Spaniards and other white foreigners; ten beds for Black women; ninety for white Americans, including women and children; and ten private rooms for VIPs and paying patients. When a visitor asked Dr. W. E. Deeks, who oversaw several wards, "Are the cases you get among the Spaniards and negroes as interesting and instructive as among Americans?" Deeks answered, "No, not nearly," explaining, "We can never get the histories of them, they are like just so many children, and their histories rarely correct." He said he preferred caring for private white patients, because they were "men of intelligence and it is important that we know what the trouble is."[9] Gorgas had hired a few Black doctors, and in 1906 Sen. John T. Morgan (D-AL) inquired about employment opportunities for Dr. Willis W. Jones, a graduate of Howard College, whose father had been valet to Jefferson Davis.[10] Gorgas explained that the Department of Sanitation paid Black physicians $50 a month in gold (compared to $100 to $250 for white physicians) to help in "ferreting out infectious and contagious diseases," but they did not practice in the larger hospitals.[11] There is no evidence that Willis did come to Panama.

## PANAMA MEDICINE

Even though Gorgas and his staff had emptied the yellow fever wards and reduced malaria cases, the hospitals remained busy. As early as 1906, Gorgas was worried about the prevalence of pneumonia among the West Indian workers, telling Kean, "We have gotten rid of tropical diseases, but pneumonia is playing hot with our negro laborers."[12] In April 1906, for example, it was the leading cause of mortality among employees, causing thirty-two deaths.[13] Initially, Gorgas attributed the high pneumonia rates to "racial peculiarity," but his thinking on race and pneumonia evolved during his years in Panama to factor in inferior living and working conditions. When testifying before a congressional committee in 1907, Gorgas described the workers' poor living conditions, how they often went to bed in wet clothes and did not take the time to buy and prepare good meals. "Of course you know how improvident the negro is," he testified, "he would never buy a whole day's food at once." When asked if he attributed the pneumonia rates "almost entirely to racial peculiarities," rather than "want of care on the part of the canal management," Gorgas replied, "Yes." But when the chairman asked again if managers "care for the negro as carefully as for the white," Gorgas hesitated. "I think so," he said.[14]

Gorgas appointed a board headed by Henry Carter to investigate the pneumonia problem, and in a six-month study it identified working conditions as the main culprit. The board found that new arrivals often developed respiratory ailments such as influenza soon after arriving in Panama and, if they were not treated quickly, could develop pneumonia. They recommended providing drying sheds for the laborers to dry out their clothes before going home, issuing each worker one or two blankets to keep him warm at night, and "feeding men instead of allowing them to feed themselves."[15] Gorgas also tried to reduce crowded housing by moving laborers out of barracks and into shacks scattered throughout the zone. This approach worked, and deaths from pneumonia fell from 416 in 1906 to 47 in 1913. Moreover, the overall death rates of West Indian workers dropped from two to three times that of white workers, to almost even by the end of construction.[16] Gorgas was proud of this record and would speak on pneumonia often over the ensuing years. In 1912 he told a correspondent, "Good environment has had a great effect on the negro."[17]

Racial disparities became awkward when the data showed that the Canal Zone white workers were as sick or sicker than Black workers. When in 1910, with a weekly sick rate for white employees of 45.18 per 1,000 compared to 16.14 for Black employees, Gorgas explained to a congressional committee that American whites actually had lower sickness rates than Blacks, but that white Spaniards had similar rates because "the environment of the foreign white is much the same as that of the black." He believed there would be little malaria if everyone lived in screened houses, but "the bulk of these people are not protected in that way, and as you get relatively lower and lower down the scale of civilization, they protect themselves less effectively."[18] Gorgas picked up this line of thought in correspondence with author and historian Charles Francis Adams. The American has "the best surroundings of every kind," he noted. "He is of a very much higher order of intelligence, and, therefore, takes very much better care of himself." Consequently, the higher hospitalization rates for whites were because "the white man goes to the doctor much more freely than the negro."[19] He did not recognize the lack of screening on housing for Black workers or that they might be reluctant seek medical care if many white doctors saw them as inferior and did not want to treat them.

In addition to infectious diseases, other kinds of noncommunicable infections and injuries showed up at the ICC hospitals. Canal construction used millions of dynamite charges and generated tons of spoil, which trains transported along the canal route across constantly shifting worksites. Explosions and landslides were a constant threat, so as disease rates fell, industrial accidents became a larger cause of admissions and mortality. Department figures showed that in January 1906, disease accounted for 95 percent of all fatalities, but in January 1912, only 60 percent.[20] The *Canal Record* reported many of these incidents. In September 1908 Rejelio Castillo, Juan Sanchez, Coementi Gonzales, and Rivio Arios were killed when two engines fell off a trestle crossing a river near Miraflores while they were on their way to meet the labor train at the lunch hour.[21] The next month, two explosions made the news in one week—one when a steam shovel struck an unexploded dynamite charge, and the other when lightning detonated a dynamite cache. The blasts killed twelve men—ten Black laborers and two white engineers—and injured eighteen.[22] The worst accident was in the cut at Bas Obispo, when forty-four thousand tons of dynamite exploded prematurely, killing twenty-six men, including three Americans, four Spaniards, two Barbadians, and fifteen "Negroes," and injured forty.[23] Working the lock gates was especially dangerous, as one song recounted:

> You get more money for that job than working in the cut
> But it all depends, honey, if you don't get hurt
> For if you ever get a drop, you surely have to die
> For the gates, Lord God, are seventy-five feet high.[24]

Gorgas spoke far less about these accidents than about disease, but in 1910 he presided at the unveiling of an ICC memorial in St. Luke's Church in Panama City dedicated to those who died in the construction of the canal.[25] That year the department saw more than twenty thousand hospitalizations for disease and injuries, 40 percent of some 50,500 canal employees. Of the 548 employees who died, 88 men perished in railroad accidents, 10 in drownings, 8 from dynamite explosions, and 35 deaths were caused by "accidental traumatisms." Surgeons performed 6,120 operations in 1910, including 140 amputations and more than 200 appendectomies. Ultimately, deaths by drowning, suicide, explosions, railroad mishaps, homicide, and accidents accounted for one-fifth of the roughly 5,600 fatalities during construction.[26]

These accidents and injuries all required attention and resources, and one thing Gorgas and Goethals did agree on was the government's responsibility to its workers. Together they made the request at a House Appropriations Committee hearing in Panama for $950,000 to pay for "medical aid and support of the insane, and of indigent persons, permanently disabled, while in line of duty and in the employ of the Isthmian Canal Commission." Gorgas told the committee that the funding was to care for "the class of people whom we have to permanently take care of, like men who have lost both legs—the class ordinarily taken care of in the county poorhouses at home."[27] The Panama Canal project thereby put in place some of the earliest American government welfare programs for workers.

## WHAT COST, SANITATION?

Gorgas and Goethals continually sparred over the ICC Department of Sanitation budget. Goethals had to request annual appropriations from Congress and was under constant pressure to keep spending down. Gorgas's budget therefore presented a big—and nonengineering—target. The year Goethals arrived, the budget for medical and sanitation operations stood at $1,950,000 for fiscal year 1907, cresting at $2,034,000 in 1908. Goethals presented this as the cost of Panama sanitation, arguing that two million dollars a year was too much. When this number started circulating in the national press, Gorgas angrily replied that the figures were misleading. He pointed out that only one-fourth of his annual budget was for sanitation, $338,178 per year on average in 1908 and 1909, and that the Department of Sanitation had many duties beyond disease mitigation. His budget paid for an organization of more than 1,200 employees, about 700 of whom worked in two major hospitals, three sanitariums, and seventeen dispensaries across the zone, as well as the quarantine service and the cemeteries. Gorgas's department was responsible for scores of people disabled by leprosy (Hansen's disease), tuberculosis, and mental illness, and he even paid the salaries of "some fifteen ministers of the gospel."[28] His budget, he argued, was modest compared to the lives it saved, the productivity it facilitated, and, ultimately, its benefits for the white race.[29] The American construction of the canal ultimately cost about $350 million, and Gorgas calculated only about 1 percent of that amount went to sanitation operations. In a 1913 *JAMA* article he wrote, "when we are through, we shall have spent on sanitation about . . . 1 percent of the total cost of the canal." [30] At $340,000 a year for sanitation over ten years, he was not far wrong.

Stung by charges of extravagance, Gorgas went on the offensive in 1910 and conducted a survey of hospital expenses in major US cities to see how the cost of running his operation in Panama compared with stateside counterparts. His office sent questionnaires to hospitals in Atlanta, Baltimore, Boston, Chicago, Cleveland, New York, Philadelphia, Pittsburgh, San Francisco, and Washington, DC, requesting information on the number of beds, patient census, medical staff, salaries, and daily hospital cost per patient. Most hospitals responded and survey results showed that hospital costs varied from an alarming low of $.30 per patient per day to $3.09 per day, compared to $1.54 to $1.96 per day in Panama. Gorgas concluded that the ICC hospital costs compared favorably with those in the United States.[31] He also liked to point out that his operations actually raised revenue for the ICC. As the Ancón and Colón hospitals developed reputations for good medical care, private patients began to use them instead of going to the United States or Europe, and fees charged to non-ICC employees generated income of about $20,000 annually, which, Gorgas ruefully pointed out, went into the general fund, not his department's coffers.[32]

During his annual visit to the United States in 1910, Gorgas used this data to air the issue in his speeches. He liked to begin by pointing out that if the Americans had experienced the same death rate as the French had during their construction effort in the 1880s, they would have lost 23,850 lives during the first five years of construction, compared to the actual 3,317 deaths under Gorgas's guidance.[33] As president of the American Society of Tropical Medicine, he told the annual convention in St. Louis that while the Panama Canal may become a commercial success, the greater accomplishment would be showing that good sanitation allows white civilization to expand. By demonstrating that the "white man can live and work in any part of the tropics and maintain good health," he announced to the convention, "the settling of the tropics by the Caucasian will date from the completion of the Panama Canal."[34] He hoped that Panama's example would "induce other tropical countries to try the same measures; and that thereby gradually all the tropics will be redeemed and made a suitable habitation for the white man."[35]

Gorgas distributed his paper to leaders in public health and government, including William Osler, William Welch, Ronald Ross, Henry Wellcome, the famed physician of Whitehall Court, Elihu Root (now a US senator), Leonard Wood, and President Taft, explaining that the "Sanitary Department of Panama has of late been accused of extravagance," and that his paper "entirely refutes this charge."[36] Gorgas also told members of Congress, "To make our work useful for the rest of mankind, we would have to show that it is within the limits of reasonable cost."[37] He developed staffing and budget plans for sanitation programs in small municipalities and calculated that proper sanitation as he had overseen in Panama would cost only $3.38 per capita per year.[38]

Over the years Gorgas cultivated a widening network of sanitarians, public health officials, scientists, physicians, and members of Congress, and put them on a mailing list so he could send them his monthly sanitary reports. These short notices reported the sickness and death rates in the zone, the distribution of various diseases among different populations, and activities of the quarantine station, mosquito brigades, and other sanitation projects.[39] Gorgas also sent out his speeches and articles to the list with the broader goal of educating people about sanitation in the tropics. *JAMA* and other medical journals regularly published the reports, often with glowing editorials.[40] This publicity campaign so irked Goethals that he sought to shut it down and in 1910, citing budget constraints, suspended publication of the monthly reports. The OTSG and Gorgas pushed back. "Goethals is crowding you to the wall," Kean told Gorgas. "I told the Secretary plainly that in my opinion Goethals' objection to your monthly report was mainly due to jealousy."[41] The AMA also launched a campaign to get them reinstated, and after a few months, under pressure from the medical world and members of Congress, the secretary of war restored the mailings. By 1911, however, Goethals had the Department of

Sanitation budget down to $1,550,000.[42] His chief sanitarian, however, continued to argue that money spent by his department saved lives.

## A CONGENIAL LIFE IN PANAMA

Despite the tension with Goethals, Gorgas loved being an army sanitarian and physician, and told Jessie that life in Panama was pleasant and the work "congenial and of endless variety."[43] He stayed out of his boss's way, enjoyed his network of family, friends, and colleagues, and savored small victories, noting in his journal in September 1912, "Was elected president of the Tivoli club. George Goethals my opponent."[44] He also maintained his sense of humor. At times he referred to his boss in code. "Our affairs down here are running along efficiently," he told Amelia. "XYZ being off on leave we have nothing to stir us up."[45] He told Mamie, "Goethals and I are getting along most lovingly. We seldom meet but write daily and are just as polite as two dancing masters." He added, "Marie and Mrs. Goethals keep up the amenities."[46] One story in particular captured Gorgas's good-natured way to push back. During a commission meeting, Goethals was complaining about the expenses of the sanitary work, especially the cost of killing mosquitoes. "Colonel Gorgas, do you realize that every mosquito you kill costs the Government ten dollars?" According to one of the doctors at the meeting, Gorgas quietly replied, "It may be expensive, but, Colonel Goethals, suppose that one of those ten-dollar mosquitoes were to bite you. What a loss it would be to the country!"[47]

Away from his job, Gorgas relished the outdoors and explored Panama on horseback, on foot, and by canoe. He and Marie brought their two horses from Havana to Panama, and in 1910 he purchased a new horse, naming him Traveler, after his predecessor. Gorgas climbed the hills of Ancón and went "orchid hunting" in the jungle. He enjoyed investigating the flora and fauna and talking to locals about their history—some of which he put in his book, *Sanitation in Panama*. He and Le Prince liked to explore the jungle. One August when they went canoeing on the Chagres with another doctor, they capsized at Gamboa, and Gorgas lost his watch and compass. He lost his watch again two years later, this time with his cousin Stanhope Bayne-Jones when they capsized on a canoe trip to Taberville. Bayne-Jones dropped his watch and camera in the river, while Gorgas lost his watch, umbrella (!), and shoes. The cousins had to walk back two miles through the jungle, Gorgas without shoes. He reported, "Took six hours and used me up." A few days later they returned to the accident scene to look for their watches, to no avail, and this time, "Motor boat broke down & we did not get back till 9 p.m."[48]

When congressional delegations came to Panama, Gorgas would take the visitors on hikes. When a senator's wife wondered at such vigorous exercise in the heat, he told her, "You can't sleep well in the tropics unless you take exercise."[49] Le Prince observed that the day after a rigorous outing, Gorgas would return to work refreshed, "as though none of the hardships and opposition to his plans and work had ever existed."[50] Toward the end of the construction period, Le Prince and Gorgas decided to be the first to traverse the isthmus by water, canoeing along the canal route from the Pacific coast to the Atlantic. They portaged over part of the Culebra Cut and then continued down the Chagres River. Approaching Tabernilla they could see workmen waving wildly at them, but before they could stop, they hit a rapids and heard a "terrific crash." They had entered a blast zone. "Rocks, stones and dirt rained about us as we went full speed ahead in the rapid boulder-strewn channel." Once they survived the torrent, Le Prince remembered that Gorgas, paddling from the rear, simply remarked that it was "a rather warm reception." With great effort and sore arms, they reached the Atlantic Coast and felt they could claim the prize. In 1914, when the first boat passed through the canal, Le Prince was amused by observers who "were under the impression that they were watching the first boat go through the canal from one ocean to the other."[51]

William and Marie were readers and had a library of some 1,800 books.[52] Amelia the librarian often sent them books. (She retired in 1906 at the age of eighty, after building the University of Alabama Library from six thousand to twenty thousand volumes.) William liked to keep a "light book and a heavy book" on hand to read.[53] He read Bunau-Varilla's *Panama: The Creation, Destruction, and Resurrection*; *The Commonwealth*, by William Jennings Bryan; and as much as he could about the Civil War, such as *American Campaign* (1909) by Matthew Forney Steele, and *The Victim: A Romance of the Real Jefferson Davis* (1914) by white supremacist author Thomas Dixon.[54] For lighter reading, Gorgas took up Mary Johnston's *Long Roll* (1909), a Civil War novel from the southern perspective. Gorgas subscribed to the *Confederate Veteran*, which one author calls "the most important organ for the Lost Cause after 1890," and purchased additional subscriptions for Old Confederate homes and veterans who could not afford it.[55]

Gorgas followed politics and political reform with William Jennings Bryan's weekly newspaper, *The Commoner*, and belonged to the American Single Tax Committee and the Henry George Lecture Association, organizations advocating for broad socioeconomic reform. But when the American Association for the Advancement of Science Committee of One Hundred, a group that lobbied Congress in support of progressive legislation, invited him to join, he drew the line, explaining that government employees could not engage in political activity.[56] Gorgas also used his free time to edit Josiah's multivolume diary and told Amelia that it was like talking to his father. He sent a copy of the journal to Mamie for her birthday.[57]

As soon as Panama appeared to be free of deadly disease, it became a tourist destination.[58] A 1906 tourist booklet noted that "the wonderful work of Col. W. C. Gorgas and his able staff of assistants has made this one of the clean spots of the earth; all sickness has been stamped out in the Canal Zone."[59] By 1911 *JAMA* suggested that Panama was an "ideal health resort" with death rates lower than in the United States, and the *New York Times* followed suit.[60] By 1912 four shipping lines were operating between Colón and New York, some offering cruises that stopped at other Caribbean islands, and encouraging people to stay in the Tivoli Hotel, visit Panama's beaches, and ride the train to observe the canal construction.[61] Full-length tourist guides appeared, such as *The Panama Guide*, by John Owen Collins, with maps and guides to hotels, shops, churches, and cathedrals, complete with advertisements for goods and services to tourists and visitors.[62]

William and Marie hosted a veritable Who's Who of the leading medical scientists and public health officials who came to study Gorgas's sanitation program, visit Darling's laboratory, and go out in the field with Le Prince. Among the first were medical men: William Welch from Johns Hopkins; Patrick Manson, the Scottish parasitologist known as the "Father of Tropical Medicine," who discovered that mosquitoes could transmit disease; and Nobel laureate Ronald Ross, who described Gorgas as a "spare, resolute man of the best type."[63] William Howard Taft came down several times, as secretary of war, and as president. Famous for his three-hundred-pound physique, when he visited in 1909, Marie had a special chair made for him to use at their dinner party. "I wished no casualty in my home for the president-elect," she explained.[64] Other visitors included Roosevelt's friend, Dr. Alexander Lambert, and Henry Wellcome, who stopped by on his way to Ecuador and afterward wrote a laudatory article on tropical medicine and research opportunities at Gorgas's department.[65] Other guests included Hiram Bingham, the naturalist from Yale, whom Gorgas had met during the Pan-American conference in Chile, and James Bryce, British member of Parliament from Dublin and ambassador to the United States (1907–1913).[66] Gorgas was also thrilled to host William Jennings Bryan when he came to Panama in 1910.

The Gorgases got to do more visiting themselves after William acquired a deputy, John L. Phillips, a medical officer at Ancón Hospital. In 1911 they traveled to Cuba for the American Public Health Association meeting and were received as returning heroes. Gorgas's former colleague Juan Guiteras met their boat, and the Cuban government paid for their accommodations. After one day of long ceremonies and laudatory speeches in both Spanish and English, Gorgas wrote in his diary, "Have had a most delightful time."[67] He told Jessie that he felt very lucky to have lived to see his work "so liberally recognized."[68]

When Gorgas returned to Panama, he received a job offer from John F. Fitzgerald, mayor of Boston, to be the chairman of the Boston Board of Health, one of the leading public health posts in the country. Gorgas was tempted, but he was also determined to see the canal project to the end, so he declined. An even more tempting offer came, to serve as the president of the University of Alabama, the position his father had held. He would have loved to live once again near Amelia and his sisters, and told his mother that Marie was "charmed with the idea of living in the old house and fixing it up and living in real old colonial style for the rest of our lives." But while "the whole romance of the thing appealed very strongly to our sentimental side," it was too soon. Ultimately, William and Marie made a political calculation. The Panama Canal project, he told his mother, "was my life work on which my scientific reputation rested," and they worried that "if I separated from the work before the canal was opened, I would lose a good share of this reputation." However, he added, "I have never given up an idea with more regret."[69]

Recognition continued for Gorgas in 1912. During his visit to the United States to spread his gospel of mosquito mitigation and tropical sanitation, he was feted everywhere he went. He met with high-ranking government officials, including Secretary of War Harry L. Stimson and several senators and ambassadors. He also gave three commencement addresses, which were something of homecomings. The first was at the University of Alabama on a visit to Tuscaloosa, then to Baltimore to speak at Johns Hopkins, and finally Gorgas traveled to Sewanee. Returning for the first time in thirty-five years, Gorgas gave the commencement address at the University of the South and received an honorary degree.[70] The son of a defeated Confederate general had done them proud.

As Goethals drove construction to completion, on time and under budget, the US Congress formalized the governance of the completed canal with the Panama Canal Act of 1912. Following Goethals's recommendation, Congress eliminated the oversight commission and put control into the hands of one position, the governor of the Panama Canal Zone. President Wilson appointed Goethals to be that first governor. Congress also mandated that only people working directly on the canal be allowed to live in the Canal Zone. At one hearing a congressman asked Goethals if this meant that after the permanent canal workforce had been hired, "all other employees may leave the Isthmus." Goethals emphatically agreed and suggested that "we use our ships for the purpose of taking all the foreign labor back to its native heath."[71] White men would now govern much of Panama. When Gorgas was consulted on the issue of who should live in the Canal Zone, he advised that allowing Panamanians to continue to live in the zone was the best way to ensure good sanitation. But he too celebrated white supremacy in his Johns

Hopkins commencement speech. "This period will be dated the beginning of the great white civilizations in these regions," he announced, and "again great tropic empires will be known as occurred in the early history of man, such as Egypt, Babylon and Nineveh."[72]

With Panama now open for business and tourism, William Gorgas turned his sights to fighting disease in other lands.

## CHAPTER 12

# Fighting Mosquitoes Abroad

> Modern sanitary measures have demonstrated the fact that even in the tropics it is possible to rid a locality of yellow fever and keep it free.
>
> —William C. Gorgas, 1909

THE LIBRARY OF CONGRESS HOLDS the only known moving picture of William Gorgas, an undated one-minute film showing him giving a tour of the Canal Zone. It opens with Gorgas sporting a white linen suit and fresh haircut, standing on the steps of a building and then nodding with the slightest smile at the camera. The camera then follows him and an unnamed member of the ICC sitting on the back of the Panama train as it travels through the countryside. Gorgas points out things of interest as the train runs alongside the canal, and when they enter Colón, we see the main streets, pass by the YMCA, and watch people cross tracks after the train passes.[1] That one minute captures the keystone of Gorgas's life and career.

The most senior man in rank and tenure in Panama, Gorgas knew his world well and loved to show it off. That world was changing by the day, however, as industrialization introduced new technology—such as the motion picture that recorded Gorgas on his canal tour—and management practices revolutionized the way people worked and lived. The Panama Canal would soon link the Pacific and Atlantic Oceans, carrying ships eighty-five feet up over the Culebra mountains along the fifty-mile canal-and-lock system, thereby reducing water travel between the East and West Coasts of the United States by more than nine thousand miles. The achievement would speed commerce and travel around the world and make the United States a powerful gatekeeper of this global passage. But Gorgas worried about how world commerce could carry *Stegomyia* and yellow fever across

Map 12.1. Schematic map of William Gorgas's overseas travels, 1898–1920.

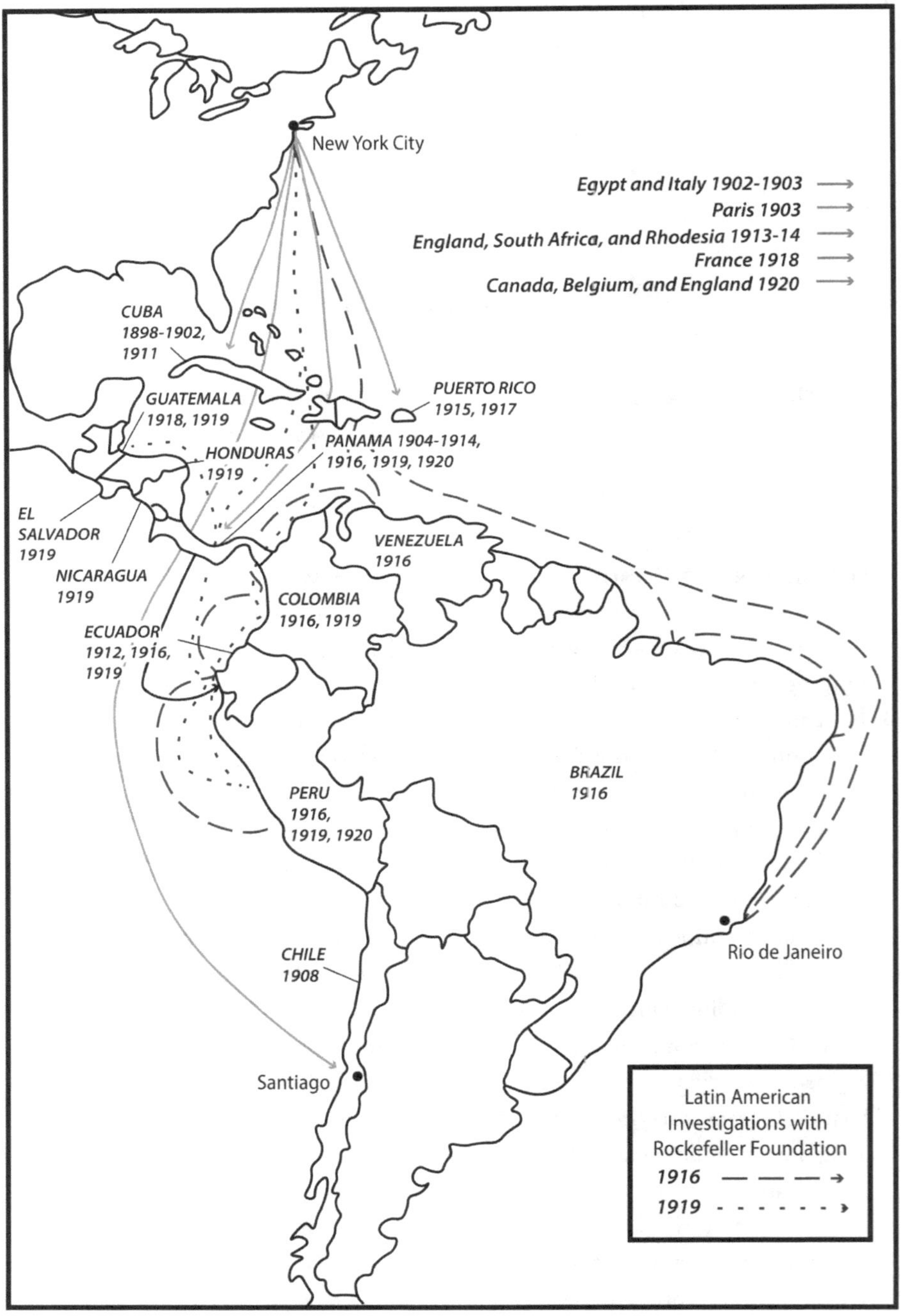
New York City
Egypt and Italy 1902-1903
Paris 1903
England, South Africa, and Rhodesia 1913-14
France 1918
Canada, Belgium, and England 1920
CUBA
1898-1902,
1911
PUERTO RICO
1915, 1917
GUATEMALA
1918, 1919
HONDURAS
1919
PANAMA 1904-1914,
1916, 1919, 1920
EL
SALVADOR
1919
NICARAGUA
1919
VENEZUELA
1916
COLOMBIA
1916, 1919
ECUADOR
1912, 1916,
1919
BRAZIL
1916
PERU
1916,
1919, 1920
Rio de Janeiro
CHILE
1908
Santiago
Latin American
Investigations with
Rockefeller Foundation
1916
1919

the continents, so he turned his gaze to that wider world in his war against disease and mosquitoes.

## GUAYAQUIL

With yellow fever now under control in Cuba and Panama, Gorgas and other public health officials pivoted to eliminate other hotbeds of infection. Some worried that regular travel through the Panama Canal could spread yellow fever to Asia. That continent had been free of the disease, but *Stegomyia* was present in China, India, and the Philippines, and people in those places were nonimmune. In 1910 Gorgas warned a congressional committee that "all that is necessary apparently to cause one of the greatest epidemics the world has ever known, is the introduction of a case of yellow fever."[2] The best way to prevent the spread to Asia, he believed, was to keep Panama free of the disease and to prevent the spread from endemic centers on the coast of South America.[3] That required investigation, sanitation, and money.

As early as 1906, Secretary of War Root told Gorgas he believed "the results which were achieved in Cuba can be extended throughout Central and South America" and asked Gorgas to advise William C. Fox, US ambassador to Ecuador on cleaning up its major port town of Guayaquil.[4] A town of 100,000, Guayaquil was one of the few large ports in Latin America where yellow fever and other fearsome diseases such as bubonic plague, typhoid, cholera, dysentery, malaria, and tuberculosis still prevailed. The annual death rate there during the 1910s averaged 45 per 1,000, three times the rate in the United States.[5] Mortality rates in Guayaquil's quarantine hospitals for yellow fever and plague were so high—50 percent—that people ignored the quarantine laws to avoid them. Guayaquil's hot, humid climate and seasonal flooding made it hospitable to diseases, and its rapidly growing population of mestizo and Indian underclasses lacked historic immunity to many pathogens. Ecuador's continual political and civil disturbances also undermined public health efforts, as did local officials who were suspicious of outside interference. As one historian wrote of Guayaquil, "the city earned and richly deserved its foul reputation."[6]

The War Department, following Root's lead, made plans for Gorgas and ICC chairman Charles Magoon to travel to Ecuador to make an assessment, but Guayaquil officials were so opposed to United States interference, the trip was cancelled.[7] Another American-led effort to develop a sanitary program for the country in 1908 also went nowhere.[8] Such hostility to the United States was not surprising. Latin American political leaders had watched with disgust Theodore Roosevelt's support for Panama's rebellion against Colombia, and the subsequent US occupation of the Canal Zone. They were wary of further colonial interference and condescension.[9]

Yet Gorgas kept his sights on Guayaquil, which, he wrote, was "permanently infected with yellow fever and had been for years."[10]

Ecuadorian officials stood their ground until 1912 when a US naval officer died of yellow fever in January, and Guayaquil recorded 147 cases of yellow fever and 124 cases of bubonic plague by May of that year.[11] Under pressure from Taft, they finally indicated their willingness to accept help from American experts, but to avoid the appearance of foreign intervention, Ecuadorian officials agreed to request US assistance and commit $500,000 to sanitation over three years.[12] They also secured assurance that if Gorgas became disabled, the United States would appoint "an equally competent person to replace him."[13] After debate about whether the United States should even be helping foreign countries, Congress approved leave without pay for Gorgas and several other army officers and allowed them to receive payment from the Republic of Ecuador.[14] The American press unhelpfully framed the mission as an example of "white man's burden" to help modernize and sanitize less-developed nations. One paper portrayed Guayaquil as "The Pest Hole of the Pacific," another as a "Menace," and another author called Guayaquil one of the dirtiest ports in South America, pontificating, "Cleanliness is next to Godliness."[15]

On December 4, 1912, Gorgas, Le Prince, and medical officer Robert Noble, the chief inspector for the ICC, trained in both engineering and medicine, sailed for Ecuador. After four days of rough seas, they arrived in Guayaquil to be met by a hostile crowd, resentful of foreign quarantines and embargoes against their city. They "threatened to mob us," wrote Gorgas in his journal, but police and an American embassy delegation escorted them to their hotel. The next day, however, he noted it was "all quiet & people as pleasant as can be" and did not mention hostility in Ecuador again.[16]

There followed what became a pattern in Gorgas's sanitation visits: meetings with government officials, water, sewerage, and hospital inspections, social engagements, and outdoor adventures. The party spent several days assessing the sanitary conditions and remediation measures required in Guayaquil. After their inspection, while Le Prince chased mosquitoes in the city, Gorgas and Noble traveled to the capital, Quito, on the new railway. At 9,350 feet elevation, Quito was the second-highest capital city in the world (after La Paz, Bolivia). Despite its location near the equator, Gorgas found it so cold that he needed "thick clothes" and could not sleep at night until he rolled up in a blanket.[17] After that uncomfortable night, they had a formal meeting with President Alejandro Cárdenas and obtained his support for their work. The next day they went to the equator for a luncheon, which probably delighted Gorgas because he always marked his crossing of that landmark in his travels. Returning to Guayaquil, the train encountered damaged rails, and they had to travel by handcar, which, Gorgas declared, was "Grand."[18] Always eager to ride, Gorgas and Le Prince went horseback riding the next day, covering thirty miles and driving so hard that they had to compensate the stables eighty *sucres* (about forty dollars) because one of the horses died. They were still able to make their departing ship on Christmas Eve at 4 p.m. and were home by New Year's Eve.

Gorgas began writing his report to the secretary of state on the voyage home and in it prescribed a stringent program. Drawing from his experience in Havana and Panama, Gorgas recommended extensive government powers and measures such as paving the streets; providing clean water, and garbage and sewage-disposal systems; upgrading building construction to prevent plague-carrying-rat infestation; and hiring a professional public health official to manage sanitation. He calculated that an annual appropriation of $150,000 would maintain the improvements. "There seems to be no reason why Guayaquil can not be made as safe a harbor from a health point of view as from any other," he told Secretary of State Knox. "The people there realize the importance of cleaning up if they want to enjoy the benefits to be derived from the commerce of the canal."[19]

Unlike the American press, Ecuadorian newspapers were skeptical of Gorgas's mission. *El Telégrafo* of Guayaquil observed that he told them nothing new about sanitation, yet they had to pay 16,000 *sucres* for it, and another paper, *La Prensa*, demanded an accounting of Gorgas's expenses.[20] *El comercio de Quito* complained sarcastically that "only the Yankees, that is the commission headed by Colonel Gorgas," were capable of bringing sanitary order to Guayaquil.[21] (Gorgas may have been amused at the Yankee sobriquet.) Ecuadorian officials nevertheless requested proposals to complete the sanitation work that Gorgas recommended, and they contracted with a British company to do it. The Great War, however, derailed the effort.[22]

## TRANSITIONS

Just days after he got home from Guayaquil, William and Marie got a cable from Dick advising that Amelia had died of influenza. She was eighty-six years old and had been growing weaker, so this was not a surprise, but it hit William hard, and he immediately sat down and wrote a meditation on his mother. "I think mother was the most capable humankind without exception that I ever knew," he told his brother. He was glad she had died before she became mentally or physically incapacitated, and he imagined her in reunion with Josiah and all her loved ones "just as if she had gone to China."[23] Minnie was with Amelia at the end and told William, not unkindly, that the day before she died, Amelia had gazed at his photograph on the mantel and said, "My Willie looks down upon me with love in his eyes, and I know in his heart." She had been very weak, Minnie had said, and "I know she often longed for the comfort and strength of your presence."[24] Gorgas did not express guilt for his absence in her last days but instead memorialized her words. When he began his new account book for 1915, he copied her words in the journal frontpiece—"My Willie looks down upon me with love in his eyes and I know in his heart"—and copied it again at the end of the volume.[25] For the rest of his life, William marked his mother's birthday or her death with letters to his sisters.

Gorgas went to Tuscaloosa to be with the family during a trip to Washington to

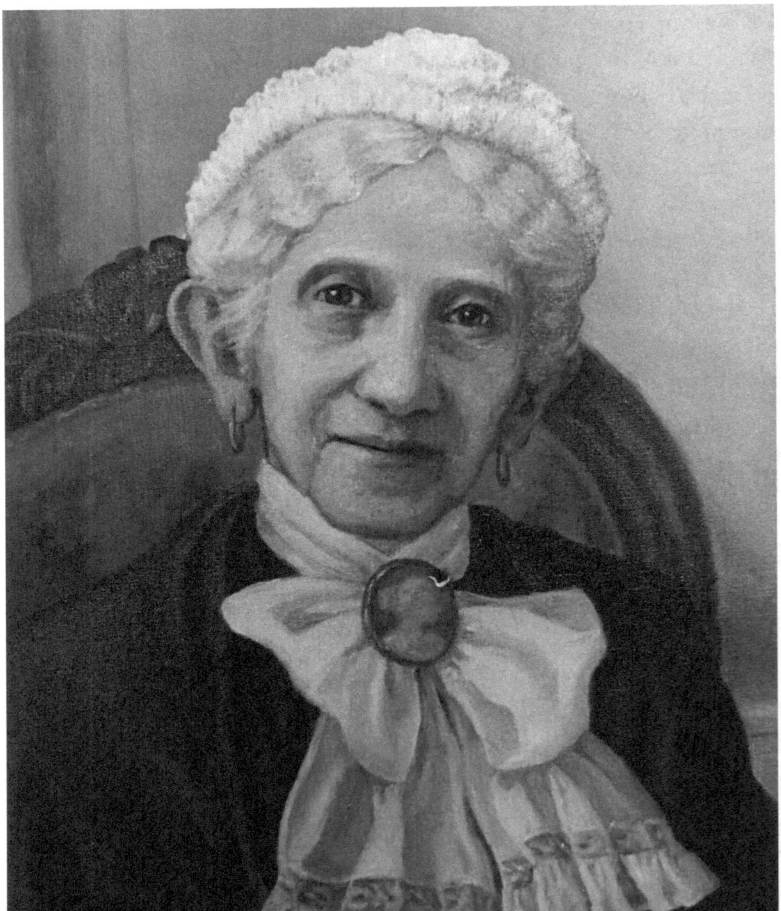

FIGURE 12.1 Portrait of Amelia Gorgas, 1890. Courtesy of the University of Alabama Libraries Special Collections.

report on his Ecuador assignment. He paid the funeral expenses and commissioned an oil painting of his mother to hang in the university library.[26] The family used one of the rare photographs of Amelia to model a head-and-shoulder portrait, with her seated in a chair, a white cap on her white hair, gold hoop earrings, a large cameo securing a scarf at her neck, looking directly at the artist with a mild expression. The University of Alabama later named its library the Amelia Gayle Gorgas Library.

William and Marie now prepared for a happier milestone, the marriage of Aileen, age twenty-three. She was a well-educated and well-traveled young woman, having lived apart from her parents off and on over the years, shuttling from New York to Cuba and Panama. Aileen helped her parents entertain the guests who came through Panama, attending dances and teas, mixing with young American engineers, doctors, army officers, and clerks in Panama for adventure. William closely chaperoned these activities and believed he had the young men "pretty well disciplined" on the Gorgas curfew rules.[27] Suitors had to be self-confident to court the daughter of Colonel Gorgas.

When it was time for Aileen to marry, she chose a man in her father's circle, William Daugherty Wrightson, a civil engineer from Maryland who had been working for Gorgas for several years. Four years older than the bride, he was serious and dutiful, and had impeccable handwriting. Before they were married, Wrightson informed Colonel and Mrs. Gorgas that he was buying life insurance for the couple and was making progress in securing a new job as an engineer for a Texas oil company.[28] Aileen joined her father when he returned to Panama from Tuscaloosa, so she and Marie could plan the grand affair. The wedding took months of preparation and would cost more than Gorgas's monthly salary. They sent out dozens of invitations to friends and colleagues at home and abroad. Aileen's cousins came down for bridal showers and all the "other events that seem to fall to a young woman about to marry," Gorgas observed, adding in a letter to Jessie, "I am rather a fifth horse in such arrangements."[29]

The April wedding was a military affair. Gorgas took Aileen down the aisle, resplendent in his uniform, and an army chaplain married the couple. St. Luke's Church was decorated with palm leaves, flowers, and "electric lights" for the evening rites, and the wedding reception was at the Gorgas home filled with flowers and music by the Tenth Infantry band. Aileen cut the cake with her father's sword, and then she and Wrightson took the train to Colón to travel the next day to Houston, their new home.[30] Gorgas recorded in his journal simply, "Wedding took place & everything passed off well."[31] Once they were gone, he admitted to Mamie that he and Marie were a bit lonely in the big house, but he could now go to bed when he wanted to.[32]

In yet another transition, Gorgas was pleased when Woodrow Wilson, a Democrat and southerner, was elected president, and he told Dick that it brought a "delightful" change in Goethals's attitude. "Goethals is as mild as a lamb. He does not feel quite as certain of this good Democratic administration as he did of the former." Gorgas was delighted when Wilson's secretary of state, William Jennings Bryan, the progressive editor of *The Commoner*, appointed his friend and colleague Richard Lee Metcalfe as governor of the Canal Zone. "It does me good to see old Goethals bare his teeth [smile] and look sweet when Metcalf [*sic*] is around," wrote Gorgas. "I did not think that he had it in him."[33] But the new administration did not suppress Goethals's ego. As construction of the canal was shaping up to be a stunning success, competition began to identify the heroes of the victory. Goethals had set the tone in a 1912 interview with the *Chicago Daily Tribune*, in which he presented construction as a triumph of executive and labor management, discounting the engineering achievements and explicitly disparaging Gorgas's work. "I do not mean that the canal has taught the world anything as to malaria and yellow fever, as far as the mosquitoes are concerned," he stated. "These discoveries were made by others, in other parts of the world."[34]

On May 20, 1913, two steam shovels met at the bottom of the great Culebra Cut, signaling the beginning of the end of the excavation. But David Gaillard, the engineer in charge of blasting through the mountain ridge, was seriously ill. He had been working nonstop for years, battling accidents and landslides, and measuring success in the tons of spoil. But now he was failing, and many people believed it was from overwork. Marie had grown close to his wife, Katherine, and in June she and William went to Colón with the Gaillards to see them off to the United States to get medical advice and treatment. Just months later, on September 26, 1913, The Gorgases went to Gatun to see the first (official) boat go through the locks.[35]

While engineers could point to giant locks and dams to show their success, Gorgas, like all public health officials, had to point to the *absence* of disease and injury as his signature achievements. He therefore used statistics to tell the story. Measuring his effort against the French disaster of 240 deaths per 1,000 in the 1880s, Gorgas reported that he had reduced the death rate by more than three-fourths (41 per 1,000 in 1906, to 8 in 1913), to a rate less than half that in the United States.[36] He estimated that he prevented the loss of seventy thousand lives, preserved the health of three times as many people, and saved $80 million, half of it in hospital costs.[37] He also proudly pointed out that by 1913 the Ancón Hospital boasted such an excellent reputation that Congress appropriated funds for a new facility. When it was completed in 1919, it would be the largest hospital in the Western Hemisphere south of the US border.[38] The medical profession celebrated

Gorgas's work. In 1913 the *American Journal of Public Health* paid a florid tribute to Gorgas's "wonderful patience and tact, and his good judgement and knowledge of men, [which] served him and his country in good stead." With a jab at Goethals, the journal noted that Gorgas's success "made it possible for every one, even for the chief engineer and down to the humblest laborer in the trenches, to live in health and safety on the Isthmus."[39]

With Aileen educated and married and the canal project coming to an end, William and Marie took another big step. They had moved around so much with the army that they had never owned a home, but now, looking to return to the United States and eventual retirement, they purchased two residential lots in Chevy Chase, one for themselves and one for Aileen and her family.[40] Rather than return to New York or Tuscaloosa, they chose for home the nation's capital, with its mild climate, quasi-southern culture, and access to national and international policy makers. But before they moved to Washington, Gorgas would have another adventure.

## SOUTH AFRICA

In 1912 the Transvaal Chamber of Mines and the Rand gold mines of South Africa sent a representative to Panama to inspect Gorgas's sanitation and medical operations, especially his methods of pneumonia prevention. Pneumonia deaths were so high among the Black gold miners that seeing the success in Panama, Rand Mines invited Gorgas to come advise them, offering to pay him $3,000 per month, expenses, and funds for an assistant. Gorgas was delighted by the invitation and told them, "Seeing South Africa was a dream I had never hoped to realize."[41] He recruited Robert Noble and Samuel Darling to join him, but Marie said she would accompany him only as far as London. "I'm afraid that she must be growing old," he told Dick. "I never knew her to refuse anything like the trip before."[42] He was also surprised when Goethals agreed to the four-month trip, telling Mamie, "He evidently had some reasons for wanting me out of the way."[43]

William and Marie departed October 15, 1913, for Washington, where Gorgas met with President Wilson, dined with former President Taft, lunched with Secretary of State William Jennings Bryan and his wife, and also met with Secretary of War Lindley Garrison to discuss the future of the canal commission.[44] The Gorgases also went to Baltimore to see David and Katherine Gaillard and learned that the engineer was suffering from a brain tumor, not fatigue, and was in serious decline. He would die within a month, at age fifty-four. Katherine would always blame Goethals's micromanagement and constant pressure for Gaillard's demise, and she and Marie would maintain a lifelong friendship.[45]

Sailing for London on November 1, on the Hamburg-American liner *Imperator*,

William told Dick that the room was as nice as one in the Willard Hotel, "with a mild earth quake thrown in every now and then." The seas were rough, but he was still able to swim in the ship's seawater swimming pool.[46] Arriving in London on November 7, as first-time visitors, they happily toured the city, visiting St. Paul's Cathedral, dining with "Sir Ronald Ross" and "Sir William Osler," and visiting the neighborhoods where Thackeray's Henry Esmond and Dickens's David Copperfield had lived.[47] Gorgas also gave an interview for the newspaper *South Africa* at his Hyde Park hotel and charmed the writer. "Colonel Gorgas is the very best type of American," the writer purred. "He is a soldierly man, with snow white hair and penetrating dark eyes." Despite his successful career, "he is of an extremely unassuming nature, courteous to a degree, and a charming conversationalist." Gorgas told the reporter that he was successful in Panama because he swore by sanitation as "the principal preventative of disease," but that he was going to South Africa "with a perfectly open mind." The writer was so impressed that he erroneously said Gorgas was an "excellent sailor."[48]

William and Marie parted when he sailed on the RMS *Briton* from Southampton on November 15, and he missed her from the very first day. The ship was fine, and they ate at the captain's table, but he wrote, "I miss you every hour. In the future you must go on all trips with me. Half the pleasure is gone if you are not with me." In another he said that he was happiest when he was near her: "So the remaining years we have in this life, let us keep together as much [as] possible."[49] The Gorgas party tracked the *Briton*'s course down the coast of Africa, helped arrange amusements for passengers during the voyage, and did background reading for their South Africa assignment. After seventeen days at sea, they arrived at Cape Town and then traveled by train 950 miles across the veldt to Johannesburg, where a large delegation met their train and welcomed the Americans with dinners, addresses, consultations, and theater tickets. They met with Gen. Louis Botha, the Boer president of the Union of South Africa, and other dignitaries and went to the Johannesburg horse races. (Gorgas did not bet.) Gorgas relished spending Christmas Day in Johannesburg, telling Dick, "Just think of spending Xmas at the heart of Africa. At the very spot which was the scene of Rider Haggard stories."[50] When asked if he wished to speak at one dinner of two hundred, he replied that he would if required but "would greatly appreciate not being called upon." He did not have to make a speech and therefore "had a real good time," he told Marie.[51]

Turning to their mission, the men went out to the Rand mining district of sixty square miles where 200,000 Black laborers drilled by hand for gold and tungsten (used to make steel). The conditions were horrible. Gorgas made no such judgment in writing but went about his task of making public health recommendations. In three weeks his team inspected the housing and working conditions and medical facilities (including more than fifty hospitals), witnessed autopsies, and at one point went two thousand feet down into the mines. They learned that the four most serious diseases for the miners were pneumonia, meningitis, typhoid, and tuberculosis. Pneumonia was the worst, with death rates averaging fifteen to twenty per thousand among the Black workers, rates comparable to those in Panama during the early years. The highest susceptibility was among new workers; more than half of the deaths occurred among men who had spent less than six months in the mine. Despite what he had learned in Panama, Gorgas attributed this difference to race rather than environmental factors. "Some races, like the white, resist [pneumonia] infection strongly," he wrote. "Others, like the negro, have less resistance."[52]

Gorgas's recommendations, which he published in *JAMA* and *Military Surgeon*, were similar to those he had implemented in Panama, such as allotting fifty square feet of living space per man instead of the fourteen square feet they found in the Rand, and "scattering" workers by allowing them to live in individual cabins instead of barracks.[53] The men's wives should also come live with them, he suggested, so they could cook more healthful meals and keep them on the straight and narrow. "A native labor force living with families near the mines," he wrote, was preferable to "keeping a large body of semisavage laborers in the community in such conditions as obviously to foster sexual crimes." Other recommendations included examinations to screen out men with tuberculosis, typhoid vaccination for new arrivals, providing water fountains instead of common drinking cups, a sewage system rather than night-soil buckets for waste, and water-spraying in the mines to dampen silicosis-causing dust. The mines should prohibit the sale of alcohol, as they had in the Canal Zone, because "alcohol for the native, I believe, is an unmitigated evil." Gorgas also recommended better equipping and staffing the hospitals, establishing a central sanitation department in the Chamber of Mines, and experimenting with vaccines against pneumonia among groups of workers to evaluate their viability. (Effective pneumonia vaccines were not developed until the 1980s.) He concluded by pointing out "the many advantages a closed compound has in the management of these semicivilized natives."[54]

Events then took a fateful turn. The governor of Rhodesia invited Gorgas to come advise his government on malaria and Blackwater fever, and he accepted, telling Marie, "I am much puffed up at the invitation."[55] Goethals approved an additional month's leave, but on returning from a dinner party on December 29, Gorgas found a telegram advising that Surgeon General Torney had died two days earlier. Cables the next day from Secretary of State Bryan and Henry Carter confirmed the news.[56] This immediately presented the question of who would succeed Torney.

The *Military Surgeon* speculated that the main candidates were Gorgas, Jefferson Kean, and Col. Merwin Maus, the senior officer of the Medical Corps.[57] Gorgas was the best known of three men, and earlier that year Medical Corps colleagues had urged him to let his interest in succeeding Torney be known. Now he was ready. He confided in a friend, "I also talked over the matter with many of my Congressional friends and let them know that I was a candidate."[58] Although support for Gorgas as the next surgeon general had been in the works throughout 1913, Kean had been spreading reports that Gorgas would not accept the appointment if it were offered. Marie and John Ross therefore cabled asking if he still wanted the surgeon generalcy.[59] Gorgas quickly confirmed that he did and then turned back to his African adventure and fighting disease.

After another two-day train ride eight hundred miles north, Gorgas's party arrived in Salisbury, Rhodesia (today, Harare, Zimbabwe). Gorgas liked to tell the story that he when he arrived for his first meeting with Rhodesian officials, his host, Sir William Milton, greeted him as "General Gorgas." Gorgas explained that he was a colonel, but Milton corrected him with the news that President Wilson had just named him surgeon general. "First news of my nomination, Salisbury, Rhodesia, South Africa," he wrote in his journal.[60] The news wires further reported that Wilson had also promoted Gorgas from colonel to brigadier general in recognition of his work in ridding the Isthmus of Panama of deadly diseases and opening it up as a "white man's country."[61]

Whether Rhodesia could also become a "white man's country" was the question the British had for Gorgas. Finding gold in the 1890s, the British had established the Shamva and Arcturus gold mines, operations that were making some white elites very rich at the expense of the lives and health of thousands of Black laborers. The day before Gorgas arrived in Rhodesia, in fact, a dynamite explosion killed twenty-nine workers.[62] Whereas pneumonia was the prevailing problem in South Africa, in Rhodesia, malaria and a deadly disease called "Blackwater Fever" were sickening thousands. Some people thought Blackwater Fever was caused by a different germ than the malaria parasite, but it is actually a pernicious form of malaria in which the *Plasmodia* cause red blood cells to burst, resulting in internal bleeding and kidney failure. Gorgas was familiar with Blackwater Fever and could therefore tell his hosts how to prevent it. The solution was mosquito mitigation, and Gorgas never tired of explaining mosquitoes, disease transmission, and control measures such as grass cutting. His party traveled by train deep into the country, inspecting conditions, meeting with farmers and giving them "sanitary talks." Gorgas spoke in town halls and in village commons, using lantern slides to show the public health work in Panama. "It was like a political campaign," he told Marie.

Upon returning to Salisbury, Gorgas explicitly recommended racial segregation to Rhodesian authorities to prevent the spread of malaria. As in Panama, a large percentage of the local people were extensively infected with malaria, and long exposure had given them some immunity to the disease. "It is important therefore to keep native habitations at a distance from the living quarters of the whites so that the mosquitoes about the whites' quarters may not become infected." Gorgas made four other recommendations as well. The government should mosquito-proof workers' homes; clear and drain within two hundred yards around any dwellings; use mosquito netting over sleeping areas; and require people to take prophylactic quinine, selling it at cost. Salisbury, Gorgas said, should also make itself a mosquito-free example as part of an educational campaign for farmers "to impress upon them that the mosquito conveys malaria." Once the locals were convinced that mosquitoes were as dangerous as cobras, "there would soon be as few mosquito bites as there are cobra bites."[63]

Throughout their African tour, Gorgas, Darling, and Noble were generally well received and wined and dined on champagne, giraffe sausage, and rhinoceros steaks; they appreciated the menus until one village served stewed monkey.[64] They were entertained with Zulu dances, visited the tomb of Cecil Rhodes at Matobo Hill, and saw a troop of baboons at the ruins of Khami.[65] But in another sense, Africa was familiar territory: a racially segregated colonial society in the tropics where Black workers suffered from industrial accidents, pneumonia, and malaria. While Gorgas's team did not formally recommend increasing wages or changing the working conditions, they did advise that improved living standards and hospital facilities would reduce disease rates. The mine owners ultimately resisted implementing even these measures.[66]

## THE ROYAL SOCIETY AND THE ROYAL COLLEGE

As the party sailed from Cape Town for London on February 28, 1914, Gorgas reflected that he was glad to return to the "dear old U.S." but also admitted, "I have had a royal six months in Africa."[67] The "royal treatment," however, was not yet over. The British were eager to honor the Americans because Gorgas had shown how disease mitigation could solve the problem of the "White Man's Grave" and enable the British to strengthen their hold on their empire.[68] British scientists and physicians therefore asked him to address the Royal Society of Medicine on his way home. His little group returned to London, sunburnt from the veldt, and were again handsomely wined and dined.[69] In his speech to the Royal Society on March 23, Gorgas began by acknowledging that the Americans had been able to succeed in Panama where the French had failed, due to scientific discoveries by British scientist Ronald Ross's work in malaria and the American Reed Commission's work on yellow fever. He then gave his standard speech on yellow fever and malaria work but took special care to encourage doctors and sanitary inspectors to use courtesy and kindness rather than orders and authority to persuade local communities. "It is very surprising to an Anglo-Saxon, accustomed to arbitrary police-court methods, to see how much can be accomplished with a Latin-American population by courtesy and kindness."[70]

A dinner in Gorgas's honor at the Savoy Hotel then followed, hosted by the Royal College of Physicians and featuring a nine-course meal.[71] He was seated between the archbishop of Canterbury and the lord chancellor, and enjoyed a program of English and American music, including both national anthems, and "Swanee River" and "Piccaninny's Lullaby" for the southern surgeon general. The 125 male attendees toasted the king, the queen, the president of the United States, and William Gorgas, and this time he did give a speech, thanking the group for their hospitality and telling them that forty-five thousand of the sixty-five thousand laborers on the canal were the "most devoted British subjects and an excellent body of men." He added, to laughter and applause, "They were inclined, however, to claim the canal—lock, stock, and barrel."[72] According to Osler, the reception for Gorgas was "the greatest ever accorded a medical man in England." The whole world, "particularly the British Empire," he continued, owed him a debt "which the Britons are proud to acknowledge."[73] Gorgas and his colleagues then went to Oxford, where he was awarded an honorary degree and had lunch with Osler and his wife. Hurrying back to London, they sailed back to New York aboard the German liner *Kaiser Wilhelm*, just months before it would be refitted as an armed cruiser for the kaiser's navy.

As Gorgas headed for his new job in Washington as army surgeon general, in Panama his deputy John Phillips reported that Marie was packing for their new home and had been "very well and gay."[74] Tranquilina, their housekeeper, stayed with Marie to the end. In anticipation of their departure, the Gorgases put money in Panama and New York banks for her and helped her find a house lot in Panama. She also found a new job in a Panama laundry.[75] Gorgas also arranged positions for his Panama colleagues who wanted to join him in Washington. His horse, Traveler, could not be transported, however, and remained on the farm at Corozal with an injured leg. It was probably just as well, because the new surgeon general would have little time for riding.

# PART IV

# TO FIGHT WAR AND DISEASE, 1914–1918

CHAPTER 13

# Public Health and the Bully Pulpit of the Army Surgeon General

That poverty was the greatest single cause of bad sanitary conditions was very early impressed upon me. If I should again go to a community such as in Cuba or Panama, and were allowed to select only one sanitary measure, . . . I would select that of doubling wages.

—William Gorgas, "Economic Causes of Disease," September 1914

At the close of his first year as surgeon general, Gorgas paused to philosophize. On Christmas Eve, 1914, it was snowing in Washington, which was strange for him after fifteen years of tropical holiday weather. As he looked out the window, he reflected on the arc of his life. When it was complete, would the "omniscient Judge" say to him, "'True you have worked & striven but your motive was in great part worldly reward and the acclamation of your fellow man.'" He should rather have followed their mother's example, he told Jessie, working "more for love of man & less for reward." That course he would now pursue and as army surgeon general would try to help the nation. He did not know when he would die but, like his granddaughter, wondered when the train trip would end or even "what the trip is or why it is."[1] Finishing the letter, he then took Marie, Aileen, William, and his baby granddaughter to Walter Reed Hospital for Christmas Eve dinner.

## THE NEW OFFICE OF THE SURGEON GENERAL

When Gorgas was named surgeon general in January 1914, it was the crowning office of his career and a position of national and international importance. But his appointment generated resentment within the Medical Corps. It must have been especially galling for Jefferson Kean to see Gorgas sweep into Washington as surgeon general. When the army leadership consulted him on Torney's successor, he had spoken against Gorgas, citing the department requirement that medical officers (like Gorgas) who had been away from troops be reassigned to service with the rank and file. "General Gorgas and General Goethals had done their work at Panama outside of the sphere of activities of the Army," he later wrote, and "it was the business of Congress to reward them both."[2] Having spent years in the OTSG trenches promoting the Medical Department, Kean believed he deserved the job more than Gorgas did. Defeated, he waited for two months to send Gorgas a congratulatory letter but then graciously admitted, "I do not think that there has ever been any time since the early days when the sentiment both within and without the service has been so unanimous in favor of one man."[3] Southern physicians were especially pleased. Seale Harris, the editor of the *Southern Medical Journal*, celebrated Gorgas's elevation to surgeon general by calling for a national department of health with Gorgas as secretary, because "our Government owes it to Gorgas to create a position of greater honor than has ever been filled by a sanitarian."[4]

But Gorgas's purview was beyond region. As a boy, he had developed an empathy for others as he watched his parents struggle with the failure of the Confederacy and the diminishment of their lives and fortunes. This empathy softened his views on American imperialism, white supremacy, and patriarchy, and he turned to public policy to find ways to help those in his charge—soldiers and their families, workers and their families, even the American population. In this endeavor, the Office of the Army Surgeon General became for Gorgas what Theodore Roosevelt called a "bully pulpit."

Gorgas was a reformer at heart. As he surveyed the political scene in 1914, he admired William Jennings Bryan's sympathy for the "common people" and told John Ross that while they both might sympathize with this class, they belonged to one that was "essentially aristocratic." If he and Ross were younger, though, they might live to see "all special privileges abolished in all civilized communities and such a condition exist where every man born in this world, and women also, would have the chance that his natural abilities give him." Furthermore, working for a living, he believed, was more virtuous than inheriting, so "large wealth which is almost certain to be dissipated" should be heavily taxed.[5] These views were gaining currency. During Gorgas's Cuba and Panama years, the Progressive reform movement to tame the laissez-faire industrializing economy had been moving from local and state governments to the national level, and in 1913 the states had ratified the Sixteenth Amendment to the Constitution to impose an income tax on the people to fund the government. Woodrow Wilson had built a coalition of southern

Democrats and northern labor unions and social reformers that would continue the work of Roosevelt and other Progressives of extending modest government protection to industrial workers; curbing free market capitalism with moral and ethical constraints; expanding democratic self-rule for certain classes of people; and using government to bring the benefits of modern science and medicine to more Americans—all the while maintaining the architecture of white supremacy. Gorgas was comfortable with these goals and, in fact, had been helping to implement Progressive reform measures in Panama.[6]

But he would also again be singled out for special treatment. On April 1, 1914, in accordance with the Panama Canal Act of 1912, Wilson had abolished the Panama Railroad Company and the ICC, and created a new agency known simply as the Panama Canal under the direction of the Secretary of War, with George Goethals as its first governor. Congress rewarded Goethals and Gorgas for their work in Panama with promotions from brigadier to major general as part of legislation that advanced one grade in rank all officers and retired officers of the army, navy, and PHS who had served more than three years in Panama.[7] Goethals demurred to his promotion, saying that he was well paid as an army officer and should not be rewarded for doing his duty.[8] Gorgas, however, was happy for the added salary and prestige.[9] The AMA added to the honors by awarding its Gold Medal in 1914 to Gorgas, "whose genius made possible the construction of the Isthmian Canal."[10]

Thus celebrated, Gorgas spent his first months as surgeon general putting together his staff and taking care of his colleagues in Panama. Gorgas offered his deputy in Panama, John Phillips, the prestigious post of the commander of Walter Reed Hospital and brought in C. L. Furbush to run his office.[11] The new OTSG then began an assessment of Medical Department programs and policies, and how they might continue reforms begun by Gorgas's predecessors to professionalize their work. In particular they sought increased support for fields such as pharmacy, dentistry, nursing, anesthesiology, and X-ray medicine. Gorgas and his colleagues also considered how to meet the increasing threat of war in Europe by creating mobile sanitary and hospital units and increasing the Medical Reserve.[12]

But just weeks after he took office, trouble emerged on the southern border. Mexico was roiled in civil war, and in April 1914, President Wilson sought to block the Germans from delivering weapons to partisans in the conflict. Opposing such European interference in Western Hemisphere affairs, the US Marines landed at Vera Cruz and engaged the Mexicans seeking the German aid and, after a short battle, occupied the port. Leery of such incursions, Gorgas was glad when William Jennings Bryan's more temperate approach of diplomacy won out over the "warlike influence" of more aggressive advisers who called for an invasion of Mexico.[13]

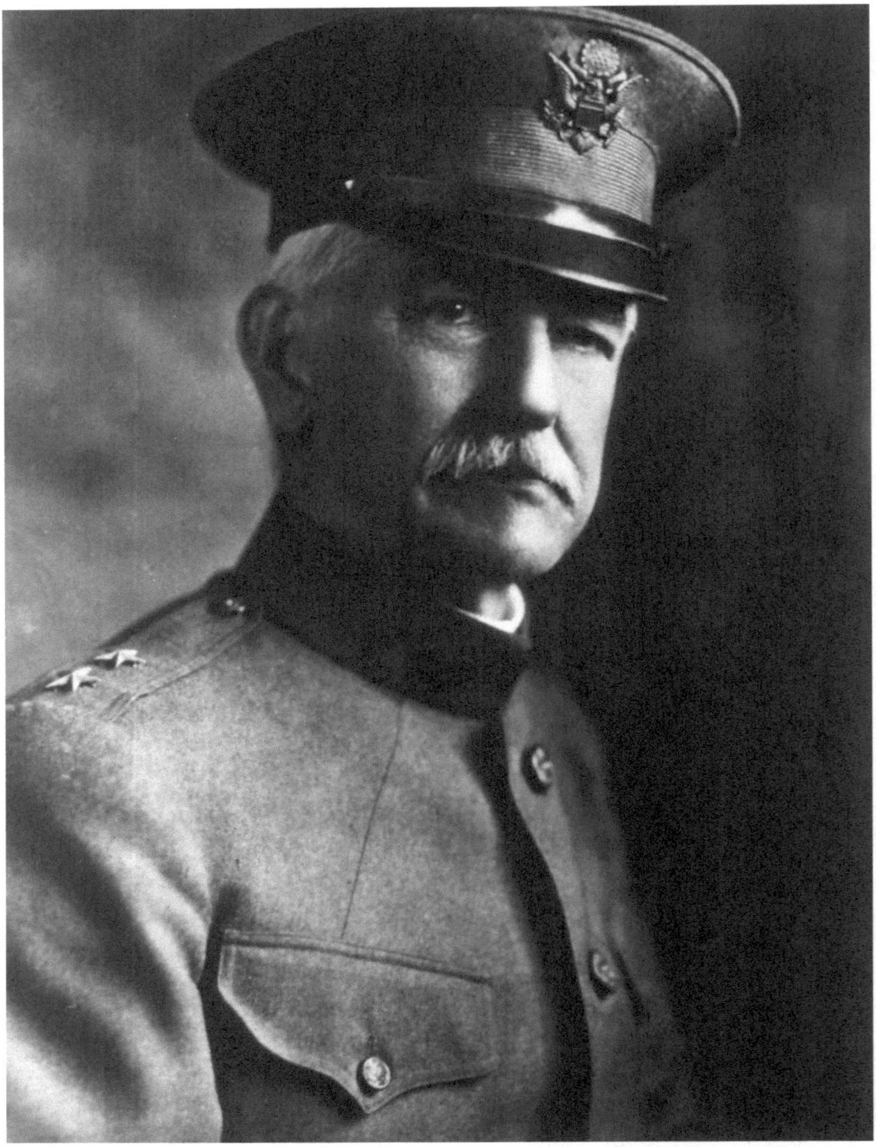

FIGURE 13.1. Major General William C. Gorgas, Surgeon General of the Army. National Library of Medicine.

Given Vera Cruz's reputation as a source of disease (and perhaps remembering it was where Josiah got yellow fever), Gorgas sent Theodore Lyster and son-in-law William Wrightson to report to him on health conditions and how to protect the occupying troops.[14] Within weeks army medical personnel sanitized the city, identified clean water sources, built a hospital, and vaccinated forty-one thousand Mexican civilians against smallpox.[15]

Months later, when war broke out in Europe in August 1914, Gorgas told a friend, "All the attention of the Department now is focused on the European War." He presaged that it would be "one of the great calamities of the century and will cause untold suffering. I have no doubt that we ourselves will feel it over here before it is through with."[16] Although Gorgas and the United States would be able to stay out of the fighting for more than two years, the Great War would color Gorgas's entire tenure as surgeon general and change the fate of the United States in the world.

## GORGAS THE SINGLE TAXER

The popular press was drawn to the new surgeon general as a medical hero who cleared the tropics of disease to make them safe for "white men" and "civilization." *Munsey's Magazine*, for example, touted him as "the international bearer of the white man's burden."[17] Gorgas used this attention and his new office not only to promote mosquito mitigation and disease fighting but to expound on his long-held view that Henry George's plan for the single tax was the single best way to reduce sickness and disease.

The single tax was a simplistic and idealistic notion, but it gained great support during Gorgas's lifetime. Henry George was a California journalist who published a broad critique of the US economy, *Progress and Poverty*, in 1879, just as Gorgas was coming into his own.[18] Disturbed by the persistence of poverty at a time of industrial and scientific advancement, George penned a ponderous book of political philosophy that became wildly popular—one of the best-selling books in the nineteenth century—and inspired a generation of reformers in the Progressive movement seeking to destroy monopoly and restore economic opportunity.[19] Instead of taxing people's labor, he called for a single tax on nonproducing land to finance the government and encourage landowners to put unused land into use. The resulting reduced rents and increased wages would enable tenants and workers to prosper. "The man who now uses coarse food, and lives in a small house, will, as a rule, if his income be increased, use more costly food, and move to a larger house," wrote George. "If he grows richer and richer he will procure horses, servants, gardens and lawns, his demand for the use of land constantly increasing with his wealth."[20] Opening up the land to the laboring classes would thus grow the economy and benefit the entire nation. It was a flawed analysis but captured the minds of many who sought a more equitable society.

Henry George's idealization of nature, his view of the family as the ideal social unit, and his calls for improved housing appealed to Gorgas even as a young man, and he discussed "Georgism" and the single tax at dances with Marie at Fort Brown and around the campfire at Fort Randall in the 1880s.[21] Gorgas belonged to the Henry George Lecture Association for years and in 1914 agreed to sit on the advisory board of the New York Single Tax League.[22] He subscribed to the *Single Tax Review*, at one point paying for four subscriptions for YMCA libraries.[23] More a panacea than a practical solution to growing inequality, the single tax concept attracted adherents in the United States and abroad, from Helen Keller and Samuel Gompers, president of the AFL, to Leo Tolstoy and the Cuban revolutionary José Marti.[24] Labor groups also welcomed this critique of the Gilded Age, and single taxers formed political parties and promoted single tax measures in at least twenty states.[25] When Democrat Woodrow Wilson became president in 1913, he appointed several single taxers to his cabinet, including Franklin Lane as secretary of the interior; Newton Baker, secretary of war; and his army surgeon general.[26] A man of the South and his nation, William Gorgas could both honor the memories of Robert E. Lee and Jefferson Davis and follow the principles of Henry George and the single tax plan for the radical redistribution of wealth.

Gorgas's socioeconomic views appeared in dozens of his speeches and articles as surgeon general. His basic message was that poverty was the single greatest cause of poor sanitation and health, and that if he could choose just one measure to improve sanitation, it would be to double workers' wages so they could afford better housing, food, and clothing. He told groups like the Business Men's Club in Cincinnati, Ohio, the Women's Single Tax Club of Maryland, and the Geographic Society of Chicago that a good standard of living was the most important path to good health. "Man in general is not dirty and unsanitary . . . [and] if you give him the means he will improve his sanitary conditions of his own accord." People cannot prosper "unless we can so change our economic laws, that this wealth will be more fairly distributed than it is now." By fair distribution he meant that "each man gets exactly what he produces—no more, no less."[27] Speaking as a true Progressive, he looked forward to a time when "poverty will be abolished from this world."[28]

The apotheosis of Gorgas's socioeconomic views appeared in a 1916 speech entitled "Sanitation and Morality," in which he posited the moral imperative of good sanitation. A model of Progressive reform, the speech suggested that sanitarians could teach morals (i.e., clean living) and hygiene all they wanted to, but if people could not afford clean water and dry, mosquito-proof homes, it would not do any good. Government officials and business leaders must "place our fellow men in such position that they can adopt our teachings." As an example, Gorgas described "a negro laborer with a wife and one or two children, living, sleeping, washing, and cooking in a room 12 by 12." Even good Christians such as his audience could not live well in these surroundings, he suggested. "What could you or I do for ourselves and our dependents in the direction of either sanitation or morals if we lived with such surroundings, getting a sufficient wage for only a bare living, knowing that when either sickness or stoppage of work occurred even that miserable wage would stop?" Therefore, he asked, "What can be expected of him in the way of personal hygiene!"[29]

Gorgas, whose family had enslaved people, compared "industrial slavery" to chattel slavery, which enabled "the robber, or the master, or the employer, whatever you choose to call him, to take all the wealth he can without any reference to the necessity of the employee." One day, he concluded, people will look upon the current industrial slavery as unjust as chattel slavery, and therefore Christians should encourage others to "adopt the teachings and morals of Christianity." The speech was well received. A single-tax organization published it in pamphlet form, and an Episcopalian journal headlined the speech, "Surgeon-General Gorgas Appeals to Christians to Help Increase Wages."[30]

## *SANITATION IN PANAMA*—GUARDING THE LEGACY

The Panama Canal was exhibit A for Gorgas's vision of making the tropics safe and productive for white people, and the stunningly successful completion of the project caused others to claim it as their legacy. No one was more energetic than George Goethals and his deputy, Joseph Bucklin Bishop, a former New York newspaper editor, political gadfly, and executive secretary to the ICC.[31] Bishop was in charge of the local weekly, the *Canal Record*, which reported on the progress of the canal work, informed members of Congress about the project, and, significantly, promoted an image of Goethals as the master of the canal.[32] In 1913 Bishop set out to cement Goethals's fame in three articles for *Scribner's Magazine*. The first, "A Benevolent Despot," profiled Goethals as the driving force behind canal construction, eclipsing the work of earlier engineers.[33] The second, entitled "Sanitation of the Isthmus," credited the engineering department for much of the sanitation work and minimized Gorgas's achievements, stating that he "had only to adopt on the Isthmus the plans of the successful campaign in Cuba to win a second and more brilliant triumph." Bishop dwelled on Gorgas's initial skepticism of the mosquito theory (still!), skipped over the early ICC opposition to his work, and with regard to malaria wrote, "the possibility of banishing that disease was too remote to be entertained."[34] These articles became part of Bishop's book *The Panama Gateway* (1913), which celebrated Goethals and, given Bishop's official position, became an authoritative interpretation.[35] Goethals's likeness began to personify the canal and to grace other books on the canal, such as Ralph Emmett Avery's 1913 volume *America's Triumph at Panama.*[36] When in 1915 Bishop produced another series of *Scribner's* articles lionizing Goethals, M. H. Thatcher, a former ICC commissioner, angrily told Gorgas, "We, who were outlawed and persecuted on the Zone, owe it, in my judgment, to ourselves and to the future to correct the falsehoods." Gorgas, he advised, should therefore "give the world an accurate account of your work on the Isthmus."[37]

Gorgas took the bit in his teeth and, in a commencement address at Washington University Medical School, St. Louis, in late April 1915, blamed Goethals for the failure of the Canal Zone government to eliminate malaria fever.[38] The surgeon general told the graduates that he had expected to "get rid of malaria" in Panama and in the first four years had cut the rate by two-thirds. But when the new commission was appointed in 1907, power was "concentrated in the hands of a single man," and "this officer," said Gorgas without naming Goethals, transferred malaria mitigation duties from the Sanitation Department to "men who had no special knowledge of anti-malarial work" and thereby retarded their program to eradicate malaria.[39] This was the most public criticism he ever leveled against George Goethals.

Gorgas's most effective and enduring effort to frame his legacy was *Sanitation in Panama*, the only book he ever wrote. He had already been working with publisher William W. Appleton, who in 1910 had approached him about writing a textbook on hygiene and sanitation. Gorgas asked Kean to collaborate with him on it, but neither of them had the time to complete the project, so it languished.[40] Now Appleton wanted to do a series on Panama, with Goethals on engineering, Richard Johnson on commerce, and Gorgas on sanitation. When Appleton dropped Goethals because Bishop would be doing the writing, Gorgas encouraged Sibert to take up the engineering story. "I think this is your opportunity for doing justice to yourself, Gaillard, Wallace, and Stevens," he advised, so Sibert and John Stevens, the second chief engineer, wrote the engineering volume for Appleton.[41]

Gorgas took the division of labor literally and wrote nothing of the engineering triumphs in his book. While he did acknowledge chief engineer John Stevens as supportive of sanitation work, he does not mention Goethals at all. Marie helped William with his volume, and during the summer and fall of 1914 they often worked until late at night.[42] The book was one part travelogue, one part history lesson, and two parts instruction in tropical sanitation and medicine. Gorgas gave Walter Reed and his commission great credit for the yellow fever work in Havana—fully 30 percent of the book is on Cuba—and reproduced much of William's correspondence with Reed during those fateful months in 1900 and 1901. Gorgas singled out Walter Reed, John F. Stevens, and Theodore Roosevelt as the people most responsible for his success and detailed the challenges he faced during his years in Panama, working under engineers and bureaucrats who neither understood nor appreciated his work. He obliquely referred to Goethals, stating, "It seems all through as though the laws were framed with the idea of making sanitation appear to have as much cost as possible, and the construction of the Canal as little as possible."[43] Gorgas carefully checked his facts and, for example, confirmed with Theodore Roosevelt the story of his conversation with Alexander Lambert regarding Gorgas's removal from office in 1905, and checked with Le Prince on the details of his mosquito-staining experiments that demonstrated how far *Anopheles* would normally fly.[44]

At the end of the book, Gorgas made grandiose claims about the war between man and disease. In man's early stages, he reasoned, people could survive only in tropical latitudes until the "two great sanitary discoveries, the most important ever made by man, namely, fire and clothing."[45] These protections enabled humans to move to the healthier temperate regions of earth and leave deadly diseases behind. That process could now be reversed. "The white man," wrote Gorgas, "of all the races of the human family, is the most eager in his pursuit of wealth." He can now return to warmer regions and make them so productive that "the great civilizations of the future will be located in the tropics." Whereas the discovery of the Americas was a great step in the history because it opened so much land to white settlement, so too, the demonstration in Panama that white people can live in the tropics "will be an equally important milestone in the history of the race."[46]

*Sanitation in Panama* found an appreciative audience. One reviewer noted that Gorgas showed how yellow fever eradication "was a fight not only against the carriers of the disease but also against the opponents of the mosquito theory."[47] Another said the book was "delightful and instructive from beginning to end, and will, no doubt, be as widely read by the general public as by members of the medical profession."[48] *JAMA* reported that amusing anecdotes and pathetic incidents made the book "read almost like a novel."[49] Gorgas sent dozens of copies to Latin American political and public health officials as a kind of sanitation instruction manual, and rather disingenuously told one admiring correspondent, "I have been rather hoping that nobody has read it. To me it does not seem a very creditable production."[50] *Sanitation*, however, continues in print, republished most recently in 2009, and is still an important source on the construction of the Panama Canal.

## MEDICAL PREPAREDNESS

As the war in Europe broadened to a worldwide conflict, many Americans continued to believe it had nothing to do with them, and President Wilson was also determined not to take sides between the Central Powers of Germany and Austria-Hungary, and the Allied Powers of Britain, France, and Russia. Gorgas and other military leaders, however, were thinking of how to prepare the country in case war came. Privately, by late 1914, Gorgas had already taken sides. "If I were a young man & my country did not go in I would shoulder a gun & join the Allies," he told Mamie. While as a scientist, he admired Germans such as Robert Koch, who had articulated germ theory, Wilhelm Röntgen, who discovered X-rays, and Paul Ehrlich, who developed a cure for syphilis, and he admired the Germans' "courage and pluck," he did not admire their kaiser. "This war will decide whether our present civilization will proceed along lines of absolutism or Democracy," he told Mamie. Everyone must therefore choose sides.[51]

Others agreed. Americans in Paris established an ambulance service, the Ambulance Americaine, financed by private funds. At the same time American surgeons, Dr. George Crile, of Lakeside Hospital (now Western Reserve Medical School) in Cleveland, a pioneer in blood transfusion and surgical techniques, and Dr. Harvey Cushing, a leading neurological and brain surgeon at Harvard, took surgical teams to France. In early 1915 Crile returned home to encourage others to join the effort and called for American hospitals to organize mobile hospital units to send to Europe in support of the Allies. Intrigued, Gorgas saw the advantage of the hospital scheme whereby hospital staff would be working with personnel with whom they were familiar. He immediately wrote to Crile to ask what it would take to put together a base hospital to send to—hypothetically, with Wilson's neutrality posture in mind—Huntsville, Alabama. He added carefully, "You understand that this letter is written purely with the object of discussion." Crile answered two weeks later in a speech outlining steps to form mobile hospitals of seventy-eight-person teams of surgeons, specialists, and nurses out of established institutions.[52] Gorgas then approached other hospitals about forming similar units, with the result that by the time the United States declared war in April 1917, the Medical Department was the best-prepared unit in the army.[53]

In May 1915 the United States came close to war after German U-boots sank the RMS *Lusitania*, killing almost 1,200 people. Calls for American retaliation challenged Wilson's neutrality policy, but the crisis passed, the country avoided war, and American medical support for the Allies continued under the aegis of humanitarian aid. By the end of the year, the American Red Cross had established a department of military relief and was recruiting nurses and organizing mobile hospitals. Gorgas met with Red Cross leaders, hospital directors, and university presidents to determine who would organize the units, how they would be staffed, and if and how they would be militarized should the country enter the war.[54] To coordinate these disparate factions, Gorgas named Jefferson Kean as army liaison with the American Red Cross.[55] This gave him a visible, national position and harnessed his administrative skills yet kept the ambitious officer on the margins of the Medical Department. The medical leadership developed plans whereby the Red Cross would enroll female nurses, and the Army Reserve organize the male medical staff, so that if and when the nation went to war, medical personnel could move directly into the army.[56] By the time the United States declared war in April 1917, thirty-three base hospitals were in the works, and the Medical Department could send six of them to England immediately.[57] As medical officer Percy Ashburn later put it, "The first contribution to the war by the United States was paid in medical officers and hospital units."[58] Years later a ceremony honoring Gorgas would unfurl the first American flag flown in Europe during the war, none other than that flown over the Base Hospital No. 4 in May 1917.[59]

If Gorgas and his colleagues were an ocean away from the violence in 1915, disease was on the move, and when typhus broke out in Serbia, the army surgeon general was willing to give up his duties in Washington and go fight it. Typhus is a lice-borne bacterial disease that thrives in the crowded and dirty conditions of armies and prisons and has mortality rates as high as 50 percent. Today it is treated with antibiotics, but in Gorgas's time the only way to fight typhus was good personal hygiene, clean clothes, clean linens, and "picking cooties," that is, delousing. The English, Russians, and French urgently needed public health measures and leadership to get the epidemic under control but were preoccupied with the immediate concerns of battle. In late March 1915, therefore, the Rockefeller Foundation, created just a few years before with the mission to fight disease, got involved. Wickliffe Rose of the foundation proposed to Secretary of War Lindley Garrison a Rockefeller mission against typhus in Serbia. When Rose invited Gorgas to sit on its advisory board, Gorgas responded that he would rather fight disease on the front lines than give advice.[60] The foundation met in May 1915 and agreed to appoint Gorgas the director of their typhus mission to Serbia, at a salary of $6,000.[61]

The Serbia mission tempted Gorgas, and he consulted with a number of people, including the German ambassador to the United States and Secretary of State Bryan as to whether he should go.[62] Secretary of War Garrison said Gorgas could join the mission if he would resign as surgeon general, and President Wilson at first agreed, writing, "I feel that we have no right to be selfish or to stand in the way in this matter."[63] Gorgas had not yet decided whether to go to Serbia when an imbroglio popped up. The *New York Times* reported that he was going to resign as surgeon general to head up a typhus commission to Serbia at a salary of $50,000 and a generous pension for Marie in case he died overseas. The journal *Science* quickly issued a denial for Gorgas, stating that if he did accept the offer, it would not be at that salary and would be due to "his sympathy with the general aims of the foundation in regard to public health."[64] This was true, because Gorgas had privately told the foundation that he would take less than his salary for the opportunity to do the work.[65] Marie supported the mission and even offered to go with him.[66] Others counseled against it. Senator Duncan Fletcher of Florida wrote, "I can see no specific call of duty there and as far as the general, humanitarian appeal is concerned, that begins at home, and we cannot spare such men as yourself."[67] Only after Gorgas accepted the appointment, on April 26, did Wilson decide that he did not want his army officers, active or retired, to take any role that might jeopardize US neutrality.[68] Gorgas accepted Wilson's decision without question but told Jessie that he had wanted to do the work because "I feel the desire of the old soldier to die with my boots on."[69]

## LIFE IN THE NATION'S CAPITAL

Surgeon General Gorgas did not like sitting at his desk and traveled often, speaking on disease fighting or the single tax much more than on military medical preparedness. In June 1915 alone, Gorgas traveled to Chicago for Red Cross meetings; spoke to medical groups in Pennsylvania, New York, and Virginia; had dinner with former president Roosevelt in Oyster Bay, Massachusetts; and traveled to North Carolina with Carter and Le Prince to inspect army grounds for malaria. Later that year, at the request of Sen. Hollis Bankhead (D-AL), Gorgas went to Alabama to answer opponents of a new power plant construction who worried that it would create a mosquito habitat, and he returned twice to testify in court on the matter of the project's safety.[70] In November, Gorgas even made a quick trip with Henry Carter to Puerto Rico to investigate a suspected case of yellow fever. When Carter, immune to yellow fever, got sick, however, they realized that it was dengue fever, another mosquito-borne disease.[71]

William and Marie enjoyed living in Washington, DC, and as a major general, Gorgas's income of $14,000 was substantial ($386,000 in 2021 dollars).[72] But living in Washington, DC, was more expensive than in Panama, where the ICC had provided government housing and other perquisites. Gorgas's account book for 1910–1914 showed that his net worth increased in Panama from $11,035.19 in July 1910 to $19,493.31 in December 1914. He felt flush enough to spend $3,200 for an electric car, which Marie drove, and, in addition to the monthly payments

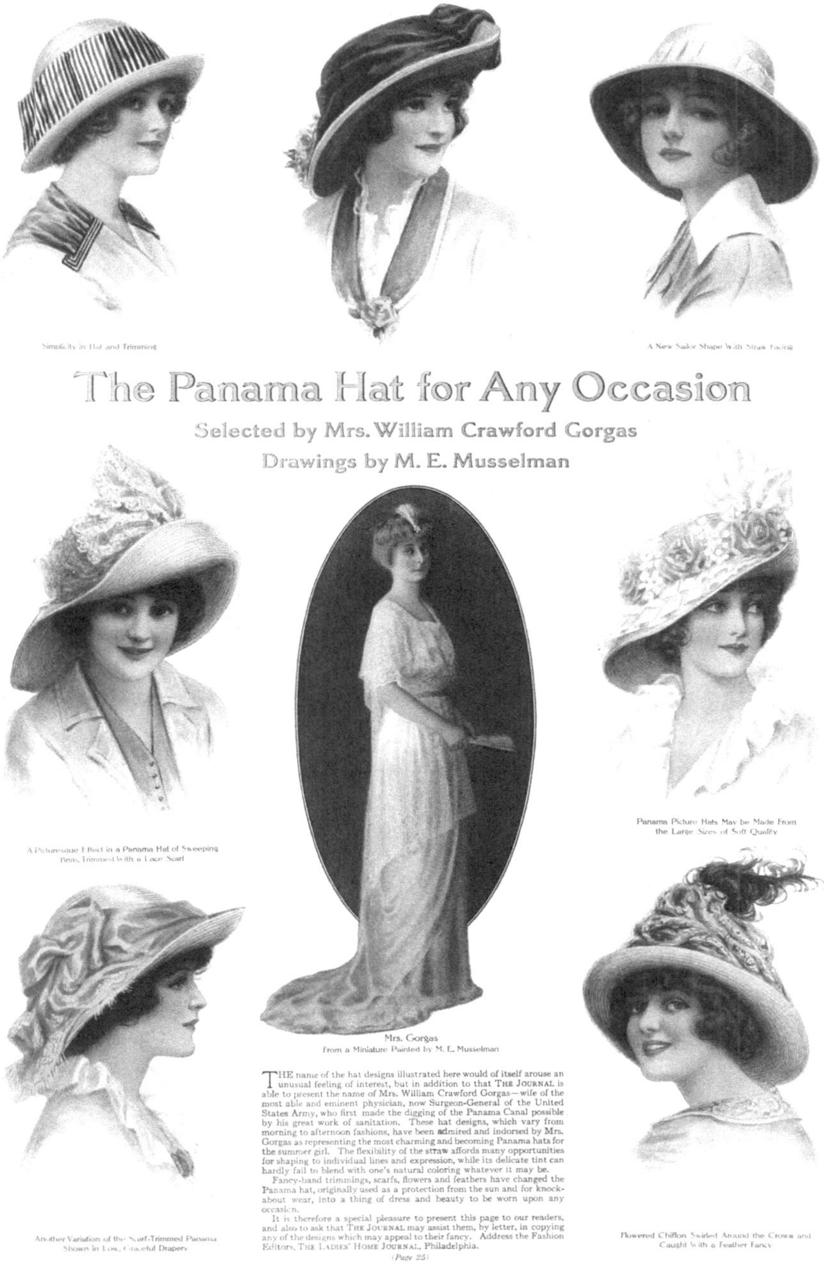

Simplicity in Hat and Trimming

A New Sailor Shape With Straw Facing

The Panama Hat for Any Occasion

Selected by Mrs. William Crawford Gorgas

Drawings by M. E. Musselman

A Picturesque Effect in a Panama Hat of Sweeping Brim, Trimmed With a Lace Scarf

Panama Picture Hats May be Made From the Large Sizes of Soft Quality

Mrs. Gorgas

From a Miniature Painted by M. E. Musselman

THE name of the hat designs illustrated here would of itself arouse an unusual feeling of interest, but in addition to that THE JOURNAL is able to present the name of Mrs. William Crawford Gorgas—wife of the most able and eminent physician, now Surgeon-General of the United States Army, who first made the digging of the Panama Canal possible by his great work of sanitation. These hat designs, which vary from morning to afternoon fashions, have been admired and indorsed by Mrs. Gorgas as representing the most charming and becoming Panama hats for the summer girl. The flexibility of the straw affords many opportunities for shaping to individual lines and expression, while its delicate tint can hardly fail to blend with one's natural coloring whatever it may be.

Fancy-band trimmings, scarfs, flowers and feathers have changed the Panama hat, originally used as a protection from the sun and for knock-about wear, into a thing of dress and beauty to be worn upon any occasion.

It is therefore a special pleasure to present this page to our readers, and also to ask that THE JOURNAL may assist them, by letter, in copying any of the designs which may appeal to their fancy. Address the Fashion Editors, THE LADIES' HOME JOURNAL, Philadelphia.

Another Variation of the Scarf-Trimmed Panama Shown in Low, Graceful Drapery

Flowered Chiffon Swirled Around the Crown and Caught With a Feather Fancy

(Page 25)

FIGURE 13.2. Marie Gorgas featured in *Ladies' Home Journal* article "The Panama Hat for Any Occasion." *Ladies' Home Journal*, June 1914.

to his sisters, began sending $50 a month to his granddaughter, "Little Marie." He could also now afford to have his father's journal printed.[73]

Regardless of their material comfort, the summer of 1915 was one of difficulty and loss. William's health was troublesome, and in May he entered Walter Reed so Theo could operate on his nose for some unspecified reason. In June, Gorgas's asthma was so bad that Marie called Theo at 3:00 one night, and he sent Gorgas back to Walter Reed for a complete physical, or what William called a "careful over-hauling."[74] And their friends were dying. In May, William Sibert's wife, Marie, died of meningitis, and John Phillips, whom Gorgas had assigned to run Walter Reed, fell down an elevator shaft and was so seriously injured that a few months later he shot himself on the hospital grounds.[75] After Carlos Finlay died, on August 20, 1915, Gorgas devoted his speech at the American Public Health Association annual meeting to his friend, telling the audience that no country "owes a greater debt of gratitude to Dr. Finlay than does the United States."[76] A happier event for the Gorgases was the birth that September of a second granddaughter, Pricilla.[77]

The ever-social Gorgases maintained a busy schedule, and Marie was gaining a public profile. Her portrait appeared in the newspaper society pages, and the *Ladies' Home Journal* published an advertisement for Panama hats "as selected by Mrs. William Crawford Gorgas."[78] A Nebraska paper featured her in its "In the Public Eye" column, in which she recounted the prominent part yellow fever had played in her life. "It even figured in my courtship!" she said.[79] Another reporter admired Marie's poise. "Her appearance is distinguished and self-possessed. Her method of speaking is direct, and her tone sustained and easy." Marie recounted how her husband's work in Cuba was "his first great opportunity to prove conclusively that an absence of these mosquitoes would mean an absence of yellow fever." Then, unfortunately, whether she was misquoted or was prone to hyperbole about William, she boasted, "It was my husband, you know, who discovered the fact that a species of mosquito carries the germ of infection."[80] Such exaggeration would rankle some in the Medical Corps.

# CHAPTER 14

# Duty to Country vs. Mission for Humanity

> We would like to call attention to the effect that the present war has had upon lessening Yellow Fever. . . . It has prevented the coming out [to the Western Hemisphere] of Europeans and has caused the return to Europe of the greater proportion of those already here. . . . It is therefore a favorable time to do anti–Yellow Fever work.
>
> —W. C. Gorgas, et al., "Report on Yellow Fever," 1916

THE YEAR 1916 WAS THE bloodiest of the Great War, leaving millions of dead and wounded: at least 700,000 casualties at the Battle of Verdun; 1.1 million at the First Battle of the Somme; and some 2 million casualties on the vast Eastern Front. As industrial warfare bled the world, Theodore Roosevelt, Leonard Wood, and some members of Congress wanted to put on their uniforms, raise a large national army, and join the fight. They called for "Preparedness" to ensure that the United States would be ready when the war came.[1] President Woodrow Wilson, however, disliked the military, was leery of war, and therefore walked a fine line between the hawks and doves. He had trouble in his cabinet. Secretary of State William Jennings Bryan had resigned in 1915 over concerns that Wilson's protest to the Germans for sinking the *Lusitania* would lead to war, while in February 1916, Secretary of War Lindley Garrison quit because Wilson would not pursue more aggressive policies against Germany. The president held closely to his neutrality stance and based his 1916 reelection campaign on the platform "He kept us out of war."

If many Americans were not sure which side, if any, to support in the war, Gorgas, who supported the Allies, was torn between two very different battles: preparing the Army Medical Department for war, and waging war against a different enemy: mosquitoes and yellow fever.

## PREPAREDNESS AND NATIONAL DEFENSE

The war in Europe nonetheless encroached on Gorgas's world. In early 1916 William Osler, seeking to further ties between American and British physicians, advised Gorgas that he would pay for two or three American medical officers to come to England and observe the British Medical Services.[2] Reasoning that a humanitarian exchange of medical staff with both the Allies and the Germans would not compromise American neutrality, Gorgas's OTSG agreed and sent six medico-military observers to Europe, including one to the Austro-Hungarian forces on the eastern front. Osler wanted Gorgas to come to England himself, but the surgeon general sent two other officers who reported regularly to him on their observations.

Trouble returned to the border with Mexico as well when Pancho Villa raided an American post in New Mexico. Wilson mobilized the National Guard and sent his best army officer, Gen. John Pershing on a "punitive expedition," March 1916 to February 1917, to retaliate against the Mexican paramilitary action. Gorgas's OTSG moved quickly, sending several ambulance units with the troops, and a sanitary train to Fort Sam Houston, Texas, to set up a temporary hospital for the sick and wounded. Many Medical Department leaders were veterans of the Spanish-American-Cuban War, including Gorgas, Kean, Robert Noble, Charles Furbush, and Merritte W. Ireland, all of whom had been in Cuba in 1898, and all were determined that the public humiliation of disease in the training camps should not happen again.[3]

The Medical Department was better prepared than in 1898 because of the reforms enacted to address lessons of the Spanish-American-Cuban War. The Congress had authorized the department to amass a year's supply of medicines and hospital equipment for an army four times its present strength. This included supply kits for two hundred physical exam stations for recruits, 373,000 individual first-aid kits for soldiers going into battle, and supplies for evacuation hospitals, field hospitals, and regimental infirmaries.[4] Bacteriology had become an ally, because a new typhoid vaccine enabled medical officers to avoid a repeat of the typhoid scandals of 1898. In 1907 the army began immunization trials with army volunteers against the disease and in 1909 made typhoid vaccination compulsory, reducing its typhoid rate from 243 per 100,000 in 1909 to 4.4 per 100,000 in just three years.[5] In 1917 Gorgas was able to tell Congress that American troops in the camps in Mexico were healthier than those in garrisons in the United States, with only one case of typhoid among the twenty thousand troops on the border.[6] While these improvements put the Medical Department in a better posture than other American military agencies, the department was still small, with only 443 medical officers in an army of 103,000. The modern armies of Europe had millions of men.

Gorgas grasped, at least intellectually, the fierceness of the fighting in Europe. Just weeks after the sinking of the *Lusitania*, he told a reporter that the new powers and reach of artillery weapons were generating more wounds and new surgical challenges due to the severity and number of wounds one man might sustain. The replacement of horse-powered ambulances with motorized ones was saving lives with speedier medical transport, and aseptic surgery was reducing deaths from infection, but heavy artillery and machine-gun fire drove soldiers into filthy trenches filled with polluted water, mud, and vermin. "Trench fighting," Gorgas said, "promotes disease." He also noted that medical personnel were being killed in unprecedented numbers because of the proximity of field hospitals to the battlefield. A field hospital located out of firing range would, after all, be of little help to the fighting forces, "so doctors and other attendants are under fire as they never were before."[7]

In this context, during the first months of 1916 Gorgas testified almost daily on Capitol Hill before various congressional committees with oversight on military affairs. He was a strong and direct advocate for his department and the Medical Corps. As he educated members of Congress on how to modernize the Medical Department and prepare it for war, his remarks provided a veritable course on military medicine. He recounted the history of military medical research, including Civil War advances in medical transport, Bailey Ashford's discovery of hookworm in Puerto Rico, the army's Tropical Disease Board's research on beriberi in the Philippines, and of course the Reed Commission's yellow fever work. In addition to caring for the wounded and sick, the Medical Department maintained sanitation around training camps and occupied territory, procured medical supplies and equipment, and screened recruits for "defectives or degenerates" who could become liabilities to the army. His department managed the Hospital Corps and Army Nurse Corps and was in charge of the transportation of sick and wounded from battlefield aid stations to field hospitals and then to specialized hospitals at home. "The duties of a military surgeon are vastly more complex than those of his civil brother," Gorgas told the Senate Committee on Military Affairs, "and no matter how capable the latter may be in civil practice he can not take the place of a trained medical officer." Medical officers needed to have specialized training in logistics regarding where to put hospitals and aid posts, how to avoid artillery and rifle fire, and how to maintain troop health "under canvas," that is, in the military camps. "Patriotic ardor," he said, was no substitute for "knowledge and skill." If and when the country went to war, the Army Medical Corps would be responsible for the health of "whatever great army we have to raise from the citizens of the country."[8]

Gorgas attended the hearings with voluminous background information, lists of recommendations, and draft legislative language to enact his proposals. He warned,

"The present war in Europe has taught the world nothing if not the lesson of preparedness," and cited the high sickness rate of the British army in Gallipoli. He recounted "the lamentable history of our own wars" whereby supply shortages and inexperienced personnel produced "calamitous results."[9] The most serious deficit, Gorgas believed, was the low number of medical personnel, and he was concerned that the proposed military preparedness legislation failed to increase the number of medical officers proportionate to the size of the army. His current cadre of 443 Medical Corps officers was only four or five per thousand enlisted men, when he needed seven per one thousand, the same ratio as in the Spanish-American-Cuban War. He also called for increasing the Hospital Corps to five men per one hundred soldiers in peacetime and twice that in wartime, and offering better pay to make the corps more attractive. To get the best doctors from the best hospitals, Gorgas wanted to increase their field pay and abolish the age limit. Some of the nation's "great operators" and "great physicians" were older, he testified, like his colleagues Victor Vaughan and William Keen. Both men were over sixty but they should be in the Medical Reserve. Congress resisted the additional cost. The Senate at first approved only 4.2 medical officers per 1,000 men, and some in Congress wanted to abolish the Medical Reserve altogether. But Gorgas continued his advocacy, describing at various medical meetings and conferences his proposal to recruit ten thousand physicians to the Medical Reserve.[10] *JAMA* supported his proposals, and members of Congress began to hear from their constituent physicians.

Despite his neutral posture, in the face of the preparedness debate and the increasing instability of the international situation, President Wilson became more willing to act and signed the National Defense Act of 1916 in June. The legislation doubled the military budget, increased regular army strength to 175,000, and the National Guard to more than 400,000, and created the Reserve Officer Training Corps. It also funded and enhanced army medical services under the aegis of humanitarian work that did not violate Wilson's neutrality policy. The act increased the ratio of medical officers to seven per one thousand, and five hospital stewards per one thousand soldiers, as Gorgas had wanted. Congress also recognized the OTSG's efforts to increase the status of medical specialties by allocating one dental surgeon per thousand soldiers, authorizing the Army Nurse Corps to staff hospitals and mobile medical units, and establishing a Veterinary Corps to professionalize the care for cavalry mounts, horse and mule trains, and other army livestock.[11] The National Defense Act also added two medical officers to the Aviation Board of the Army Signal Corps, the body which operated the aerial war service from 1914 to 1918. Gorgas assigned Theo Lyster to the board to assess the candidate fitness to be airmen, and this appointment would put his nephew in a position to be a pioneer in aviation medicine.[12] In his 1916 annual report, Gorgas judged that the National Defense Act placed the Medical Department "for the first time in its history, upon a satisfactory basis."[13]

Perhaps most importantly, the act also created a Council of National Defense and a series of advisory committees to guide American war preparations. Dr. Franklin Martin, a leading surgeon at Chicago Medical College, was named to the council, heading up the General Medical Board to advise on the nation's wartime medical needs. Martin, a founder of the American College of Surgeons and editor of the *Journal of Surgery, Gynecology, and Obstetrics*, had been advising policy makers since the beginning of the war and became one of the most informed observers of the Medical Department's performance during the war years.[14] He met Gorgas after a congressional hearing in 1916 when the surgeon general invited him to his office to discuss ways to expand the Medical Reserve Corps. "I need all the help I can get," the surgeon general explained. Of that first meeting, Martin wrote that Gorgas's "kindly but direct approach to the purpose of the interview, is a never-to-be-forgotten incident."[15]

Gorgas returned to Congress regularly on behalf of the Medical Department, most often regarding budget matters, and was extended the courtesy of floor privileges to the US Senate chamber.[16] Among the issues he testified on were funding for dogs to locate and comfort the wounded on battlefields, similar to German canine units, which Congress denied, and proposals regarding the inclusion and status of various medical practitioners in the military. No doubt to his great satisfaction, he was also able to get language inserted into a military appropriations bill that transferred mosquito-mitigation operations in Panama from the Quartermaster Corps back to the Department of Sanitation.[17]

Despite the time and effort devoted to Medical Department preparedness, Gorgas continued to be torn between his work in military preparedness and his fight against disease. All of the six articles he published from July 1915 to June 1916 concerned yellow fever and tropical sanitation. When he addressed the Second Pan-American Scientific Congress convening in Washington, DC, in late December 1915, rather than report on the American military medical posture, he spoke on yellow fever eradication.[18] And when the AMA asked the surgeon general to speak at their annual meeting in San Francisco in June 1916, Gorgas drafted remarks on yellow fever, not on preparedness or the military medical challenges of the war. Thus, during the first half of 1916, he was the highly engaged surgeon general of the army, but in the second half of the year, he declined to attend the AMA meeting in California and asked a colleague to deliver his remarks.[19] He instead took leave from government service and sailed for South America to continue his campaign to fight mosquitoes and eradicate yellow fever from the face of the earth.

## ROCKEFELLER FOUNDATION

What may be seen as an inexplicable dereliction of duty was in Gorgas's mind an equally important mission. The year before, he had written an essay, "The Two Greatest Events of 1915," describing the first as the war in Europe, which would determine the future of world power, and the second, the discovery that white men could live in the tropics. Both events, he wrote, promised the greatest change for "civilized man" in three or four thousand years.[20] The essay, though never published, reveals why Gorgas continued his campaign against tropical disease despite the impending national emergency. Not only could he put an end to the human suffering caused by yellow fever, but the work could also, he believed, free up new lands for production and relieve the poverty of millions of people.

In this quest he found support from one of the richest men in the world. John D. Rockefeller had accumulated a massive fortune in oil and mining and was now heeding Andrew Carnegie's warning in *The Gospel of Wealth* that "the man who dies rich dies disgraced." Seeking to do good works, and perhaps atone for the rapacious exploitation of his industries, in 1901 he founded the Rockefeller Institute for Medical Research in New York with the goal of helping American science compete with the best in Europe. He named William Welch as president and Simon Flexner, a well-respected physician and scientist at the University of Pennsylvania, as director.[21] In 1909 Rockefeller also established a $50 million trust, calling it the Rockefeller Foundation, with the lofty purpose to "advance the civilization of the peoples of the United States and its territories and possessions and of foreign lands in the acquisition and dissemination of knowledge, in the prevention and relief of suffering, and in the promotion of any and all of the elements of human progress."[22] The foundation invested in schools of public health, gave scholarships to students around the world, and created the International Health Board (IHB) with the vision that eliminating communicable disease would be the single greatest measure to improving human health. Under the motto "a partner but not the patron," the Rockefeller Foundation distinguished between charity and philanthropy. Rather than provide direct aid to the sick and the poor, the Rockefeller Foundation intended instead to identify problems and train local people on how to deal with them, thus aiding governments and not individuals.[23] The IHB's first project was a brilliantly successful drive between 1909 and 1914 to help state and local governments fight hookworm in the American South. It was led by Wickliffe Rose, an educator from the University of Nashville (now Vanderbilt), and the first IHB director, from 1913 to 1923.[24]

The Rockefeller Foundation yellow fever program was born in July 1914 during a meeting between Rose and Gorgas. Rose had been to Malaya to investigate the hookworm situation, and during his visit, public health officials had expressed concern that commerce through the Panama Canal would spread yellow fever to Asia. Gorgas shared this concern because he, Henry Carter, and others theorized that yellow fever existed in endemic "key centers" or "seed-beds" in South America and Africa from which it could spread to other regions. That was why Gorgas had gone to Guayaquil in 1912, after all. They believed that the yellow fever germ existed only in humans and mosquitoes, and that endemic yellow fever therefore required "a continuous supply of *Stegomyia*, a continuous supply of non-immune human beings, and a continuous supply of infection." Mosquitoes could carry the germ for 180 days at most, so destroying the *Stegomyia* would break the cycle and stamp out endemic foci. If these centers were cleaned up, the disease would be completely eradicated and the threat to Asia eliminated.[25] Yellow fever had already been eliminated in Rio de Janeiro and Vera Cruz, both "key centers," and as Gorgas told one audience, sanitarians felt they were on the eve of destroying all such centers.[26] He even compared the "extinction" of yellow fever to the extinction of the dinosaurs and other prehistoric animals, writing that once they had done their job, "The yellow fever germ can no more be redeveloped than can the mastodon, or the saber-toothed tiger."[27] The disease, he assured Rose, could be "eradicated from the face of the earth within a reasonable time and at a reasonable cost." No undertaking could be more rewarding for the Rockefeller Foundation—or Gorgas.[28]

Some scholars argue that Rockefeller Foundation sanitary efforts were largely an extension of the self-interested public health policy to prevent disease from spreading to the United States.[29] Gorgas had broader goals, however, and told Rose that he hoped to have the privilege of writing the final chapter in the history of yellow fever. "To this I propose to give up the rest of my life," he declared.[30] Rose adopted this view in a memo, "Yellow Fever: Feasibility of Its Eradication," and the Rockefeller Foundation agreed to take on yellow fever as well as malaria and hookworm as its "major objects of attack."[31] The IHB created a yellow fever commission with Gorgas as chair, with a mission to pursue the disease in specific endemic centers: the Yucatán of Mexico; Guayaquil, Ecuador; the north coast of Colombia; the north coast of Venezuela; Trinidad; the Amazon valley; Rio de Janeiro; and the West Coast of Africa.

War, however, threatened to prevent the project from getting under way. Gorgas told Rose in March 1916, "You can understand that it would not look well in me to just at present to bring up the question to the Secretary of my taking leave, but I hope this Mexican flurry will be like the others that have gone before." When things calmed down, he wrote, "I may feel justified in talking over with Mr. Baker the South American Trip."[32] The "flurry" in Mexico never did amount to much, so

Gorgas finally approached Secretary of War Baker about taking leave. The prospect of his fighting mosquitoes in the Western Hemisphere did not seem to threaten American neutrality in the European war, so on May 24, 1916, Gorgas recorded in his diary, "Had talk with Sec. Baker about going to South America. He is willing."[33] The yellow fever commission left three weeks later.

Before they sailed, a newspaper reporter asked Gorgas how he would know when he had achieved eradication. "The campaign will continue until the last germ is dead," he replied. "And how will you know when the last germ is dead?" he was asked. "When men cease to fall sick of yellow fever," said the surgeon general.[34]

## SOUTH AMERICA, 1916

The group that departed from New York Harbor on June 14 was a study in nepotism. Gorgas could not convince Dick to join him, but Theo Lyster and his son-in-law William Wrightson, did, as did Henry Carter and Juan Guiteras, who were as good as family. Eugene Whitmore, a pathologist from the Army Medical School, was the only "outsider."[35] He and Guiteras would focus on the etiological and pathological aspects of the disease, Carter on the epidemiology and the broader development of outbreaks. Wrightson, the engineer, would advise on water and sewerage systems, while Gorgas handled the political and policy aspects of sanitation and public health, with Theo as his deputy. Marie came too, as did Theo's wife, Lua.

The commission's travel for the Rockefeller Foundation was a mixture of privilege and privation, luxury and hardship, and continuous adventure. In a time before government ethics were carefully outlined and codified, Gorgas traveled with family members and received gifts and free accommodations on many of his visits. The international corporation United Fruit had long given the Gorgases passes on its shipping line in exchange for medical advice on travel in the tropics. Now Gorgas benefited from the imprimatur of Standard Oil and the Rockefellers. The party met with high officials and wealthy hosts everywhere they went and sometimes stayed in luxurious accommodations. Government officials often smoothed their way through port quarantines and customs.

Still, travel in Latin America in the early twentieth century was neither easy nor comfortable. They often traveled on small ships loaded with livestock or in hot, crowded boats and trains, and they could find themselves stuck because of bad weather, train wrecks, or shipping delays. The work was not glamorous, either, as the Gorgas party inspected water and sewerage works, stockyards, and abattoirs. They visited hospitals looking for yellow fever patients, advised on diagnoses, and attended autopsies of suspected victims. They were constantly on

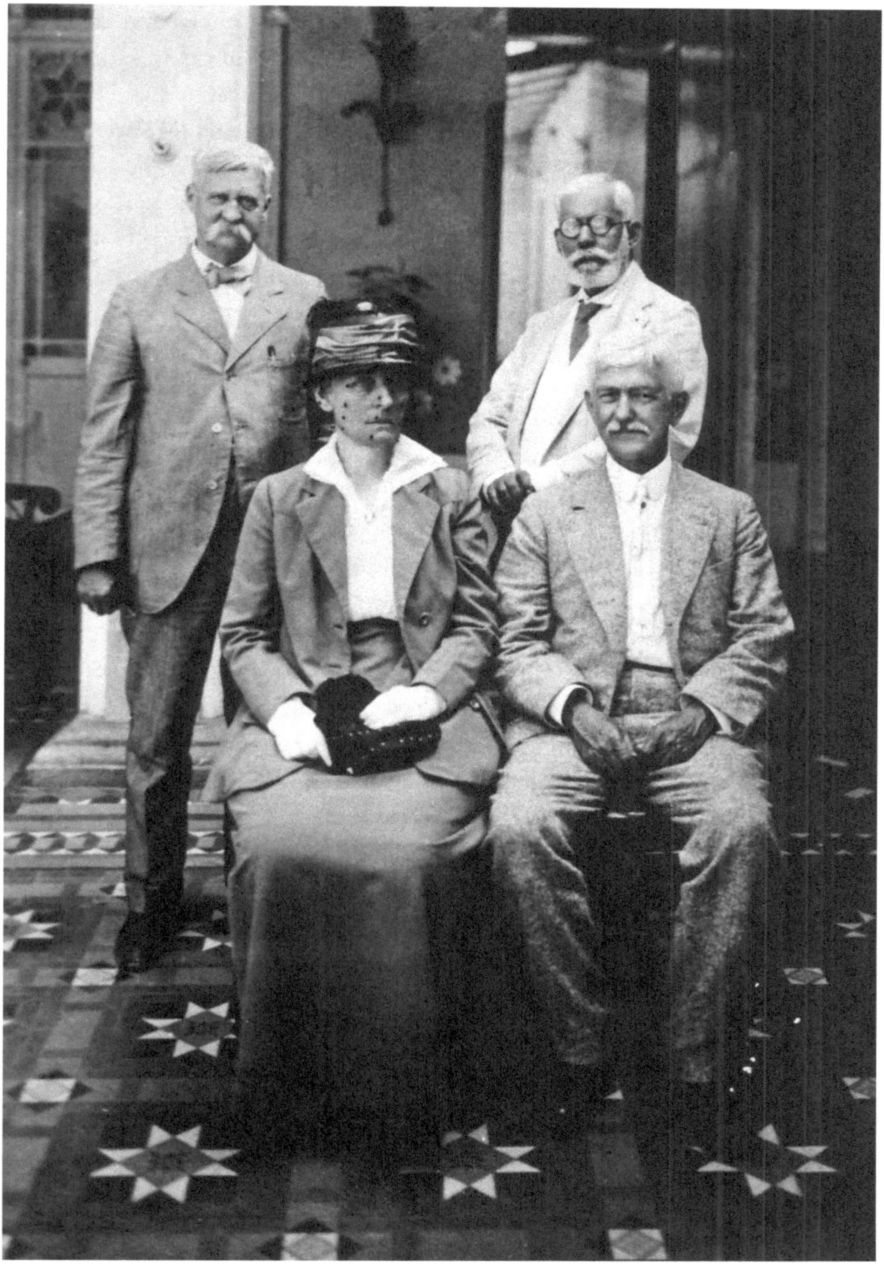

FIGURE 14.1. Rockefeller Foundation Yellow Fever Commission members, clockwise, from top left, Henry Carter, Juan Guiteras, and William Gorgas, with Marie Gorgas, c. 1916. National Library of Medicine.

the move, perhaps staying a week on a ship or in a city, but rarely more than two nights in hotels during their inspections. Their luggage was unwieldy, with clothes for all seasons, instruments, field cots for their field investigations, and boxes of government reports, reference books, and public health laws and regulations from Cuba and Panama to guide South American officials.[36] But the group was game and would wear themselves out one day and be ready for more the next. Gorgas's travel journal reported to his family on their experiences, including the weather, people's health, transportation arrangements, their food and accommodations, and the people they met.[37]

### *Ecuador and Peru*

The commission practiced a blend of public health and diplomacy. They first went to Ecuador, visiting many of the same officials and localities from Gorgas's 1912 trip. Arriving at Guayaquil in early July they first stayed in the Wellington Hotel, "the best in town," but encountered so many rats and mosquitoes that they moved out the next day. Neither Wrightson nor Whitmore was immune to yellow fever, so Gorgas told Wickliffe Rose, "I shall feel relieved when we are able to say 'Good-bye' to Guayaquil." Happily, this visit to Guayaquil was more productive than the previous one. "The whole attitude of the Ecuadorian Government has been most cordial and satisfactory and I feel very much encouraged," Gorgas told Rose. "There is no evidence whatever of suspicion on their part as to our motives or intentions." He credited it not only to their public health mission but also to their nongovernmental status. A few days later, he reported that while "the feeling against the United States on account of the Mexican trouble is at present very strong," the Ecuador officials "consider us entirely in the light of a scientific commission, sent by the Rockefeller Foundation."[38] Gorgas and the foundation, however, had different views of their mission. Whereas Rose and Rockefeller were focused on eradicating yellow fever, Gorgas as a physician and public health official had broader aims of modernizing Guayaquil's sanitation system. When he suggested that the foundation finance a new water and sewerage system as the quickest way to improve health in the city, Rose and the Rockefeller Foundation insisted that the local community pay for such improvements. Their aim was disease eradication, not "charity" to another country.[39]

Gorgas's group split up to visit different yellow fever centers, getting a history of the disease in each area, checking diagnoses, and evaluating mosquito populations and possible transmission routes. After a meeting in Quito with the outgoing president of Ecuador, they met with the president-elect, Alfredo Barquerizo, and agreed to join him on his rail tour of the country. Barquerizo invited Marie to join the party, and when she acted as an interpreter for the group, Gorgas was so pleased that he made her an honorary member of the commission.[40]

Continuing south to Peru, the commission stopped at several ports along the coast to inquire about yellow fever cases. As their boat took on a load of sugar at Guadalupito, Peru, Gorgas went down to the hold to see some other passengers—fifty cattle, or "beeves," as he called them, who "raised their heads and smelled me eagerly as I passed along." Ever the doctor, he inquired as to their welfare, and when he learned that the animals had not been fed or watered for three days, complained to the steamship company.[41]

The party found a warm welcome when they arrived in Lima. President José Pardo y Barreda assured them of his support, and the mayor of Lima asked them to examine their water system. After Wrightson and Whitmore made proposals on how to modernize city sanitation and medical systems, the Peruvians asked if the men would stay on to oversee the improvements. Gorgas therefore asked the PHS and the army to give Wrightson and Whitmore leave so they could do so. "Sending these men down here will be of great assistance to the Peruvian Government, and would be excellent for the men themselves," he wrote. "The tendency would be to make cordial relations between the two Governments." He concluded that Ecuadorian and Peruvian government officials were "much pleased at the action of the Foundation in sending to them a commission with the objects we have in view."[42] Public health was good diplomacy.

### *Colombia and Venezuela*

The visits to Columbia and Venezuela offered adventure. The Colombian ports of Cartagena and Barranquilla were both suspected of being seedbeds of yellow fever, but finding no recent cases in either locale, the team instead inspected the water system as a suspected source of childhood deaths from diarrhea. Then, to get to the capital Bogotá in the interior, they traveled up the Magdalena River on a riverboat. Gorgas was impressed that Marie could sleep on a cot with no pillow or sheets and was "learning to rough it like a soldier," he wrote in his journal.[43] He was amused by a man named Beltrán who shot alligators lying on the riverbanks and was happy that the mosquitoes on the river were not troublesome. "I rather think the mosquitoes did not know who I was; having found out they are treating me with more respect," he quipped.[44]

Gorgas found their reception in Bogotá "most gratifying." The Colombian officials were cordial, and "no anti-American feeling has been shown us, either in public or in private."[45] Hearing reports of a case of yellow fever in Muzo, an emerald mining district in the mountains above the capital city, they decided to investigate.

Gorgas, Whitmore, and Wrightson set off on horses, with pack mules handled by Indian guides who went on foot, for a three-day trek to the mines. They rode twenty miles to their first stop, much of it in the rain. The next day they switched to mules and covered thirty-five miles, riding into the night. It was "anything but pleasant," wrote Gorgas, as he contemplated falling off the trail into the darkness, but he marveled at the Indians' stamina as they climbed thousands of feet up and down the mountains. "I do not see how they can stand it, yet they evidently consider it no particular hardship," he wrote. They reached their destination at 10 p.m., and the next morning went to the Muzo mines accompanied by local doctors to track down the yellow fever cases. They found neither yellow fever nor *Stegomyia* there but diagnosed the seriously ill people with malaria instead. Gorgas figured that the doctor who had reported yellow fever was a "bright and intelligent man but is not a trained observer."[46] There was so much malaria, though, that contrary to the Rockefeller practice of no individual charity, Gorgas distributed $600 to these "poor people for the purpose of getting medicine [most likely quinine] which we had prescribed."[47]

Returning to Bogotá, William found that Marie was not well, so the party split up, and the Gorgases retraced their steps back to the coast while Wrightson and Theo went on another mule train to inspect more mining areas.[48] It must have been a hard trip, because when they arrived in Cartagena, Gorgas wrote, "Never thought that I would be so glad to see the dear old dilapidated place."[49] At the ages of sixty-two and fifty-two, traveling in an era before light-weight fabrics and air conditioning, William and Marie were exhausted.[50] While they recovered, Gorgas asked Rose to send copies of his book, *Sanitation in Panama*, to the officials who had hosted the commission, and he sent along slips of paper with his autograph to be enclosed in each volume. He explained, "I think it will show a little more appreciation than simply a letter."[51] Guiteras and Carter soon arrived in Cartagena, and, comparing notes, the commission concluded that yellow fever was no longer endemic in Colombia but that vigilance was needed in the Pacific port of Buenaventura, because disease could spread there from Ecuador.[52]

Although the commission was far from the war in Europe, its impact was felt now and then. In Ecuador, the Muzo emerald mines had been idled because the war had closed off the European markets. In Peru, talk of the war generated spirited discussion at a dinner when the host said he supported the Germans. While in Medellín, Colombia, Gorgas noted the "startling news" that German agents had attacked a munitions plant at Black Tom pier in New York Harbor, sparking an explosion that killed five, destroyed $20 million work of military goods, and damaged the Statue of Liberty.[53] Now, on the way to Venezuela, Gorgas's party were among only ten passengers on a ship with a capacity of three hundred, because people were afraid to travel, and they could not use the telegraph for fear of attracting German U-boats.

They nonetheless steamed safely along the northern coast of Venezuela, inspecting health conditions at a couple of ports along the way, arriving outside of Caracas on August 31. There they were met by a delegation of doctors who drove them to the city in a hair-raising trip, whereby "anywhere at a hundred points along the road a swerve of the wheel would have sent us over a precipice five hundred feet below." Once safely in Caracas, the Venezuelans accommodated the group with a house and servants, but a few days into their visit, all engagements were cancelled because the Venezuelan secretary of the interior had died of typhoid. Gorgas the sanitarian observed that the death made a "deep impression" and would probably hasten the installation of proper sewage and water supply systems in Caracas.[54]

After Caracas, the Gorgases and their colleagues joined up with Theo at Curaçao, but instead of sailing directly to Brazil, they found that the quickest route would be through New York, so they booked passage and arrived in New York on September 25. They immediately went to Washington, but it is surprising that Gorgas was not more concerned about his OTSG when he arrived home. He made very little comment in his journal or correspondence. The acting surgeon general, H. P. Birmingham, had submitted a positive annual report for the Medical Department, reporting that medical mobilization for the Mexican campaign had been excellent practice for future campaigns, with only eight cases of typhoid and no deaths, and that a hospital train of ten Pullman cars designed by the OTSG operated smoothly between the Mexican border and the East Coast.[55] Gorgas did go to the office once and "got a welcome that warmed the cockles of my heart," and when he went to Secretary Baker, he received compliments on the Medical Department's work on the Mexican border.[56]

After meeting with Wickliffe Rose and others at the Rockefeller Foundation in New York, the Gorgases attended a few plays and bought William a new suit. About the latter he had been reluctant. "I always have a feeling towards old clothes as if they were old friends." The yellow fever commission then sailed for Rio on the Norwegian ship SS *Vasar*, on October 7.[57]

### *Brazil*

Gorgas, like many Americans, continued to be naive about the violence of the war in Europe. As the *Vasar* steamed out into the Atlantic, Gorgas sought to "poke fun" at the captain for not reporting their location, for darkening the ship against a possible German attack, and for keeping their location a secret in radio transmissions.

The captain then told him confidentially about recent German submarine attacks upon vessels off Nantucket, which sobered the surgeon general. The next day, when he learned that the captain had a son in the trenches in France, he confessed in his journal, "The patriotism and self-sacrifice of all the people engaged in this war impresses me strongly." A week later off the coast of Brazil, they heard about more German attacks near American coastlines. "This interference with neutral commerce on our shore," Gorgas wrote, in a stunning understatement, "must seriously complicate our relations with Germany."[58]

When the ship docked at Rio de Janeiro, they were met with much ceremony by the surgeon general of the Brazilian army and several high-ranking officers. They soon had a meeting with President Venceslau Brás, who spoke highly of the Rockefeller Foundation and gave his approval for their mission, offering to contact various governors on their behalf. Gorgas also met Dr. Oswaldo Cruz, the famed public health officer who had launched a yellow fever eradication campaign for Rio using the techniques developed by Finlay and Gorgas as well as Dr. Carlos Chagas, who in 1909 discovered the cause of the insect-borne disease that bears his name, Chagas disease. William and Marie found Rio as beautiful as they had heard and had so many invitations that they had to decline quite a few of them. They did, however, accept a visit from Dr. Pyles, the son of an "old Confederate," whose family had migrated to Brazil after the Civil War and formed a colony of such southerners in Rio.[59]

Inspecting the national mortality records, the commission found that there had been no yellow fever in any large Brazilian city during the previous year but that a survey had turned up cases in several regions in the north. They prepared to sail north along the coast, planning to stop, as usual, at port cities along the way to look for possible yellow fever centers. Gorgas was less casual about the war when they departed Rio on November 1, writing in his journal, "I hope we shall escape being blown up by German submarines."[60] Stopping at ports along the way in the states of Bahia and Para, among others, they asked about yellow fever, searched for *Stegomyia*, and examined all fever patients in the local hospitals but did not find any yellow fever. Impressed with the investment the Brazilian states had made in sanitation and mosquito control, the commission members determined that yellow fever would not regain a foothold in the region.

The commission returned to New York in early December and set about preparing a comprehensive report to the Rockefeller Foundation. After chasing down every rumor of yellow fever in five countries, they concluded that the only endemic center lay in Guayaquil, Ecuador. They recommended eliminating yellow fever from that port and maintaining surveillance on the southern coast of the Caribbean and

Brazil's east coast in case new outbreaks should arise. The war made it impossible to conduct their investigations in Mexico or cross the Atlantic to West Africa, so the commission advised postponing inspection of those regions until conditions allowed.[61]

Marie described the trip through South America as "something of a triumphal progress" for William and "among the most delightful and enjoyable" times of his life.[62] At a time when many Latin American countries were wary of if not angry at the United States for its interventions in Central America and the Caribbean, the Rockefeller Foundation's IHB campaign showed the power of public health to make connections instead of divisions between nations. This dynamic, in addition to killing mosquitoes, had been very much on Gorgas's mind as he traveled around the continent. Thus, when John Rockefeller offered Gorgas a permanent position as a director of the foundation, he was tempted to accept and went to Secretary of War Baker in January 1917 to discuss retirement.[63] Baker was initially willing to release his surgeon general, but relations with Germany were deteriorating by the day, and as the United States edged toward war, they dropped the matter.[64] The war had come to Gorgas.

## CHAPTER 15

# Mobilizing the Nation for War

I am a Crusader and believe in War. And in all history
I think there never was a holier war than this.

—William Gorgas to Daniel Kiefer, April 1917

THE 1917–1918 YEARBOOK OF THE Medical Officers Training Camp at Fort Riley, Kansas, was dedicated to "Major General W. C. Gorgas, who, above all others, has been responsible for the high standing of the Medical Corps of the United States Army and who now represents to the people of the Country the Ideal of an Officer and a Gentleman."[1] A photograph shows him handsome and smiling, but with some wear and tear: his face has well-earned laugh lines and wrinkles, his mustache and hair are a bit unruly, his officer's cap looks too big for his head.

If Gorgas was revered in many corners, most histories of military medicine during World War I are not as generous, relegating him to the sidelines of the war and deeming him a weak administrator who had seen better days. Mary Gillett, author of an official history of the Army Medical Department, acknowledged his contributions in disease prevention and in drawing talented men to service during the war but described Surgeon General Gorgas as "past his prime" and "more interested in a worldwide battle against yellow fever and other epidemic diseases than in administration." While she also recognized that the American refusal to consider the possibility of entering the war "doomed the [Medical] department to bear an essentially unbearable burden once war had been declared," she characterized Gorgas's OTSG as confused and chaotic.[2] Another historian wrote that Gorgas "had always been more interested in disease prevention than in office administration."[3] The Rockefeller Yellow Fever Commission trip to South America in 1916 would be exhibit A for such allegations. Gorgas's contemporaries were also critical of his leadership. Kean wrote that Gorgas served "at the head of the vast and turbulent machine" that was actually run by his OTSG staff, and that Gorgas "would have been a happier man if he had retired in January 1917."[4] Even more harshly, Merritte Ireland, the chief surgeon of the American Expeditionary Forces in France (AEF), told Secretary of War Baker in 1918 that he thought Gorgas's OTSG was "rotten" and wanted nothing to do with it.[5]

A closer look at Gorgas's tenure as surgeon general, however, shows that despite his distraction—if not obsession—with tropical-disease fighting, he was in many ways well suited to lead the wartime Medical Department. As the United States strove to increase its armed forces from 270,000 in 1917 to more than four million in just eighteen months, the Medical Department had to scramble to find and train the medical personnel to care for them. Gorgas had the reputation and access to the nation's leading medical institutions to serve the country in this effort in a number of ways. As a respected sanitarian, he attracted good doctors and built up the Medical Department to protect the health of recruits from across the country; as a physician he endeavored to ensure that medical judgment and personnel were included in military policy up and down the War Department bureaucracy; as a public health educator, he spoke, wrote, and testified to government officials, professional groups, and civilian audiences about the importance of sanitation and scientific medicine in the army and the nation; and as a man he was secure and modest enough to let others take the limelight and credit for success. In these roles he took risks and made mistakes, and his tenure was at times controversial, but he guided the continually growing and changing Medical Department during the worst war the world had ever known.

## MOBILIZATION

When Gorgas returned from South America, the war still seemed distant. American voters had even just reelected Woodrow Wilson under the banner "He Kept Us Out of War." By late 1916, however, the war was drawing troops and supplies from every continent into the Western Front caldron, and bloody battles raged in Eastern Europe, the Alps, and East Africa. After the horrific battles of Verdun and the Somme, the year 1917 held even more deadly drama as the French Army mutinied, the British Army became mired in the mud of Flanders, Italy suffered severe defeat at Caporetto, and Russia convulsed in revolution. The United States too was becoming increasingly enmeshed economically, sending food and supplies to the Allies. Wilson knew that neutrality would be difficult to maintain.

Just days after Gorgas decided against retirement, the Germans renewed submarine attacks on American and British ships, and the British decoded the

Zimmerman Telegram, revealing that the Germans were urging Mexico to attack the United States in exchange for territorial rewards in California, New Mexico, and Arizona. On April 2, 1917, Wilson was finally compelled to ask Congress for a declaration of war against Germany, and Congress complied within days. The United States, long protected from enemy attack by two oceans, and historically reluctant to have a large standing army, would now mobilize its huge, industrialized economy to send young American men to fight and die in Europe.

Gorgas, like many Americans, had confused feelings about the war. At one point he joked with Carter about it: "Things look very war-like this morning. Are you prepared to go after a German submarine? I am quite sure that Guiteras is just boiling over to tackle one."[6] The next day, he reflected soberly on how his life had been bracketed by war. "You and I have witnessed the greatest event that has occurred in the history of our own country; I refer to our War between the States," he wrote to surgeon William Polk. "Now we are seeing settled the greatest event that has ever occurred in the history of the world. I think we can count ourselves as fortunate."[7] Still, he could not completely turn away from fighting disease. Just days after the United States declared war, he told a colleague, "I am going into the yellow fever work in South America just as soon as [we] whip the Germans."[8]

Turning his attention to medical preparations, Gorgas wired George Crile on April 28, 1917, to mobilize his Base Hospital #4. Crile with a staff of seventy-seven departed for France within a week, followed by Cushing's Base Hospital #5 out of Harvard on May 11. These two units were among the first American military personnel to join the Allies. Then, inexplicably, in May, just weeks after the United States had declared war, Gorgas boarded a ship to Puerto Rico to investigate a possible yellow fever case there. This decision earned him the reprobation of colleagues and historians alike. Henry Carter joined him, and as in their 1915 trip to the island, the case turned out to be dengue fever. While they were there, Gorgas asked Carter to go back to Brazil and Venezuela on another Rockefeller Foundation tour, adding, "I would expect to join you whenever my work in Washington is finished."[9] Carter, however, chose to fight the Germans instead and stayed with the PHS throughout the war.

American military mobilization was slowed by the absence of a strong central government. Rather than employ the European approach of national planning and the rationing of food, fuel, and other goods, Americans sought to mobilize the economy through business and government cooperation to balance military and civilian needs. The Wilson administration and Congress created a system of both coercion and voluntarism, such as financing the war with a combination of taxes (coercive) and "Liberty Bonds" (voluntary), and creating a patchwork of public and private institutions to meet the war needs. The War Department furnished soldiers with clothing, room and board, health care, and twenty-five dollars a month, but it augmented its operations with goods and services from other government agencies and private, voluntary organizations. The PHS, for example, took responsibility for health conditions around the training camps, enlisting the Boy Scouts to help with mosquito mitigation.[10] The Red Cross was a quasi-governmental agency, organizing hospitals, recruiting nurses, and raising funds and in-kind donations for the Allied cause. Its membership exploded during the war, from fewer than twenty-two thousand members in 1915 to more than twenty million adult members by 1918.[11] Marie worked in her local Red Cross chapters sewing bandages and collecting supplies to support the troops. Other voluntary organizations, like the YMCA and the Jewish Welfare Board, provided recreation and other support for soldiers, sailors, and marines in the camps at home and in France.

## TRAINING CAMPS

Mobilization also offered opportunity for broad reform. In the war to "Make the World Safe for Democracy," many Progressives, Gorgas and President Wilson among them, saw an opportunity to improve the world. Training camps could acculturate recruits, especially immigrants and rural trainees, to the prevailing American middle-class culture and reinforce patriotism.[12] An Allied victory could extend American democracy and capitalism overseas. Gorgas shared these aspirations and saw the war as an opportunity to educate the country on public sanitation, personal hygiene, and even economic reform with the single tax. When labor leader Samuel Gompers solicited Gorgas's support for various tax measures to finance the war, Gorgas responded that he especially liked the land tax idea, because while "future generations are going to get some benefit from this war," they should not be burdened with the debt.[13] When Daniel Kiefer of the National Single Tax League expressed reservations about the war, Gorgas countered that the war offered an opportunity to point out the "desirability and efficiency of levying some of these taxes on land value." Kiefer, he suggested, should send his single-tax pamphlets to the YMCA libraries in the training camps.[14]

Gorgas also favored compulsory service, because it was for a "holy cause" and was "the only fair and democratic way of raising an army."[15] Unwilling to rely on volunteerism to build an army, Congress quickly approved a draft, but the first year was difficult, because no one knew how large a force the Americans would need. General Pershing, in charge of the AEF in France, at first called for a million soldiers, then two million, then three; during 1917 the army strength increased from 217,272 in January to 1,538,203 in December. By the November 1918 armistice, there were 4.8 million men in the American armed services.[16]

One of the Medical Department's first responsibilities was to screen the recruits for health. The Selective Service ultimately had a system of some 4,600 local draft boards and ten thousand physicians who conducted physical examinations of 10 million of the 24 million men ages eighteen to forty-five registered for military service.[17] The boards rejected millions of young men for poor health, family responsibilities, or jobs considered vital to the war effort. But when the process was over, the US Army reflected the diversity of the society. About 20 percent of the draftees were foreign-born; they spoke at least forty-six languages and at least 5,700 Mexican aliens and 12,500 American Indians were in military service.[18] By 1918 the War Department had fifty training camps across the country to prepare these men to join the Allies in France. Gorgas's Medical Department was responsible for their health.

One of the department's early challenges was that the physical exams revealed thousands of health problems. Hundreds of young men had tuberculosis, so they could neither be placed in military units nor be sent back to infect their communities. When these men began to flow into the army hospitals, Gorgas called upon the army's tuberculosis specialist, Col. George Bushnell, to head up a special tuberculosis division. Bushnell established a system for keeping the disease out of the ranks and caring for those cases that developed in the training camps. Gorgas sent another specialist to France to identify tuberculosis cases among the US troops in the AEF.[19] This one disease ultimately required the Medical Department to establish eight additional tuberculosis hospitals to care for the 18,500 men in the training camps and 3,500 men in Europe diagnosed with the disease.[20]

Gorgas and his colleagues knew that they were up against difficult odds, because disease thrives on mobilizing armies. They therefore sought to make the Medical Department a model of public health and implemented sanitation and preventive measures in the camps such as vaccinations, water purification and sanitary waste disposal, diets to prevent deficiency diseases such as scurvy and pellagra, and "foot surveys" to examine boot fittings. Periodic physical examinations checked for infectious diseases, vermin, and sexually transmitted infections. Medical officers quarantined sick recruits; treated curable ailments such as hernias, troublesome tonsils, and dental problems; and referred men who violated sanitary regulations to their superior officers for discipline.[21] Many enlistees also arrived addicted to drugs and alcohol. Rather than bar them from service, Gorgas suggested that they be retained and treated for addiction in order to preserve "many thousand competent soldiers" for service and prevent others from malingering by claiming addiction to avoid military service.[22] On the eve of Prohibition in the United States, however, this idea did not gain traction.[23]

Gorgas especially cautioned his medical officers, the War Department leadership, the public, and anyone else who would listen that respiratory diseases, in particular pneumonia, would be a problem in the camps during the winter: "We must now give renewed and most extraordinary attention to our precautions against 'this greatest of all the captains of the men of death,'" he wrote in one report.[24] He recruited Victor Vaughan, dean of the University of Michigan Medical School and his colleague and patient in Siboney, to run the Medical Department's infectious disease division. Vaughan issued a similar warning: "The mobilization of raw, untrained men and their hurried transformation into effective soldiers have always been accompanied by marked increase in morbidity and mortality." The camps, he said, acted like "drag-nets" for infections, and overcrowding and poor personal hygiene among recruits exacerbated the conditions.[25]

Such problems soon became evident. When Secretary Baker had asked Gorgas, Franklin Martin, William Welch, and Vaughan (the latter three now in uniform) to examine housing plans for trainees, they found "two grave sanitary defects": too many men in each dormitory, and insufficient floor space per person. The camps allowed 338 cubic feet per man, where the minimum should be 500 cubic feet. This was dangerous, they warned, because spinal meningitis, pneumonia, tuberculosis, measles, mumps, scarlet fever, and whooping cough were all transmitted through human contact, and "the degree of transmission is inversely in proportion to the distance between individuals."[26] They called for more medical personnel, more hospitals, warmer clothing, observation or detention camps to monitor recruits for diseases before they joined other trainees, and a gradual ramp-up to military training to reduce the stress on civilian recruits. Gorgas also wanted increased military rank and authority for medical officers so they could ensure healthy conditions for soldiers.[27] Few of these recommendations were adopted by the War Department, because they required money, time, and space in training camps and troop ships, and interfered with the army's urgent drive to get troops to France.[28] Medical officers therefore lacked the resources and authority they believed they needed to protect the health of the men in the camps. They treated the sick and advised on medical issues, but the power in the army resided with the General Staff and the line command.

## THE ARMY MEDICAL DEPARTMENT IN WARTIME

As a wartime surgeon general, Gorgas sat atop a ballooning government agency. The War Department underwent numerous reorganizations as the army grew, creating new offices and agencies, and additional levels of authority to meet the expanding needs. The Medical Department likewise underwent myriad reorganizations.

The OTSG headquarters grew from a suite of three rooms in the Army Navy Building to a couple of buildings covering two square blocks. One organization chart for the OTSG from June 22, 1918, shows twenty-four divisions reporting to the surgeon general, including "General Surgery," "Medicine," "Army Nurse Corps," "Psychiatry," "Food Division," and "Publication Board."[29]

The department's most urgent need, however, was for doctors to care for the men. While Gorgas was in South America, Franklin Martin and the AMA surveyed the medical profession and estimated that there were 146,500 doctors in the United States, 2 to 3 percent of them African Americans, and 3 to 4 percent women.[30] As Pershing demanded more and more soldiers for the AEF, it seemed the war might require mobilizing them all. Applicants had to be US citizens between the ages of twenty-two and fifty-five, graduates of approved medical schools with at least one year in a postgraduate hospital internship, in possession of a state license, and "of good moral character and habits." They also had to pass physical fitness and professional competency examinations.[31] But the Medical Corps remained an old boys' network. Gorgas and his staff prevented osteopathic physicians from getting commissions in the Medical Corps, opposed legislation to establish a pharmaceutical corps for druggists in the army, and raised requirements for medical officer commissions above those for most state medical licenses.[32] And, unlike the US Army rank-and-file, which included thousands of African Americans, and men from every region, race, and ethnic group in the country, Gorgas's Medical Corps generally maintained a white, male, largely allopathic profile.

The War Department figured it needed twenty-one thousand medical officers to support an army of three million, but by November 1917 newspapers were reporting that only twelve thousand physicians had signed up.[33] Federal officials considered drafting physicians, but Gorgas and others assured them that the profession would meet the emergency. They launched a public relations campaign vaunting patriotism, adventure, manliness, honor, courage, and "doing one's bit," as well as the opportunities for research and professional advancement war medicine offered. The AMA mailed sixty-nine thousand letters, and *JAMA* editorialized on the need for medical officers, appending blank application forms in two issues. When physicians finally began to sign up by the thousands, the Medical Department established four medical officer training camps across the country to accomplish the enormous task of training new officers. Unfortunately, personnel were so desperately needed in the camps and the AEF that men were often deployed before they had completed their training.[34]

Gorgas and his OTSG recruited the best talent in the country for the Medical Department. In addition to Cushing of Harvard, Crile of Case Western, and

Vaughan of Michigan, Gorgas was able to get other leading medical men such as William Welch of Johns Hopkins, Simon Flexner of the Rockefeller Institute, and the Mayo brothers, William and Charles, of the Mayo Clinic.[35] George Bushnell, the tuberculosis specialist, observed that Gorgas appreciated expertise and freely delegated responsibility, believing that it contributed to the success of the OTSG. Gorgas provided initial guidance, he said, then left the experts to work and "rejoiced over the results which so amply justified his course."[36] Gorgas also fostered research, and in late 1916 the OTSG established a Research Division in the Army Medical School to employ scientists full-time to investigate the causes and prevention of disease.[37]

As he had throughout his career, Gorgas brought his friends and family to work with him. He appointed his old advocate Alexander Lambert director of civilian relief of the American Red Cross in France, recruited Marie's surgeon William Keen into the Medical Reserve, and appointed Theo Lyster to numerous offices and boards.[38] By the end of the war, he had helped Theo win a promotion to brigadier general at the young age of forty-three, jumping rank over Jefferson Kean, fifteen years his senior. Gorgas's son-in-law, William Wrightson, also rose in rank during the war, promoted to lieutenant colonel in February 1918, and to colonel just before Gorgas retired. At Gorgas's urging, in 1917 Congress created a new Sanitary Corps of officers without medical degrees to relieve medical officers of administrative and research duties, and in an egregious act of nepotism, Gorgas named Wrightson head of the new corps.[39] The surgeon general got his brother Dick an administrative job at Camp McClellan in Alabama, too, explaining to the chief medical officer there, "After a short course at your hospital he will be assigned as adjutant to one of the hospitals going overseas."[40] Dick did not go to France but worked in the hospital at Camp Lewis in Alabama, close to family.

Gorgas did not recruit everyone he favored. When he was in Puerto Rico in May, Bailey Ashford, the army medical officer who discovered that hookworms caused anemia, said he wanted to go to France. "What?" cried Gorgas. "Do you think I am going to send a high-class laboratory man, on whom we have spent a lot of money by leaving him in Porto Rico so many years, to get butchered up in France? No, sir, you will *not* go to France."[41] Tropical medicine held precedence in Gorgas's esteem, but Ashford did get to France and taught at the Army Medical School at Langres.

### *A Medical Corps Segregated by Race and Sex*

Despite the initial physician shortage, Gorgas and his colleagues did not recruit African American physicians and barred women physicians from the army entirely. The army awarded medical commissions to only 356 of the 3,000 to 4,000 African American physicians, surgeons, and dentists in the country, and required some of them to serve as rank-and-file infantry privates instead of in their fields of expertise. The OTSG held Black physicians to the same professional requirements as white medical officers but marked their race on their records and established a segregated training camp for them at Fort Des Moines, Iowa. Although white dental and medical officers treated troops of all backgrounds, African American dental and medical officers treated only Black troops, often with inferior equipment and supplies.[42] This double standard often resulted in poorer nutrition and substandard medical care for Black units.[43]

A series of letters between Black medical personnel and Gorgas's OTSG in May and June 1917 shows the OTSG's tortured policy. After the United States declared war, Maj. James R. White of the Eighth Illinois Infantry, one of the few Black officers commanding troops, petitioned Gorgas to appoint Black physicians to the Medical Corps. The surgeon general put him off, responding that the matter was "being given consideration in this Office and will be decided when the organization of colored regiments is authorized." When he heard no word, White inquired again, and the OTSG admitted that it was "dodging the issue" because there was no place to assign Black officers, explaining that "it would be a cause of dissatisfaction and an embarrassment" for them to be assigned with white troops. In June, Gorgas reiterated the army's policy not to call "colored men" to active duty except with "colored troops," and only "as the exigencies of the service demand."[44]

Even earlier race-neutral policies were reversed. Before the war, it had not been practical for small army hospitals with only a hundred patients already separated by rank and illness to segregate by race. But in an irony of the "war to save the world for democracy," the increase in patients enabled the Medical Department to resegregate hospital wards. After Gorgas's OTSG received complaints about integrated hospital wards, it issued a memo in March 1918 stating that "it would be a better procedure, and for the best interest of all concerned, to arrange for the care of white and colored patients in separate wards or separate rooms, so far as possible."[45] The Gorgas administration thus commissioned African American physicians in small numbers to care for Black patients but allowed Jim Crow to prevail in army hospitals as it did in much of the United States.

Women physicians had even less access to the Medical Corps.[46] There is no record that Gorgas employed women physicians or scientists in Panama or in his inner circle in the Medical Department. While working in Panama, however, he did tell a friend that Aileen had considered studying medicine like her father, so he did not outright oppose women doctors.[47] Women physicians constituted only 3 or 4 percent of their profession in 1917—5,000–6,000 total out of 146,000—but when they conducted their own survey, almost one-third of their cohort wanted to serve in the war.[48] One group pointed out to Gorgas that since the National Defense Act of 1916 required medical officers to be "citizens . . . [and] physically, mentally and morally qualified to hold such commissions," they were surely qualified for the Medical Reserve Corps.[49] The Judge Advocate General's office ruled, however, that soldiers were specified as "men" in army regulations, so Gorgas lamely told the women that while he personally supported their petition, he had to abide by the ruling. The continuing physician shortage through 1918, however, persuaded the OTSG to admit fifty-five women physicians to serve in the Sanitary Corps and as civilian "contract surgeons," working as bacteriologists and pathologists in laboratories or as sanitarians for army installations. Eighty other women physicians, two of them African Americans, served overseas with voluntary organizations such as the Red Cross, but women physicians could not formally serve in the army until World War II.

*Nurses*

The women in the army were the nurses. Having long worked with female nurses, Gorgas did not need to be convinced of their competence and value. Although Congress had established the Army Nurse Corps in 1901, female nursing did not come of age in the army until the war. This corps also emerged as a single-sex, white, professionally trained organization. The American Red Cross ultimately recruited twenty-one thousand female nurses for the Army Nurse Corps, all single and from approved nurse-training schools.[50] The military status of army nurses remained unclear, however, because the War Department did not grant military rank or privileges to the women. Most were not commissioned but instead held "relative rank," a vague term that one congressional committee defined as "above a sergeant major and below a second lieutenant."[51] Gorgas maintained inconsistent positions with regard to military rank for nurses, supporting the rank of major for the head of the Army Nurse Corps, several captains as her assistants, and the rank of first lieutenant for hospital head nurses, but opposing commissions as second lieutenants for all army nurses.[52] The British, after all, did not commission their nurses, he reasoned, and besides, "I think we are getting along well enough."[53] Gorgas did support the professionalization of nursing, however, and in 1918 approved the establishment of an Army School of Nursing to hone the expertise of military nurses. By the end of the year, the school had accepted more than five thousand students, but none of them completed the three-year course before the war was over.[54]

Black nurses were not recruited, and when African American leaders called for enlisting them in the army, Gorgas gave them a bureaucratic runaround. In February 1918 he explained that the government was not calling Black nurses because "there are no separate quarters available for them, and it is not deemed advisable to assign white and colored nurses to the same posts." He referred them to Jane Delano, head of the Red Cross nursing program. She told the petitioners, "There has never been any question in regard to our willingness to enroll colored nurses." The question was rather where to assign them to duty, and that, "after all is a matter for the Surgeon General to decide, rather than our office."[55] Only at the end of the war during the extreme emergency of the influenza pandemic did the Army Nurse Corps admit eighteen Black nurses to serve at Camp Sherman, Ohio, and Camp Grant, Illinois, to care for sick Black soldiers.

Gorgas's call for one thousand women to serve as reconstruction aides and the establishment of training schools across the country opened a new employment avenue for women, especially in the field of rehabilitation medicine.[56] In August 1917 his OTSG authorized "women war workers" to support the Medical Department's hospitals as dieticians, occupational therapists, and physical therapists who would help rehabilitate soldiers suffering from fractures, burns, amputations, and other wounds.[57] Such developments might have occurred without Gorgas in the OTSG, but he was often an advocate for an increased role for women in military health care.

## THE OTSG IN WARTIME

The Americans in 1917 were playing catch-up in all aspects of modern warfare, and as soon as the United States entered the war, Alfred Keogh, director general of the British Royal Medical Service, sent one of his best officers, Col. John Goodwin, to Gorgas as liaison. Goodwin had been on the front, and Keogh wanted him to impart to the Americans the medical needs of modern warfare and "the practical knowledge he has gained in the field where he has been since the commencement of the war."[58] Gorgas responded enthusiastically, "It pleases me beyond measure to be Surgeon General of the United States Army at the time when we join England in this great work. I have felt from the beginning that we were shirking our duty and that this fight was as much ours as yours."[59] The arrangement created another one of Gorgas's great friendships. The surgeon general gave Goodwin a table in his office, and "from that hour until I left the United States in January 1918," the British officer wrote, "I was in the closest possible association with him, seeing him daily in the office and accompanying him on tours of inspection, etc."[60] Goodwin tried to educate American medical officers on what they would find on the Western Front, such as how industrial warfare was causing horribly severe wounds from artillery and chemical weapons, generating new diseases like trench fever (from lice), trench foot (tissue deterioration from long immersion in the water of the trenches), and shell shock, now known as Post-traumatic Stress Disorder.[61] Many American specialists seized the opportunity to gain the new medical knowledge from their European counterparts. The British high command recalled Goodwin in late 1917 to succeed Keogh as surgeon general of the Royal Army Medical Corps, jumping him over dozens of senior officers, due in part to his Washington experience. Gorgas rejoiced in his promotion. "If Washington were not so strong for prohibition," he told him, "we would all meet tonight and drink to your success."[62]

If Goodwin appreciated his desk in the OTSG, Gorgas avoided his and saw his role more as an advocate for the Medical Department and medical profession in the War Department and as a cheerleader for public health in the broader society. He left much of the management of the OTSG to his second-in-charge, Robert Noble, and deputies H. P. Birmingham and Charles Richard, all brigadier generals, with Gorgas's longtime executive assistant, Charles Furbush, running the office.[63] Gorgas instead attended scores of congressional hearings and government meetings, personally inspected training camps, and spoke to reporters and audiences across the country. The most important committee on which Gorgas served was the General Medical Board of the Council of National Defense, formed just days before the

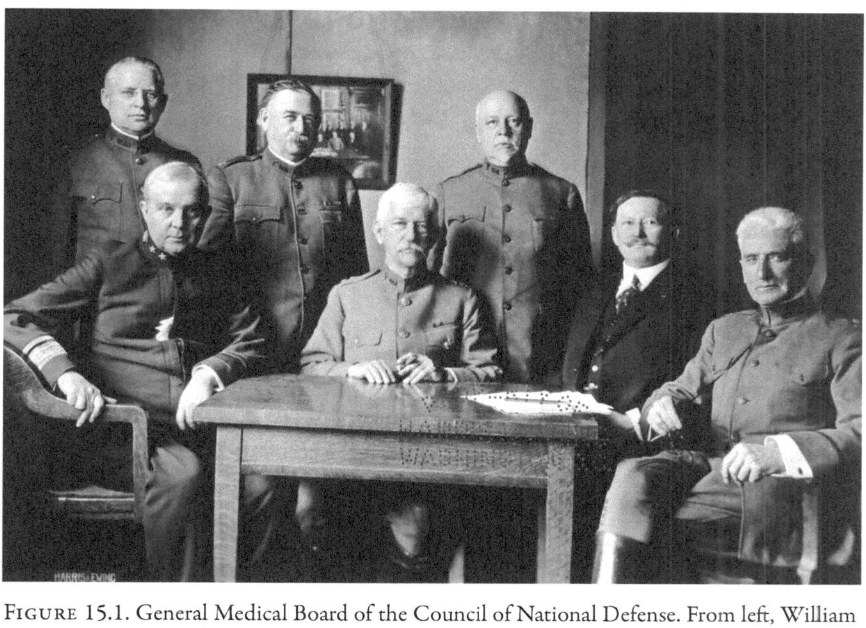

FIGURE 15.1. General Medical Board of the Council of National Defense. From left, William Braisted, Josephus Daniels, Victor Vaughan, Gorgas (with cigar), William Welch, Rupert Blue, Franklin Martin. National Library of Medicine.

United States entered the war. The board's eleven-member executive committee, chaired by Franklin Martin, the Chicago surgeon, included the surgeons general of the navy and the PHS; the AMA president; Jefferson Kean; William Welch; and the White House physician, Cary Grayson. They met Mondays at 8:00 a.m. in Martin's office on Pennsylvania Avenue. Martin's secretary, Florence O'Brien Donnelly, later remembered that each time Gorgas arrived, his attendant, William, handed him a cigar, because Gorgas was asthmatic and believed that "smoking afforded him relief." One morning before a committee meeting, Gorgas turned to Donnelly with an unlighted cigar to ask her, the only woman in the room, if she minded if he smoked. She was nonplussed. "Knowing of the necessity for his smoking and feeling so insignificant in the presence of the first real general I had ever encountered, I was quite overcome and faintly stammered: 'Certainly not.'" With that, he had won her heart, she told Martin. "No one was too insignificant for his consideration."[64]

In addition to the huge task of medical mobilization, the OTSG handled some of the most sensitive issues in the army, such as vaccination policy and sexually transmitted diseases among the troops. Immunization had a long, proud tradition in the army, beginning with Gen. George Washington's inoculation of the Continental Army against smallpox in the winter of 1777 to combat a virulent epidemic. In the early twentieth century, well-trained physicians prized immunizations as efficient public health tools. Gorgas, of course, vaccinated for smallpox in Cuba and Panama, and sponsored Juan Guiteras's ill-fated yellow fever inoculation trials in 1900. While immunizations had been required for army troops and people in occupied regions, the war now brought millions of civilians into the military medical arena, and not all of them were compliant. Immunization was not risk free, and smallpox vaccination, for example, could leave nasty wounds. Opposition to army vaccination arose immediately. Some church groups believed that vaccination was against God's will and claimed, "We would rather be imprisoned, put on bread and water diet, or be shot than to disobey God."[65] One citizen petition against vaccination was accompanied by a rather gruesome photograph of twenty trainees showing angry sores from vaccination.[66] Gorgas's office easily batted these objections away with confidence in science, the War Department's legal authority, and statistics showing that vaccination had all but eliminated smallpox and typhoid from the ranks. One memo to Secretary Baker simply stated, "To protect our allies and ourselves against these diseases, compulsory vaccination in the army is necessary."[67] Baker agreed.

Gorgas was equally enthusiastic about stamping out sexually transmitted diseases, which were the greatest cause for sick report in the army and took longer to cure than many injuries and other illnesses. Physicians encountered thousands of these infections as men entered military service, and national leaders worried that others might acquire new infections on camp furloughs and take them home to their wives and girlfriends with dire consequences such as blindness, sterility, and insanity. That would be a national scandal.[68] Doctors did have new tools against syphilis: the Wasserman blood test enabled them to diagnosis a syphilis infection, and Salvarsan, an arsenic-based injectable medication, was the first effective treatment. Developed in 1906, it was a pioneer in chemotherapy, and although treatment took several weeks and had harsh side effects, it could cure the disease.[69] Leaders thus exhorted soldiers, sailors, and marines to remain "Fit to Fight" for their country, clean for their wives, and, as Woodrow Wilson wrote, "straight in everything, and pure and clean through and through."[70]

Unlike many Americans at the time, the army surgeon general was not afraid to talk about sex and health. In a rambling speech to the American Public Health Association, "The Venereal Diseases and the War," Gorgas outlined the army's four-pronged attack on sexually transmitted disease. The first was recreation to distract men from activities involving alcohol and sex; next, law enforcement and penalties for men who got sick; third, medical treatment; and finally, education on the causes and dangers of infection.[71] Gorgas explained that his thirty years in sanitation taught him the importance of education—including moral education—on the causes and consequences of disease. He then segued to the importance of mosquito mitigation against yellow fever and malaria. Upon returning to the subject at hand, he suggested that if men could be more like women and use less tobacco and alcohol, and not try to be so manly, "venereal disease prevention would be far on the road to success." He closed the speech remarking that "like the Irish potato and turkey," yellow fever and syphilis were brought to the Western Hemisphere when Columbus discovered the Americas.[72] Gorgas could relate anything to yellow fever.

## OPTIMISM AND UNEASE

Gorgas understood that the physical welfare of men in the army fell to his Medical Department "from the time of their entry into active service until they are discharged."[73] While the duty of the military doctor was to care for the wounded and the sick, and return them to duty as soon as possible, Gorgas knew that an even more important mission was to prevent soldiers from getting sick in the first place. In speeches, interviews, and columns, he became adept at reviewing how the Army Medical Department's medical screening, sanitation and personal hygiene, good nutrition, vaccinations, and modern medicine were making American soldiers healthier and stronger than the general population. All of the old terrors of the army, he liked to say, "had been forced to surrender to science and sanitation."[74]

But fifty training camps of twenty thousand to forty thousand men presented a serious challenge. Despite the Medical Department's efforts, fatigue, exposure, and crowding made them easy targets for infections. "And the infections came," wrote one medical officer, explaining that as recruits moved from camp to camp by the thousands, they took with them "such diseases as they were incubating, thus infecting all camps."[75] Getting these men to France was equally difficult and dangerous, with crowded ports of embarkation and thousands of troops cheek-by-jowl on ships. Moreover, efforts to mobilize the economy to prepare a modern, industrialized army and navy were faltering, because the Wilson administration was reluctant to pivot from its domestic policy agenda and put the government fully on a war footing. The first draft call-up was in May 1917, but as men arrived in the training camps in September, uniforms, shoes, or blankets were in short supply, as were weapons and ammunition with which to train. Some trainees used sticks instead of rifles for practice maneuvers.

The War Department was struggling to mobilize, because its nineteenth-century organization was built on independent combat divisions whose commanding generals competed for weapons and supplies in the decentralized, free-market American economy. The lack of national economic coordination led to chaos as industries and government agencies struggled to secure raw materials and goods such as steel and flour and even typewriters. Civilian and military sectors of the economy were competing over resources as well. The railroads' lack of coordination almost paralyzed transportation, so that by late 1917 the industry asked for government regulation. That fall, with only one American unit, the First Division, training with the French in the trenches on the Western Front, some members of Congress began to discuss legislation to create a special "war cabinet" to manage the effort.

With the War Department in disarray, when Pershing wired the army leadership repeatedly for more personnel and weapons, the unwieldy bureaucracy often failed to meet his demands. Tensions developed in the medical services as well. Pershing and the War Department created a Chief Surgeon's Office, separate from the OTSG, to support the AEF in France, but problems developed between the two offices from the outset. Gorgas, loyal to a fault, recommended the aging H. C. Bradley to be AEF chief surgeon. Pershing wanted Merritte Ireland, but Gorgas insisted on Bradley, who was already with the British medical services as an observer and was the senior Medical Corps officer, so Pershing accepted him, with Ireland as his second-in-charge. Although Gorgas gave Bradley authority over AEF medical personnel and operations similar to that which he held over the Medical

Department at home, things did not always go smoothly.[76] In one small example, Ireland requested food inspectors to improve the food supplies in the camps and made the initial request to Gorgas's office January 18, 1918, but Pershing cabled the request again on February 15, and not until March 1 did Gorgas advise that six inspectors would be sent. The offices also disagreed on the number of ambulance companies for the AEF. Ireland requested forty-eight, but Gorgas said he could send him thirty-one, until Ireland again enlisted Pershing and the additional ambulances were sent.[77] Ireland also complained that the OTSG's organization plans for the mobile hospitals were not sent to him for several months, so that he had to develop his own plans.[78] Also contributing to the tension between Gorgas and the AEF medical services was the problem of Gorgas's divided devotions. "Even during the busiest periods of the war," wrote Franklin Martin, putting a positive gloss on it, "the officials of the International Health Board could count upon [Gorgas's] enthusiastic co-operation and advice pertaining to epidemics in different sections of the tropics." Gorgas's hope, Martin explained, was "that when the war ended, he could have a part in abolishing yellow fever from the earth."[79]

In October 1917 Gorgas ordered Robert Noble to inspect a number of training camps, and he reported back that the majority of the camps were doing the best they could. Most of the medical staff was competent, and the only serious medical problem was that large numbers of men were arriving at the camps with syphilis and gonorrhea. Much of the barracks and hospital construction, however, as well as procurement of supplies for the coming cold weather would not be completed in time for the arrival of thousands of draftees.[80] The next month the government's information bureau, the Committee for Public Information, created to rally support for the war effort, delivered an upbeat assessment under the heading, "General Sanitary Inspector in Report Shows That Health of Soldiers in Camp Averages Better than That of Civilians."[81]

But in December 1917 the war news darkened. With revolution in Russia and the collapse of the Russian Army on the Eastern Front, the Germans were redeploying their troops to the west while the US mobilization effort faltered. The Allied cause was therefore in the balance when several congressional committees began hearings on the stalled mobilization. Their inquiries at first focused on supply shortages and problems with military procurement of small arms and ammunition.[82] Then the boys in the training camps started getting sick.

# CHAPTER 16

# Doctors vs. Officers

## *Challenging the Army Hierarchy in the Name of Medicine*

You know, I am just an advisory officer. I have
no direct authority anywhere.

—William Gorgas, before the Senate Committee on Military Affairs, March 1918

GEN. WILLIAM GORGAS, THE CAREER army man, respected the chain of command. Franklin Martin remembered how the surgeon general was unwilling to go to Secretary of War Baker's office without an invitation. Baker himself told Gorgas to feel free to come see him whenever he had something to discuss, but Martin had to get Baker's secretary to phone Gorgas, asking him to meet with the secretary. Gorgas kept the relationship formal, but not everyone was as deferential.[1] As thousands of civilian doctors and scientists joined the Army Medical Corps, they chafed at the military regimen and resented having to obey orders from superior officers whom many considered their social inferiors. They complained so much that the *Military Surgeon* published an editorial exhorting physicians to be good soldiers and obey their superior officers. "Whatever our age or former position in civil life may have been, however superior we may feel ourselves to those of higher rank, socially or intellectually, it is not for us to argue or to question, but to obey," pleaded the journal.[2]

Gorgas also defended the chain of command. The United States had been born in rebellion, creating "a species of men and women who could think and act for themselves without reference to other people," he wrote. The current emergency, however, meant "we are all of us public servants . . . to be of use to our country in its hour of need." He recognized that many of the medical officers in his department were civilians, new to the military, and had left family and home and sacrificed lucrative practices to serve their country. They must nevertheless give up their individuality and learn to be "wheels and cogs in the great military machine." Although doctors had to be competent and think for themselves, they must also "do whatever is asked of them without question and with all their might and main."[3] Gorgas's own ability to submit to his superior officers, however, would be tested.

## MEASLES

Just as medical officers feared, in late 1917 epidemics of communicable diseases—measles, mumps, scarlet fever, meningitis, and pneumonia—seized the training camps, sickening thousands of trainees, killing hundreds, and igniting a political storm. While measles and mumps regularly circulated in large populations, conferring immunity to people as children, many rural communities—which comprised fully half of the country in 1917—could go untouched for years. Consequently, when measles arrived in the training camps, the virus found fertile ground. The disease began to appear in October, and by mid-November case rates were as high as 30 percent in some camps. In Camp Wheeler in Georgia, the hospital admission rate reached 534 per 1,000 men.[4] Scientists had not yet identified the measles virus, but medical officers knew that it was highly infectious, transmitted through the respiratory tract, and that one attack conferred lifetime immunity. They also knew the illness could be complicated by secondary bacterial pneumonia, which killed one in four patients and debilitated survivors for weeks. As Vaughan observed, "measles and pneumonia are so closely associated in military camps that it is well to consider them together."[5] In 1917 measles-associated-pneumonia constituted 30 percent of army mortalities. During the entire war period, measles caused more than ninety thousand hospital admissions, 2,200 deaths, and more than 1.7 million "non-effective days" among soldiers.[6]

Medical officers attributed the epidemics not only to the virgin soil of rural trainees who had no immunity but also to the army's rejection of Gorgas and his colleagues' recommendations to improve trainee living conditions.[7] Vaughan charged that insufficient clothing, lack of heat in the housing, and overcrowding in tents, barracks, and hospitals "have been potent in the development of the pneumonia among our soldiers, and for these deficiencies the medical corps is not responsible."[8] The War Department was not being economical, either, because treating infectious patients required a great deal of resources. Medical Department instructions included segregating patients by disease; providing 1,000 cubic feet of air space per patient; screening between beds to prevent cross-infection; equipping medical attendants with gowns and face masks; rigorous ward hygiene; and keeping patients in the hospital for ten days after their fevers subsided.[9]

Without direct authority over troops, Gorgas and the Medical Department used sanitary inspections as levers to convince the War Department leadership and line officers to follow their advice, much as he had done regarding mosquito work in Cuba and Panama.[10] His staff made more than a thousand inspections during the war, visiting every medical station at least once, and camps and hospitals many times. As measles burned through the camps, Gorgas went on an inspection tour with Vaughan and Welch from November 26 to December 17, inspecting camps in seven states: Wheeler in Georgia, Sevier in South Carolina, Bowie in Texas, Beauregard in Louisiana, Pike in Arkansas, Funston in Kansas, and Doniphan in Oklahoma.[11] They visited sick wards, interviewed medical personnel, attended autopsies, inspected camp latrines and kitchens, and everywhere measured the square footage in the barracks and tents. During these inspections Gorgas made it a point to share at least one meal with patients in the hospital mess to sample the food they were served, and he insisted that his inspectors do the same.[12] After each visit he fired off telegrams with recommendations to the army chief of staff, followed by pointed memos of his findings.

Gorgas and his team found that recruits were arriving at training camps that were still under construction. Army quartermasters were building armories before hospitals, so that many of the hospitals were without heat, running water, and well-managed kitchens when they admitted the first patients. Most camps also fell short of the recommended fifty square feet floor space per man, and Gorgas reiterated his recommendations for quarantining the sick, halting the arrival of new men into a camp during an epidemic, and establishing observation camps for new recruits to avoid bringing in new infections.[13] From Camp Beauregard in Louisiana Gorgas recommended "that no more men be sent to this camp until the division commander is prepared to care for them along the lines of the above recommendations." At Camp Wheeler, in addition to measles and pneumonia, they found meningitis, scarlet fever, and mumps. Camp Sevier had 2,000 cases of measles, 60 deaths from pneumonia, and no wool clothing for the men. The weather was cold, and "the whole command is still in khaki," Gorgas reported. At Camp Funston in Kansas, he charged that the post commander was delaying action on their recommendations.[14] Despite such problems, Gorgas remained upbeat, assuring his superiors that the situation could be brought under control if the army would follow his advice. Many commanders, however, were reluctant to adopt such measures, because they cost time and money, and the exigencies of military mobilization demanded speed and efficiency. This time, however, the conflict between the surgeon general's Medical Department and the War Department's line command would be aired in congressional conference rooms.

## THE "GORGAS REPORT"

Returning from their inspections, Gorgas and his colleagues combined their field notes into a final report to Secretary Baker, "Sanitary Conditions at Army Camps." Once it became public, it was dubbed the "Gorgas Report" and became a political football. The report could not have come at a worse time for President Wilson's administration because his War Department was clearly not prepared to manage a modern, industrial, million-man army, and the French and British armies, bloodied and depleted from three years of war, were waiting desperately for American troops. With fewer than 150,000 in France, Pershing was constantly cabling from Europe for men, weapons, and supplies.

Gorgas's report therefore received extensive coverage in the national press. The *Cincinnati Enquirer* announced, "Fear Is Shown by Gorgas over Danger of Pneumonia in American Army Camps," while a *New York Times* headline announced, "Gorgas Reports Troops at Camps Crowded, Ill-Clad."[15] Secretary Baker sought to blunt the criticism the next day by announcing that the army had already complied with most of the surgeon general's recommendations; Gorgas did not make any statements to the press to the contrary.[16] But as new recruits arrived home in caskets just weeks after they had enlisted, horrified families wrote and wired their elected officials, demanding information and better care for their sons, brothers, and husbands.[17] The Gorgas report offered a powerful critique of the mobilization effort and provided ammunition to members of Congress who were determined to find out what was going wrong. The congressional hearings that had begun regarding the inefficiencies of Wilson's war mobilization now focused as well on health issues. Measles and pneumonia took center stage.

Members of Congress who visited the camps did not like what they saw. After a trip before Christmas to Camp Mills on Long Island, where men from Montana and other western states were quartered, Rep. Jeanette Rankin (R-MT), the first woman member of Congress, found "shocking conditions of sanitation and health" and called for an inquiry.[18] Other members did the same. To make matters worse, the winter of 1917–1918 turned out to be one of the coldest in years. When members of Congress went home for the holidays, they encountered constituents angry about the poor conditions in the camps, and when they returned to Washington, several took up Gorgas's call for more clothing, less crowding, and more medical personnel. Members read parts of the Gorgas Report in the House and Senate chambers, and the House published it in the *Congressional Record* on

January 8, 1918, as House Document 806, "Sanitary Conditions at Army Camps," with thirty-three thousand copies printed.[19]

Wilson and Baker resented congressional interference with the war effort and resisted reforms, but by mid-January, events were forcing them to act. In addition to food and fuel shortages, the first member of Congress to join the army, Rep. Augustus Gardner (R-MA), died of pneumonia in Camp Wheeler.[20] Former President Theodore Roosevelt even weighed in with a speech at the Washington Press Club criticizing sanitation in the camps and war mobilization.[21] Then, in late January, Sen. George E. Chamberlain, Democrat from Oregon and the powerful chairman of the Senate Committee on Military Affairs, launched a public critique of the Wilson administration's conduct of the war mobilization. In a three-hour speech on the floor of the Senate he charged that the military establishment of the United States had "fallen down," because of "inefficiency in every bureau and in every department of the Government of the United States."[22] He cited shortages of coal to heat the camps, of clothing, bedding, and other supplies for the trainees, as well as the lack of rifles, mortars and other ordnance for training. The president did not know the true conditions in the camps, he suggested, because the War Department had misinformed him.

The most explosive charges concerned the health of the soldiers, and Chamberlain turned to Gorgas's inspections, saying that "nearly all of the deaths and the epidemics at the cantonments could have been avoided if the War Department had been efficient and effective." Brandishing Gorgas's report, he charged that "the hundreds and thousands of young men who are dying in all of these encampments, [are doing so] due to the inefficiency of the War Department itself."[23] Chamberlain read letters from families who found their sons lying in filthy beds in the camps or received their sons' remains in "mortified" condition, not even in uniform, and charged that if the War Department had complied with Gorgas's repeated calls for fifty square feet of floor space per person in the camps, "I doubt if there would have been one-half of the deaths that there have been."[24] The *New York Times* carried the full text of the chairman's speech, and scolded Wilson when he tried to brush off the criticism. "This is not, after all, the Administration's war; it is the people's war, supported by their blood and treasure," the *Times* stated. "Since they pay the cost, . . . their criticism cannot, with safety, be disregarded."[25]

## DUEL

When Congress called on Gorgas and Baker to testify, their responses opened a rift between the two men personally and revealed tensions between the Medical Department and War Department leaderships. Appearing before a Senate committee on January 25, Gorgas avoided blaming soldiers' sickness and mortality on individual camp commanders' failure to take his advice but seemed eager to have Congress intervene on his side against the War Department brass. When asked what caused the epidemics, Gorgas blamed overcrowding and said that memos he had sent to the General Staff recommending sixty square feet of floor space per man in army housing had been ignored. As to why his recommendations to increase housing facilities at Forts Oglethorpe and Riley had not been acted upon, Gorgas responded, "I know of no reason except getting a decision on it from the General Staff."[26] The *New York Times* declared the next day: "Gorgas Ascribes Deaths to Haste," reporting that "in its haste to answer the call from France and England the Government sent many young Americans to their death from disease."[27] Papers across the country had similar headlines. The *Atlanta Constitution* reported, "Soldiers Dying in Camps from Lack of Clothing and Being Overcrowded"; the *Hartford Courant* charged, "Overcrowding and Poor Sanitary Conditions Blamed for Epidemics in Camps"; and the *San Francisco Chronicle* reported, "Camp Greene Is Unsanitary Says Gorgas."[28] As the surgeon general questioned the judgment of his superior officers, members of Congress began to take sides. Rep. Philip Campbell (R-KS) suggested that the report was "very offensive to the Secretary of War," while Charles Reavis (R-NE) captured the dire nature of the conflict. "If we have boys in the encampments who are being sacrificed, they ought to be sacrificed for the country and not by the country."[29]

Amid the outcry Baker offered his resignation to Wilson but, after the president refused it, threw himself into defending the administration's mobilization policies.[30] He did so at the expense of Gorgas and the Medical Corps. While Baker acknowledged problems with war mobilization, he told the Senate investigative committee on January 28 that he wanted to correct any view that the War Department was not up to the job of conducting the war. He conceded that some camps were crowded but insisted that he had consulted Gorgas and other army medical leaders on the housing problem, and they had agreed with him not to halt construction but to provide more tents to relieve crowding.[31] When senators asked Baker why the construction of camp hospitals was postponed, he said they had first thought that men would not be in the camps long enough to get sick, but then that view changed.[32] He spoke of the seriousness with which he and the War Department took the welfare of the soldiers and asked that the Senate view the problems as exceptions, "not a sign the whole effort had fallen down." He claimed that it was he, after all, who had sent Gorgas to inspect the epidemics in the camps and he who then released the report to the newspapers, showing that, "in the first place, I wanted no concealment; and in the second place, I wanted the help of the country in correcting those conditions."[33]

But Baker was not done. He pivoted to blame the Medical Department for health conditions by pointing out that medical officers were primarily responsible for the health (and sickness) of the recruits. In an extraordinary move, he brought up two courts martial in late 1917 in which army physicians had been tried and convicted for the deaths of recruits from pneumonia. The courts having determined that the patients had died from medical neglect, the physicians were summarily dismissed from the army. But Baker sanctimoniously told the committee that he and Wilson had recommended imprisonment. "I want the country to know," he declared, "that the lives and welfare and the illnesses of these soldiers are a responsibility which I will not permit to be dodged or handled in any cavalier fashion."[34] Taken aback, Gorgas reviewed the court-martial proceedings but did not defend the officers. He promised to "weed out 'medical incompetents'" in the training camps and told the committee that the department had discharged 854 physicians who were "not equal to the work."[35] When Congressman Ashton Shallenberger (D-NE) asked Gorgas, "Have you ever tried shooting medical officers for neglecting their men? Have medical officers ever been executed for such things as that?" Gorgas calmly replied, "The medical officer is subject to the same articles of war as every other soldier."[36] But the damage was done. One representative finally asked Gorgas, "If there has been any lack of health conditions there, and any blame is attached to anyone, it would be chargeable to you, would it not?" Gorgas replied, "Yes."[37]

The Senate and House interrogations dragged on over several days. The most difficult were inquiries about individual soldiers, when committee members brought telegrams and letters from grieving parents about sick or dying soldiers and asked for Gorgas's response. Private Albert Hestwood had died of meningitis at Camp Doniphan, Oklahoma, and his father, a minister, requested an inquiry. Gorgas looked into it and found that Hestwood had been sent to the wrong hospital ward, so did not get the proper care.[38] Another member brought up the case of a Texas man who buried both of his boys in December 1917; one of them had died in his summer clothes at Camp Bowie, near Fort Worth, during one of the coldest winters on record. "My poor son died, but he didn't die for his country; he died for want of care and nourishment." All Gorgas could say was that he had recently been to Camp Bowie and that conditions were improving.[39] As Congress investigated the Wilson administration's war effort, Gorgas also testified on Medical Department appropriations for the next year, and House committee members were also rough on him. He told one committee that "while we have made mistakes and may make other mistakes, I can assure you that we will endeavor not to the make the same mistake twice."[40]

The congressional investigation was the worst professional experience Gorgas had ever had. He told Mamie, "Just at present I am having a pretty hard time. All my friends seem to have deserted me & everybody is giving me a kick as I pass by."[41] He commiserated with his British counterpart, Keogh. "I am just in the midst of a Congressional investigation in which all sins, sins both of omission and commission are being shown up." Of the criticism, he said, "I had never before believed that I could be quite as bad as it appears that I am."[42] Keogh sympathized. "We have to bear these crosses," he said, because administration was a mystery to medical men and bureaucrats knew nothing of medicine, "so we have to bear with two sets of ignorant people."[43]

The political tension continued into February as Gorgas and his staff pursued their inspections, and members of Congress continued to use their reports to criticize the War Department. Touring Camp Greene, North Carolina, on February 12, Gorgas found that sick rates were not high among the forty thousand trainees, but conditions were unsanitary, with knee-deep mud, a fuel shortage, no sewage system installed, and overcrowding, with eight or more men in tents designed for five. Congressman Edwin Webb (D-NC) took Gorgas's inspection report to the floor of the House on February 22 and demanded action. He too had visited Camp Greene and found "the pick and flower of the young manhood of this country, ready to lay down their lives, if necessary, for their country." But, he cried, to applause on the House floor, "the Government of the United States has no right to ask the boys to die ignominiously like rats in a mud pen."[44] Gorgas and the OTSG kept the pressure on and went so far as to recommend that the next draft be delayed until the camp hospitals were prepared to receive the sick. The adjutant general denied the request, due to the "urgent needs for men in organizations high on the priority list for foreign service."[45]

By March health conditions in the camps were improved, and the Wilson administration was gaining control of the war effort by imposing more national economic planning on American industries and agriculture. Even in December 1917, Baker had begun to address the problems by naming George Goethals acting quartermaster, to bring his administrative prowess to the army's struggling construction, supply, and transport programs. He also recalled Gen. Peyton March from France to be the army's new chief of staff, and he immediately began to reorganize the War Department to be more efficient. Baker and Wilson thus fended off legislation to create a war council and a munitions bureau, and instead Congress gave Wilson new executive powers to conduct the war effort.[46] Mobilization soon accelerated so that by the spring of 1918, a year after the United States entered the war, 300,000 well-equipped American soldiers were arriving in France every month.

While the Medical Department had suffered blows during the hearings, it emerged from the controversy strengthened, because the public attention on health conditions had forced army officials to improve living conditions in the camps and increase medical personnel. The department report for 1918 nevertheless concluded that many of the deaths from disease could have been prevented "if the country and the department had been willing to purchase that advantage by delaying the calling and training of the soldiers until thoroughly satisfactory arrangements for clothing, housing, and caring for them had been matured."[47] These were serious charges. The public outcry and finger-pointing had also scarred Gorgas and damaged the relationship between the secretary of war and his army surgeon general.

## MEDICAL DEPARTMENT, MEDICAL BUREAUCRACY

As the army grew, so too did the Medical Department. The Medical Corps increased from 443 officers to more than 30,000; from 400 nurses to more than 21,000; and from 7,000 enlisted men such as hospital stewards to 281,000. The number of army hospital beds increased more than fortyfold, from about 9,500 beds in 1917 to more than 400,000, with 120,900 beds in the United States, and almost 290,000 in hospitals in Europe.[48] Given this constant growth, one of Gorgas's most important roles was presenting budget requests for the Medical Department to Congress, and this was a moving target. In his first years as surgeon general, the budgets were less than one million dollars; the Army Medical Department appropriation for fiscal year 1916 was $750,000, based on a military force of 100,000 officers and men, or an allowance of $7.50 per man per year for medical services.[49] Gorgas's OTSG developed formulas for the various medical units, such as the supplies and equipment required for a hospital of 1,000 beds, or the medical field supplies required for an army division, which could then be multiplied by the number of hospitals or divisions the War Department deployed. As the army grew, the medical requirements grew accordingly. Thus, when the OTSG made estimates in March 1917, it calculated $24,780,000 for an army of one million, about $25 per year per man, and then a few months later submitted an additional request of $29,800,000 for the second million men.[50] During the war, Medical Department appropriations therefore grew from $35,000,000 for fiscal year 1917, to $134,000,000 for 1918, and then $297,000,000 for 1919. These funds accounted for less than 3 percent of army war expenditures.[51]

The Medical Department also acquired more responsibilities as new fields of medical care emerged out of the Great War, and William Gorgas went to Capitol Hill with his notebooks and calm demeanor to ask congressional committees to allocate funds for these new fields. The war saw the advent of chemical weapons that caused severe injuries to skin, eyes, and lungs, even death, and the Medical

Department became responsible not only for caring for the injured but for selecting and distributing gas masks for men and horses to fend off attacks of chlorine and mustard gas. In 1917, therefore, Gorgas added a new line item of $10,000,000 for the Gas Defense Service in his department.[52] Another new field was military psychiatry. Some military personnel were so severely traumatized by violence that they could no longer function or go into battle. British and French medical officers had been trying to better understand the psychological injuries of war and develop ways to treat patients, rather than punish them as criminals for cowardice. Gorgas therefore sent three distinguished civilian psychiatrists to Europe to study the problem of mental and nervous disorders in war, especially "shell shock," known today as Post-traumatic Stress Disorder. The AEF consequently established rest camps to care for men near the battlefields, and the Medical Department designated specialized hospitals for shellshock victims in the United States.[53]

Gorgas's Medical Department was also instrumental in the establishment of reconstructive medicine during the war.[54] Medical and surgical advances meant that soldiers were surviving wounds that would have killed them in earlier wars, but they also required plastic surgery, prosthetics, and physical reconstruction to restore them to active, productive lives. In August 1917 Gorgas established a division for physical reconstruction, and the OSTG staff developed plans for a system of hospitals dedicated to different disabilities, and the facilities, staffing, and training required to operate them.[55] For its part, Congress passed the War Risk Insurance Act in October 1917 to provide "rehabilitation and re-education of all disabled soldiers." This, however, created a benefit without a government apparatus to deliver it; the Veterans Bureau had not yet been established. Gorgas therefore had to explain to a House appropriations committee, "The War Risk Bureau has informed us that they will expect us to take care of such men."[56]

Historian Beth Linker describes how prior to the establishment of the Veterans Bureau in 1921, the Army Medical Department and Gorgas took the lead in reconstruction and rehabilitation. "Rehabilitation was born as a Progressive Era idea," she writes, "and took shape as a military medical specialty, and eventually became a societal norm in the civilian section."[57] Gorgas and his OSTG quickly adopted the multidisciplinary nature of reconstruction medicine, believing that education and medicine could work "hand in hand" for the benefit of the patient.[58] His goal was a "maximum cure" for patients under the Medical Department's care, and he directed that "physical reconstruction be defined as the completest form of medical and surgical treatment carried to a point where maximum functional restoration, mental and physical, had been secured."[59] This was an early recognition that care for disabled soldiers and sailors was a matter for government, not just the individual.

Gorgas gave several speeches on this topic. In late 1917 he told businessmen in Chicago that for every million men in the army, he expected that each year about 100,000 men would come home because they "will never be able to return to the firing line." His department was therefore establishing special reconstruction hospitals for men who had lost limbs or been blinded or whose lungs had been damaged by gas or tuberculosis, so that they could be healed as much as possible and gain new skills to enable them to make a living. "The care that will be given them will be principally to fit them for their avocations in civil life," he explained, and thus the hospitals "will be more teaching centers than surgical or medical centers."[60]

But all of these new programs and the exploding size of the army took a toll. The OTSG was under siege. Arriving at Gorgas's office one day, Harvey Cushing, the surgeon who had taken the Harvard mobile hospital to France, was alarmed to see piles of unopened mail on Gorgas's desk and the surgeon general "still answering his own telephone which is not even in reach of his chair." Acting as his deputy was William Welch, seated at a desk "answering the telephone and helping in other ways to handle the mounting volume of correspondence."[61] This did not seem to be the best use of the venerable pathologist. But there was a mountain of mail because the war unleashed a firehose of government reports, military orders, and letters from people across the country. By mid-1918 Gorgas's office was handling over 150,000 pieces of mail and 9,500 telegrams a month.[62] Letters came from physicians and citizens asking for information on their loved ones or on Medical Department policy. Others offered their services to the Medical Department or prescriptions for "medicines" and "treatments" for ailing soldiers. The White House and other government agencies also "bucked" queries concerning medical issues and social welfare to the OTSG for response. One of many odd proposals was from a man from Pennsylvania who called for a tax on dogs to encourage the destruction of unnecessary mouths to feed and to help pay for the war. (Gorgas was not a supporter).[63] When Senator Benjamin Tillman (D-SC) alleged that English and French army surgeons were conducting surgery without anesthesia, Furbush replied that it was "absolutely untrue," and that the OTSG was, in fact, "being constantly annoyed by receiving copies of the chain letter referred to in your communication."[64]

Gorgas turned to the national media to assure the public of his department's commitment to soldiers' health. He told *JAMA,* for example, that while parents whose sons were killed in battle may reconcile themselves to death for a worthy cause, he recognized that "if they have reason to fear that their sons have been neglected when sick or wounded, they develop a spirit of bitterness for which there can be no antidote."[65] Dashing in his dress uniform, trim and white-headed, he appeared in the *Leslie's Weekly* series "Men Who Are Winning the War," which declared that because of his record in conquering disease, "the health of our men in the field will be safe-guarded better than that of any other army in the world."[66] Gorgas apparently agreed, answering the *Ladies' Home Journal* question, "Is my boy really healthy in camp?" with soothing words. "No safeguard is omitted. The result is that the American army is the healthiest, best cared for army in the world today."[67]

When reporter Mary Mullet interviewed the surgeon general in March 1918, for *American Magazine*, she found "just what every father and mother of a soldier would have him be—simple, human, direct; unhurried yet efficient; a man of few words but with a fact behind every word." Gorgas believed that army life was improving American manhood. "I've seen these sallow, pasty young clerks get out and turn into Men! I've seen young chaps who were little more than flabby human jellyfish transformed by their life in the trenches into husky fellows that were grit clean through." He asserted, "It was their life as soldiers that gave them this new possession."[68] Gorgas also eagerly reviewed advances in medicine that were improving the treatment of the wounded. Americans had benefited from the Allies' medical experiences over the last three years, and survival rates were improving with the advent of antiseptic surgery, X-rays for finding bullets and fractures, antitetanus serum, surgical expertise, and specialization such as bone-grafting and plastic surgery. In an article entitled, "The Credit Side of Our War Ledger," Gorgas wrote that "the stupendousness of the task of properly safeguarding the health of our soldiers" was making young men healthier and providing physicians with new medical and surgical knowledge.[69]

Home life also provided a haven for Gorgas from the hard work and congressional criticism, with Marie working at a Red Cross unit in Washington, and Aileen and the grandchildren close by.[70] His eyes continued to bother him, though, and Theo was treating him for asthma. Unable to hunt or hike in Washington, Gorgas got his exercise by walking more than a mile to work and climbing seven flights of stairs to his office instead of taking the elevator.[71] Several times a week, he also joined a group of federal officials for morning exercise sessions. It was a high-powered group including the attorney general and the secretaries of interior, labor, and treasury. They met at the Washington home of a former congressman at 7:30 a.m. to work with a trainer for fifteen minutes, walk (and no doubt talk) for thirty minutes, and then have breakfast.[72] Gorgas also kept his sense of humor. When his cousin George Denegre gave him a watch with an alarm, Gorgas told him that he was in a New York hotel the first time it went off, and he feared that his startled reaction was "unsoldierly." It reminded him of the children's play [*Peter Pan*] about the alligator who swallowed an alarm clock and when it sounded convulsed in contortions. "I felt very much like the alligator," he told Denegre.[73]

Another day he teased Victor Vaughan after a meeting to hammer out an important medical policy. "This is your judgement and it is mine," Gorgas said with a twinkle in his eye. "But remember that your judgement and mine have at times been at fault. Do you recollect the burning of the village of Siboney in 1898 in order to stamp out yellow fever? I have often wondered how many infected mosquitoes were killed in that conflagration."[74]

## RANK AND PROMOTION FOR MEDICAL OFFICERS

If Gorgas was getting pressure from the Congress, from Pershing and Ireland in the AEF, and from regular citizens, some of the greatest tensions developed between Gorgas and the General Staff concerning the promotion of career Medical Corps officers and increased rank for officers of the Medical Reserve. Military rank ordered everything in the army and was the basis for pay, living conditions, authority, and status in the army. The National Defense Act of 1916 had authorized seven medical officers per thousand soldiers, but now the military rank of those officers was at issue. As thousands of civilian physicians swelled the Medical Department, career Medical Corps officers in the United States and the AEF expected to rise in the ranks like officers in other army departments. New medical officers were commissioned as lieutenants and with time and experience advanced up the ranks to captain and major. Only 3 percent of the Medical Corps could rise to colonels and majors, however, and they had to wait for colonels to die or retire before they could be promoted to those rare positions. There were only nine brigadier general positions and one major general in the corps.

But disagreements among the upper brass, administrative snags, and outright mistakes stymied the promotion process. Some career officers blamed Gorgas and his OTSG for the problems even years after the war. Kean charged that while they were "busy making promotions at home, they showed no very great concern for the medical personnel in France."[75] This was not the case. Historian Mary Gillett spreads the blame, writing that "for unexplained reasons" Pershing's headquarters was slow to forward promotion recommendations to the War Department, that one list of promotions was lost in the mail, and that the delays were also due to conflicts between Pershing and Army Chief of Staff Peyton C. March.[76] Kean harbored resentment for years, but another officer in the OTSG credited Gorgas's efforts, remembering his frustration when the General Staff approved only 30 of the first 225 names he submitted for promotion, only after Gorgas brought the subject to Baker's attention. "The narrow mindedness evidenced in this matter by certain members of the General Staff," the officer wrote, was "repugnant" to Gorgas's sense of justice.[77]

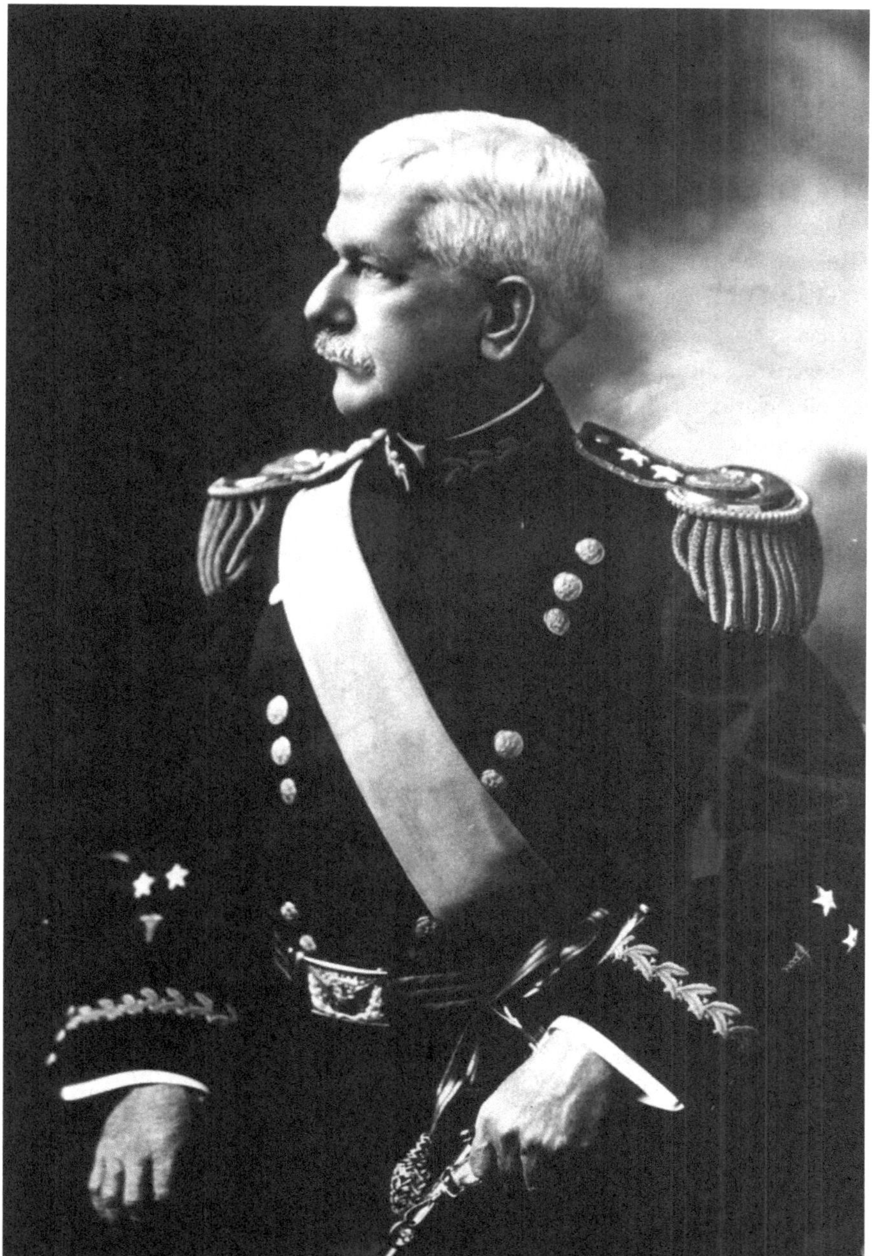

FIGURE 16.1. Major General W. C. Gorgas, Surgeon General of the Army, July 22, 1917. National Library of Medicine.

Gorgas was especially rankled that Medical Reserve Corps officers of the stature of his National Academy of Science physicians like Mayo, Cushing, Welch, and Vaughan, and others would be mere captains or majors.[78] This made them subordinate to English and French medical officers who were colonels and generals, a situation Franklin Martin described as a "humiliation to the Americans." The General Medical Board proposed legislation to increase rank, pay, and benefits for medical officers to make the Medical Corps more attractive to civilian physicians.[79] They had a powerful ally in the US Senate, Robert L. Owen (D-OK), whose brother, William O. Owen, was a medical officer. He introduced legislation in the Senate to make 5 percent of all medical officers generals, and 12 percent colonels, adding fifty generals and 120 colonels per thousand medical officers. The purpose, Owen explained, was to ensure that "the sanitary regulations and recommendations made by the medical officers should not be lightly set aside by a line officer of superior rank."[80] Rep. Leonidas Dyer (R-MO) introduced a similar bill in the House, but Baker, Chief of Staff Peyton March, and the General Staff opposed the legislation, arguing that medical officers did not need additional grades and that they did not command troops like line officers did, anyway.[81]

Gorgas disagreed. Medical officers may not have regiments or brigades under their authority, but running a hospital of five hundred beds and dozens of doctors, nurses, and orderlies was indeed a matter of command. Testifying before Congress, he explained that because medical officers can only advise army line officers with regard to sanitary, medical, and surgical services, they need enhanced military rank in addition to their professional knowledge to convince the commanders of the importance of such measures. He had to assure worried members of Congress that army surgeons would not leave the operating room for administrative duties once promoted.[82] He also pointed out the number of illustrious physicians in the Medical Reserve Corps and that six members of the Reserve had already been killed in the war. It was not fair that "these men, thousands of them coming in from civil life, should be given so much less reward than the men in any other branch of the service." It was a matter of "justice."[83]

Baker and March did agree to fix responsibility for camp health and sanitation on post commanders to clarify accountability but disapproved most of Gorgas's recommendation, such as including medical officers in military planning.[84] At one hearing Gorgas agreed that medical officers should not be able to overrule line commanders regarding camp conditions, because "we are to fight, and we have to whip the Germans, and everything has to be secondary to that." But increased rank would give "weight" to their role as advisory officers. When a senator asked Gorgas how often their advice was discounted, he replied, "Very frequently," and offered the example of a medical officer at a port of embarkation who had cautioned against bringing men to the camp until the hospital was ready. When troops arrived anyway, he "was overwhelmed with sick and they were not properly taken care of."[85] Medical officers, including Gorgas himself, wanted respect and the authority to do their jobs.[86]

Gorgas had at times been reticent to challenge his superiors, but after the measles and pneumonia outbreaks in the camps and the ensuing criticism of his department, he became more willing to speak up and rally public support for the promotions bill. The AMA and other medical organizations supported increased rank, as did newspapers across the country.[87] When the General Staff continued to oppose the bill, Gorgas engaged in what the *Washington Post* called "sharp warfare" and went directly to Congress and President Wilson to ask for their support.[88] "Gorgas Appeals Direct to Congress; Goes over Heads of Superiors in Fight for Higher Rank for the Medical Reserve," wrote the *New York Times*. The surgeon general, the paper explained, was bringing the medical community in against the "old antagonism of the line officers to what they consider unjustifiable and harmful interference with their conduct of military operations." But by appealing to the president to support a policy opposed by Baker and General Staff, the *Times* observed, Gorgas had overstepped "the bounds of discipline" and thereby "invited punishment for insubordination."[89] Wilson, however, rewarded Gorgas's boldness on March 5, 1918, with a presidential endorsement of the "Owen-Dyer bill."[90]

Chief of Staff March was furious and summoned Gorgas and Martin to the War College to discuss their "pernicious activity in behalf of the Owen-Dyer bill." Gorgas, however, made no apologies, reiterated his case for the bill, and asserted that he was "in favor of the passage of the Owen-Dyer Bill, and would consider myself disloyal to my corps if I did not do everything in my power to bring about its passage."[91] Owen framed his bill dramatically as a matter of "the health and the sanitary, medical and surgical care of our beloved young men we are sending to battle" and attached the Owen-Dyer language to the military appropriations bill.[92] After Gorgas conceded that he would not insist on the specific number of officers, which was troubling some members of Congress, Owen trimmed the bill to approve almost two thousand colonels but limited general officers to just six. Peyton March then threatened a presidential veto of the whole military appropriations bill unless Gorgas dropped his demand for more generals—an extraordinary move in time of war. Gorgas held his ground. When he asked Franklin Martin what he would do, and Martin said he would not back down, the surgeon general responded, "I hoped you would say that. In my own mind I had already decided on that course."[93] He was therefore gratified and relieved when White House physician Adm. Cary Grayson advised Martin that the president would sign the bill. Gorgas had gone over and around Baker and March and had won. Congress passed the Owen-Dyer bill as part of an emergency war funding measure on July 9, 1918, and Wilson signed it.

This success, however, further frayed relations between Gorgas and his superiors. "A lot of us in the war department spent our time gathering up the ravelings where he cut red tape," Baker said of Gorgas two years later, "but we never restrained him."[94] That would not be entirely true. Gorgas had directly challenged army policies regarding mobilization, sanitation, the treatment of soldiers, and even military rank. He had also gone around the chain of command to Congress and the president to advocate for the Medical Corps and for the care of the soldiers. Although he won some battles, Gorgas's political machinations angered the War Department leadership, and they would find ways to punish his audacity.

PART V

# THE FINAL CAMPAIGNS, 1918–1920

CHAPTER 17

# General Gorgas Is "Retired for Age"

No medical officer can acquire fame in war, but every medical officer has the opportunity to do good.

—William Gorgas in 1918, quoted by Victor C. Vaughan

FRANKLIN MARTIN ALWAYS ADMIRED GORGAS'S open-door policy for staff and the public. Furbush had even set up three different offices for his boss to make it more difficult for people to find him.[1] One day late in August, the twenty-ninth, Martin went to the OTSG and found it empty except for Gorgas, who was meeting with a physician from Indiana about a Sanitary Corps commission for his son. After the man left, Gorgas greeted Martin, looking "a little distracted." Martin knew Gorgas had been ordered on an inspection tour of AEF medical services and asked when he was departing. Gorgas responded cryptically, "Doctor, at 3 o'clock I am going fishing." Martin asked, "General, when will you return?" and Gorgas replied, "Doctor, I don't know; when I am through with my fishing." Wrote Martin, "There were tears in the dear old fellow's eyes, and it was evidently a very trying moment for him." Gorgas "was leaving his desk, in all probability never to return as Surgeon General." He added dramatically, "His last official act was a kindness to a country doctor."[2]

Gorgas's retirement from military service was the culmination of his strained relations with the General Staff. The official line, which historians have followed, was that Gorgas retired because he had reached the customary retirement age of sixty-four.[3] It is more likely that Gorgas was eased out of office. Martin's story about "going fishing" and Gorgas's comments in his journal and letters to Marie show that he was reluctant to go.[4] Just eighteen months earlier, the Wilson administration had discouraged his retirement, because war was imminent, and they needed an experienced army surgeon general. Now they had four million men in uniform, half of them in the battlefields of France trying to drive back the deadly German offensive of 1918. Changing surgeons general in the middle of the war could be destabilizing, and firing a national hero would be politically delicate. Secretary Baker and the War Department therefore did it in a circuitous manner and kept Gorgas in the dark about his future until the very last.

## "RETIRED FOR AGE"

As early as February, during the contentious hearings in Congress, Gorgas told Carter, "I have had no intimation as to whether I'm to be retained after October the 3rd, the date when I retire by statute, or not. I am ready to serve anywhere in any capacity until the war is over." He added, "How, or where I serve, is the Secretary's business, not mine, and I am glad I have nothing to do with the decision."[5] In May 1918, however, as Gorgas was pushing the increased-rank bill, physicians across the country were lobbying to retain him in office. *JAMA* lauded Gorgas's work in recruiting physicians to military service, noting that men left their homes and practices to serve their country "due not only to patriotism, but also to their respect for and admiration of General Gorgas."[6] The *Birmingham Age-Herald* demanded that Gorgas be reappointed, and Seale Harris of the *Southern Medical Journal* asserted that Gorgas was "second in efficiency only to President Wilson."[7] If the president would not reappoint him, Seale argued, Congress should. Sen. Robert Owen, author of the increased-rank bill, did his part, telling Wilson that Gorgas was "admired and respected by the whole United States" and had "extraordinary capacity," unimpaired by age. "I believe it would serve the public interest if you intend to retain him in office," and, he wrote, "you should indicate it to him at an early date so he might adjust himself accordingly."[8] Wilson, however, would not be hurried.[9]

Baker and Wilson consulted with a number of people about who should succeed Gorgas but did not ask Gorgas himself. The two leading candidates were Merritte Ireland, whom Pershing had appointed as his chief medical officer for the AEF in May 1918, and Robert Noble, Gorgas's deputy. One morning in July, as they were riding in a car over to the War Department, Gorgas brought up his retirement with Martin. He "seemed to doubt that he would be retained as Surgeon General," Martin remembered, "as the Secretary had informed him that it had been his policy not to retain men in their old positions beyond the retiring age." Martin could not understand "why a man of the popularity of General Gorgas, and who in their opinion had made good in a magnificent way, should not be retained in office during the period of the war." He may, however, have sensed Gorgas's physical decline, because when Baker sought his counsel, Martin proposed keeping Gorgas on at least for the duration of the war or reappointing him surgeon general with two assistant surgeons general, Noble in the United States and Ireland in France.[10]

In August the *Military Surgeon* extolled Gorgas in editorials lauding his work in recruiting the medical profession to the war effort and in behalf of the men in the rank and file. "The country has given its sons into his keeping," stated the journal, "in every confidence that its trust will not be betrayed, and with firm resolve that this brave, able, modest soldier-physician shall in no way be unnecessarily hampered in his work for them, but heartily supported by all until this war is won."[11] That month Gorgas told John Ross that he had asked to serve to the end of the war, but feared he was to be retired on October 3. Nevertheless, he told his friend, "It is the Government's business and not mine as to how I serve."[12] Instead of speaking directly to Gorgas about his future, Baker ordered him on an AEF inspection tour.

## INFLUENZA

Before he left Washington on August 29, Gorgas told the *Ladies' Home Journal* that the American army was the healthiest in the world, and "I have no fear of its becoming less so."[13] He was tragically wrong, because at that very moment a highly infectious and virulent influenza virus was arriving from Europe that would generate the worst epidemic in modern history. In just eighteen months, influenza swept the globe, infecting from a quarter to a third of the world's population and killing at least fifty million people worldwide before it burned out in 1919 and 1920.[14] The 1918 influenza toll was more than three times that of World War I, killing more American troops in the United States, France, and military outposts around the world than died in combat on the Western Front. But in a perverse stroke of luck, ousted from his job, William Gorgas avoided being at the helm of the Army Medical Department during its most deadly period in history.

Although the actual origin of the pandemic remains unclear, many scholars believe it began in the spring of 1918 when influenza appeared in Camp Funston, Kansas, and spread with troops to several other training camps.[15] The outbreaks were not deadly but serious and widespread enough for medical officers in several of the camps to write them up. After Gorgas's office received multiple reports of "fever, type undetermined" or "influenza," Victor Vaughan investigated.[16] He and Gorgas reiterated their calls for isolation camps, less crowding, and better camp conditions, but influenza soon disappeared, so the problem subsided. By summer, however, the virus reared its head again, now spreading among troops on both sides of the Western Front. In June news came of influenza in the German army.

Philip Gibbs, *New York Times* reporter with the AEF, reported that "influenza is now epidemic all along the German front," and some reports were of a fatal strain.[17]

By August, just two days before Gorgas left Washington, this new, more virulent influenza landed in the United States. The navy surgeon general pinpointed the arrival of the second deadly wave in the navy on Tuesday, August 27, at Commonwealth Pier in Boston. That day three cases of influenza among naval personnel were recorded on the sick list. The next day there were eight cases, and the next, fifty-eight cases, fifteen of whom were so ill they were sent to the nearby naval hospital. Three medical officers who had seen the patients also fell ill, and by September 8 influenza had reached civilians in Boston and soldiers at the army's Camp Devens. Within ten days the base hospital and infirmaries were overwhelmed with a thousand sick trainees. From Massachusetts influenza swept across the country, east to west, hitting cities, towns, and rural areas equally hard. The *New York Times* began tracking the flu's death toll in the camps daily, and on October 16 reported that influenza had reached epidemic proportions in "practically every State in the country."[18]

With the departure of Gorgas and no announcement of his replacement, one of his deputies, Brig. Gen. Charles Richard, served as acting surgeon general, and he sent the OTSG's team of disease experts to investigate the outbreak at Camp Devens—Vaughan, Welch, and Rufus Cole, an expert in respiratory diseases. Attending autopsies of victims, they were shocked by what the flu was doing to young men's lungs and realized that this was the uncontrollable respiratory disease epidemic they had feared. They reported that "the situation remains grave and many more fatalities are expected before the epidemic has run its course."[19] Vaughan later wrote, "The realization of the utter helplessness of man in attempts to control the spread of this disease depressed me beyond words."[20] Despite his temporary status, Richard was not timid and mobilized the Medical Department to respond to the epidemic in Camp Devens. He recommended sixteen measures to control the epidemic in the camps, including the Gorgas standard of fifty square feet of living space per man, additional medical personnel, and screening around hospital beds and dining tables to prevent contagion. He also recommended to the General Staff reducing the camp populations by ten thousand each to ease overcrowding and suspending all transfers into or out of Devens until the epidemic passed. Influenza left Camp Devens after six weeks, having produced more than fourteen thousand cases of illness—more than one-quarter of the camp population—and 757 deaths.[21]

Charles Richard and the OTSG watched in horror as their worst fears of an airborne epidemic unfolded.[22] This influenza's symptoms shocked medical officers. While the usual infection gave patients a fever, chills, aches and pains, and often a sore throat and cough, this influenza produced fevers of 105, even 106 degrees, which made patients delirious, rendered some incontinent and others nauseous, and caused some to bleed from the nose and ears. Some victims coughed up bloody sputum, which one pathologist described graphically as "foamy and bloody, and sometimes mixed so completely as to resemble tomato puree."[23] Medical officers found cyanosis, or blueness of the skin from lack of oxygen in the lungs, to be one of the most alarming symptoms.[24]

The pattern of high morbidity at Devens was repeated in camps across the country as influenza swept from the northeastern seaboard south and west, following wartime transportation routes.[25] It arrived in Camp Dix, New Jersey, on September 18; Camp Funston, Kansas, on September 20; Camp Kearney, California, on September 27; and Camps Wheeler and Greenleaf in the interior of Georgia on October 11. Feverish patients flooded hospitals at the huge camps of thirty thousand to forty thousand, with sickness rates of 20 to 40 percent. Camp Wadsworth in South Carolina had noneffective rates of more than 50 percent in late September and reached a shocking 100 percent the first week of October.[26] The annualized death rate in the training camps increased almost a hundredfold, from 2.3 per 1,000 the week of September 13, to 206 per 1,000 the week of October 11.[27]

Influenza was equally devastating in the civilian population, and the situation was exacerbated by a shortage of health care personnel due to the Medical Department's recruitment of so many physicians and nurses from civil life. Cities and towns across the country appealed to retired doctors and nurses and to medical students to help, and PHS Surgeon Gen. Rupert Blue pleaded with Americans to keep the sick at home to relieve overwhelmed hospitals.[28] Such penetration into all corners of the country gave influenza the power to reduce American life expectancy for 1918 by about twelve years.[29]

## GORGAS IN FRANCE

Jefferson Kean was in France as Ireland's deputy chief surgeon of the AEF. A careful diarist, he created a telegraphic record of the emergence of deadly influenza among the troops. In late May Kean had noted a "mild epidemic of 'three-day-fever' causing no deaths." On August 9, however, he recorded new outbreaks of "three-day-fever" that were becoming "more virulent," and he amended the entry with an ominous notation: "Influenza." A week later Kean wrote, "Influenza increasing and becoming more fatal." On September 4 he recorded "influenza appearing again, with severe pneumonia." He also noted that on August 26 Merritte Ireland was promoted to brigadier general, a prelude to being named surgeon general.[30]

On August 29 William and Marie departed Washington for New York, leaving by train at 5:00 p.m., still hoping he would be retained as surgeon general but fearing the worst. As usual, he kept a journal, labeling this one, "Notes on trip to France with Secretary of War Baker." He began, "Never have gotten from Sec. Baker the information as to what my future is to be after my retirement on October 3rd. This is August 29th, so I will probably be retired while in France." He added, "I do not understand why he makes such a secret of the matter."[31] The Gorgases met Charles Furbush and his wife at the Hotel Astor in New York, and after a day of preparations and dinner and the theater, the men told their wives goodbye at the hotel and boarded the *Northern Pacific*. They joined four thousand men on their way to France, including Secretary Baker's contingent of senior officers of several army departments. The convoy included the *Leviathan* and other ships transporting twenty thousand troops to the war, and, Gorgas noted, "The greatest secrecy is observed about our departure."[32]

Now he felt the danger of war. During the crossing passengers were "called to quarters" several times for submarine attack drills. "This is a grim business," he wrote. "At the call every man dresses just as if he were going over board. Puts on his life preserver." Within five minutes everyone made their way to stand on deck by their boats. "Each time that we get the call to quarters we know that it may be the real thing and we stand at our posts wondering whether the fatal call to abandon ship is coming this time or not." Once it seemed especially real, because the ship's guns commenced firing as everyone hurried to their posts.

There were also speeches and meetings. On Tuesday, September 3, Baker and Gorgas addressed a labor battalion of eight hundred African Americans on the ship. "Sec. Baker made a beautiful speech. A good part of his speech was devoted to my life & work of which he spoke in the most flattering terms." He added, "Furbush is much elated. He feels sure now that the Secretary is going to continue me as surgeon general." Gorgas was less sure: "The Secretary has not mentioned the matter to me. I think it queer that he is so secretive. I do not intend to say a word to him about it till he broaches the subject himself."[33] Still at sea literally and figuratively, neither Gorgas nor Furbush knew that Ireland had already been promoted to brigadier general. A few days later, Gorgas recorded, "Sec. Baker and I are getting along first-rate. He is an agreeable and attractive man. He has not yet given me an intimation as to what he is going to do with me after my retirement."[34] Gorgas had to endure rough seas, and on the last night, passengers slept in their clothes in case of emergency. As they approached the coast of France, five destroyers arrived to escort their convoy into Brest Harbor.

When they landed, Baker and Gorgas went to Pershing's headquarters in Paris, where, without Gorgas's knowledge, Baker had summoned Ireland as well. There, before meeting with Gorgas, the secretary advised Ireland that the president was going to make him surgeon general upon Gorgas's retirement, but, Ireland wrote, Baker was not announcing it yet because that was "the President's privilege." Ireland responded that he was happy in his current position as chief surgeon of the AEF, responsible for an army of two million men in the field. Moreover, he believed that "the present Surgeon General's Office was rotten," and he wanted no part of it. But he did accept the appointment and, sworn to secrecy, joined the meeting with Gorgas. Ireland found Gorgas "far advanced in old age, as Mr. Baker had told me I would find him." In fact, he continued, "I think it is fair to say that General Gorgas did not know what was going on. The only real subject he could discuss during my visit with him was the fact that he wanted to continue as Surgeon General during the war."[35] Gorgas, either hopeful or oblivious, did not sense Ireland's disdain and thought him "very polite and cordial to me."[36]

Gorgas may have been aging, but he was also sick, suffering from the voyage and rheumatism in his shoulder.[37] But after a day in bed, he rallied and was ready for his tour. He and Furbush would have the privilege of seeing the operation of the AEF medical services at the height of their work during the two greatest American battles of the war, at St. Mihiel and the Meuse-Argonne.[38] Gorgas had access to every level of AEF medical services, as well as the British and French operations along the 250-mile front where stood at least twelve million soldiers on both sides of no-man's-land. He and Furbush set out to develop a comprehensive overview of modern medical and surgical practices on the biggest and bloodiest battlefield in history. They began to compile an alphabetical list of all AEF medical units in France, from the dressing stations and field hospitals at the front, to the evacuation hospitals and hospital trains that followed the troops, to the fixed base hospitals that received the seriously sick and wounded behind the lines. The stamina required for the six-week tour belies reports of Gorgas's decline, but various individuals who saw Gorgas at the front were acutely aware of his aging and fatigue.

Leaving their bags at the hotel in Paris so they could return periodically during their tour, they first ventured to the Toul headquarters and La Justice.[39] There, Gorgas made an official inspection of a "gas hospital" for victims of chemical weapons during the AEF's first big battle at St. Mihiel (September 12–16). He spent his thirty-third wedding anniversary, September 15, on the battlefield near Thiaucourt. But instead of his usual romantic musings, he described for Marie how the landscape was riven with shell holes and towns that were "pretty well knocked to pieces." He saw his first dead German in the doorway of a dugout the Americans had bombed; he told Marie, "I almost stepped on the body." The next day Gorgas went right up to the front lines near Pagy, where they could hear the shelling and see German shells exploding in the distance. They encountered a man whose hand had been blown away by a grenade, and when they visited a field hospital, a German shell passed overhead, causing them to duck. When the shelling increased, they moved back away from the fighting, but as they left the town, shells fell to the right and left. They saw two horses killed by a shell, and when they stopped to watch an artillery unit return fire, Gorgas was "impressed by the utter indifference the men had for the shell fire." As they observed the battlefield from a hill, a German plane flew overhead, causing them to put on their steel helmets.[40] After years working behind the lines, the old medical officer was finally on the battlefield.

Dr. Gorgas wanted to visit the wounded, so that evening, he returned to the gas hospital for an unofficial visit. It was a busy night of the St. Mihiel offensive, and Harry Goodhall, a young medical officer, was there. As they received dozens of wounded, Gorgas visited the triage, where they assessed each person for care, and then reviewed the wards. "His interest seemed to be entirely in the soldier," Goodhall wrote, "making special note as to the methods of keeping them warm, feeding them, and of the initial medical treatment that they were receiving."[41] Another officer made a similar observation when Gorgas inspected his hospital in Bazoilles. "He wished to speak with every one of them, talk with them about their injuries, about their plans." He was less interested in the hospital, he wrote, than in "the ordinary soldier."[42]

After that Gorgas did not write in his journal for a week, explaining that their days were so long and he was so tired that he just wanted to "go to bed as soon as I can." But he and Furbush continued their inspections. At Neufchateau, Gorgas, still working as the surgeon general, met with Harvey Cushing, in charge of one of the base hospitals, to discuss postwar medical plans. Cushing painted a poignant scene of their meeting. "G. is a fine chap, though visionary" [meaning he had his head in the clouds.] But, wrote Cushing, "He came down to earth for a moment . . . [and] in this process he observed that my garden needed weeding, and, stooping casually, pulled three varieties of weeds." The famous neurosurgeon admitted, "I have long known it needed weeding, but [. . .] I couldn't tell the dwarf nasturtiums from French weeds." Chagrined about his weedy garden, he "surreptitiously" put aside the plants Gorgas had pulled to guide his future weeding. A few days later he wrote, "With the aid of these specimens, I have just weeded my southeast quadrant and it's quite wonderful."[43]

At Langres, Gorgas and Furbush visited the medical officers' training school, and on September 20 they continued to Dijon to inspect the AEF's central medical laboratory. The day of Gorgas's visit, laboratory personnel were in the midst of a crisis, with calls from numerous hospitals to investigate influenza and pneumonia outbreaks. Gorgas toured the facility and later described the activities of the laboratory in detail but, perhaps distracted with wondering about his fate as surgeon general or focused on war injuries rather than diseases, said nothing about the influenza. Ward McNeal, a bacteriologist at the laboratory, however, would publish the first comprehensive paper on influenza in the AEF.[44]

Back at AEF headquarters, Gorgas dined with Ireland and Kean. "We had a very pleasant evening, but no allusion was made to the fact that a new Surgeon General was due to be appointed two weeks from that date," wrote Kean, adding, "Gen. Gorgas was carefully chaperoned by Col. Furbush."[45] Gorgas's report to Marie was, "If Ireland knows anything about his future, he keeps it very quiet"; and he added, "On the contrary he talks as if he thought that I am to be continued as Surgeon General; constantly asks me to attend to this, that or the other thing when I get back—such things as only a Surgeon General can do." Gorgas did not get a chance to talk to Baker, though. "He is so much on the go that he is difficult to catch," he told her.[46]

As Gorgas visited field hospitals, he was especially interested in seeing how the American care for the wounded compared with French and English methods. He inspected Allied hospitals with John Goodwin, who had been the British observer in Gorgas's office and was now in charge of the British medical services, and saw how the Americans had adopted much of the knowledge and practice the British had developed since 1914. Gorgas also sought out family and friends during their inspections. His cousin Stanhope Bayne-Jones was a medical officer with the Twenty-Sixth Division at the front near Verdun. To reach him they had to pass through trenches and the former no-man's-land, where a dense forest had been "knocked to smithereens." Bayne-Jones was at a dressing station in an old German dugout. Gorgas found him "in the pink of condition & . . . happy in his work."[47] The younger officer was alarmed, however, at his cousin's appearance. "A week or so ago, General Gorgas paid me a visit. He came a long way out a muddy ravine when we were in the line and must have taken a lot of trouble to find me," he wrote to his family. "I was happy to see him but was distressed at his appearance. He looks older and rather badly—and was limping—I don't know why?" He speculated, that "the work of the huge medical department that we now have must have been a big task for him during the last winter."[48]

From Verdun, Gorgas and Furbush went to the Argonne Forest to observe the American offensive there. As the artillery fired, the commander offered lunch, and they dined on bread, meat, and coffee out of a private's kit. Gorgas was cognizant of the extraordinary moment. "I think it quite an event to have eaten in the trenches while the greatest battle of all time was going on. Artillery and small arms firing on all sides." Then, as the wounded came into the dressing station, a chaplain asked for assistance in carrying the body of a Colonel Smith. Never squeamish, Gorgas assisted and even took the covering off the man's face to see if he knew him, but "I could not be sure." Returning to the dugout, Gorgas observed, "This was much the severest cannonaid [cannonade] I have had pass over me."[49]

"I have heard nothing from the Secretary," Gorgas wrote to Marie on October 2, the day before he was due to retire.[50] But he did learn his fate the next day—his birthday—when Furbush found an army paper at Bar la Duc announcing that Ireland had been made surgeon general. "Col. Furbush was much upset—he had expected that I would be continued," Gorgas wrote in his journal. It must have been embarrassing for a man who had enjoyed such public acclaim to be so unceremoniously replaced. But Gorgas was philosophical: "I was not anxious to be continued as S.G. though I would have felt complimented at being asked." And, he reflected, "This is a very fitting way to retire. In the battlefield of the greatest battle ever fought—or ever likely to be fought."[51] Gorgas later told Baker that he had thought it would be "ideal" to die on his sixty-fourth birthday, "being killed in battle," yet, when he actually came under shell fire that day, "he found all his old desire gone and was quite content to go to a place of safety and keep on living!"[52] The matter settled, Furbush gave his chief a birthday party before they continued their inspections and then returned to Paris. Never having felt secure financially, William told Marie that Baker had said "to continue my investigation as long as I saw fit, and that as soon as he got to Washington, he would issue an order placing me on active duty." This, he assured her, "will cover the matter of full pay till I get back."[53]

The inelegant end of Gorgas's distinguished career was curious. Secretary Baker and Chief of Staff March were wary of firing a national hero and setting off an outcry in the press and medical profession. But given their disagreements over health policies in the camps and medical officers' status in the army, they took that risk and replaced Gorgas as quietly as possible. Baker's appointment of Merritte Ireland was not in itself controversial. One medical journal, for example, editorialized that "perhaps no army appointment in recent years has met with such universal approval in the regular service as that of Major General Merritte W. Ireland to be Surgeon General of the Army."[54]

But if Baker, Ireland, and Bayne-Jones saw Gorgas as an old man, he and Furbush also completed a rigorous trip of 3,500 miles by car in six weeks to battlefields and AEF and Allied hospitals along the Western Front. Throughout the tour he maintained the respect of the troops and was welcomed everywhere he went. "They always treat my coming as an event," he told Marie. "When I visit a hospital I talk to a number of the wounded and am surprised to find that most of them know me and tell me that they have often heard of me."[55] He also felt well enough, given his age and vision problems, to do some of the driving, but on one leg of the trip, ran into some plate glass windows trying to avoid another car.[56]

After one more inspection of French hospitals near Avize, he and Furbush left for Brest and the ship home. In one final misadventure, their car broke down on the way, so they had to take the train.[57] Sailing on October 16, Gorgas began to write his final report on the inspection tour. It represented something of a valedictory and a handbook on military medicine in the AEF. The bulk of the report, which remained classified until the 1980s, was devoted to the medical transport and surgical treatment of the wounded, but it also lauded the programs to control venereal diseases, noting President Wilson's "courageous stand, . . . supported by his medical and line officers, in protecting in every practical way the physical conditions, health, and morals of the men." Gorgas had few criticisms, but said the delousing system needed to be improved, noted that several divisions arrived in France without any evacuation hospitals, and called for more robust litter bearers, explaining that they needed "physical sturdiness and staying qualities, alertness of mind, moral stability and stamina, courage, resourcefulness, and adaptability to unusual conditions."[58] Baker had asked Gorgas for his personal observations, and Gorgas thanked him, saying, "No medical officer ever had a better opportunity for investigating the functioning of the Medical Department in the field." He commended the work of the army doctors and nurses, and concluded with fourteen recommendations for additional personnel, medical supplies, and medical transport, as well as the perennial call for more space for hospital patients. He assured the secretary of war, "I would not hesitate to assure any wife, mother, or sister that her husband, son, or brother, when wounded in France, would receive the very best professional and nursing care."[59]

## WHERE WAS INFLUENZA?

Gorgas was in France during the very height of the influenza pandemic. But despite the fact that he had been warning of the dangers of respiratory disease outbreaks for months, he mentioned influenza only twice in his official inspection report, simply observing that influenza deaths were compounded by crowding.[60] Influenza was nevertheless exploding in the AEF, where Kean continued to record its progress. On October 6 he wrote, "Influenza and pneumonia have increased by thousands of cases. Case mortality of pneumonia, 32 percent. The situation is very serious," and then on October 11, "Pneumonia mortality this week 45.3%."[61] The peak army influenza-related death rates in the United States came during the first week in October with 6,160 officially recorded deaths. Among US soldiers in Europe, such deaths peaked a week later, during the American Meuse-Argonne campaign.[62] One medical officer reported First Army losses during the Argonne offensive as 17,647 killed, 69,832 wounded, and 68,760 "medical cases, largely influenza."[63] As many men fell sick as were wounded. Case rates among soldiers in France were lower than in the United States; one army report set hospital admissions for influenza at 167 per 1,000 in the AEF compared to 361 per 1,000 in the United States camps.[64] This difference in morbidity was most likely because many of the men in France had already been exposed to the flu in the training camps by the time they went to Europe.[65]

When Gorgas arrived back in New York on October 23, influenza was still wracking the country. Once again, he was a lucky man and escaped the brunt of the pandemic even as it was all around him. Marie did fall ill in November, most likely from influenza, but the rest of the family escaped serious illness and death from the disease. And, absent from Washington during the peak of the pandemic, William Gorgas did not have to read the mounting sickness and death reports coming into the OTSG every week during the fall of 1918, nor he did have to report that influenza and pneumonia were the leading cause of death for army medical officers, enlisted men, and nurses. Even though many men stayed in their tents or barracks when they fell ill and did not seek medical care, by the end the of the war, the War Department had recorded 1,125,401 primary hospital admissions for influenza, bronchitis, bronchopneumonia, and lobar pneumonia (791,907 for influenza alone) meaning that some 26 percent of the army had been sick enough to be hospitalized.[66]

Given Gorgas's long concern about respiratory disease outbreaks, why did he virtually ignore influenza? Perhaps he saw his tour as an opportunity to learn and report on combat wounds and war surgery and focused on that. Or perhaps he was so familiar with epidemic diseases that he took them for granted or did not take influenza as seriously as he did yellow fever, typhoid, or plague, which had higher case fatality rates than the typical flu. Once home he did acknowledge in a speech that influenza and pneumonia had been "very fatal" in the camps, but instead of blaming a virulent germ, Gorgas cited the failure to follow two important "sanitary laws"—setting up detention camps to prevent cross-infection and avoiding troop crowding. "The breaking of these two laws has been the cause of our excessive death rate in measles and influenza."[67] Or it might be that Gorgas, like other American leaders, wanted to avoid revisiting an experience in abject failure in the face of a deadly disease.[68] Modern science, bacteriology, medicine, and sanitation had all failed to contain the influenza of 1918.

He was not alone. Despite the fact that American physicians and health authorities published hundreds of scientific papers on influenza epidemiology, treatment, and pathology, they said little about the pandemic in their memoirs or speeches. In his memoir Victor Vaughan, Gorgas's chief epidemiologist, stated flatly, "I am not going into the history of the influenza epidemic," and summed it up in one vivid sentence: "It encircled the world, visited the remotest corners, taking toll of the most robust, sparing neither soldier nor civilian, and flaunting its red flag in the face of science."[69] General Pershing did not mention flu in his report to Congress on AEF operations, and Secretary Baker's final report characterized health in the AEF as "marvelously good."[70] Congress fell silent as well; in contrast to its anger and concern about the measles and pneumonia epidemics the previous year, aside from funding for PHS influenza activities, there were no investigations or recriminations of the far worse influenza disaster.[71] The entire world had suffered, after all, civilian as well as military populations, so who could blame the army or its Medical Department for the disease?

After the hostilities ceased with the armistice on November 11, the second deadly wave of influenza subsided as well, and Americans, eager to return to their normal lives, began to turn away from the war. The War Department quickly brought troops back home, and the army shrank to prewar levels within a year. A third, less virulent wave of influenza swept the world in 1919, but the deadly scourge soon became but a ghost of a pandemic, marked only by the graves of young adults in cemeteries across the country, and absent from history books for the rest of the century.

## DENOUEMENT: ASSESSMENT OF SURGEON GENERAL GORGAS

In late October, perhaps to soothe any wounds, Secretary Baker released to the public a highly laudatory letter he sent to Gorgas, noting his long career of service as a soldier and a doctor. "Even the gracious modesty which is part of your habit of thought cannot keep you from realizing that your career has been one of brilliant distinction." Baker also acknowledged "the cordial and helpful relations which have existed between us officially" and the "many personal courtesies and kindnesses which I have received from you during our most happy association."[72] Gorgas was so pleased (and relieved) that he sent a copy to Welch, who thought the letter "splendid."[73] After Gorgas formally retired on December 1, March and Baker awarded him the Distinguished Service Medal for "especially meritorious and conspicuous service."[74] It was a high honor. President Wilson and Congress had just created the medal to recognize outstanding wartime service, and among the first recipients were General Pershing and other commanding officers of the Allied Armies.

The subsequent judgment on Gorgas's leadership of the Medical Department has been mixed. Contemporaries and historians have shared the view that Gorgas preferred fighting disease to working at a desk, and as surgeon general was out of his office more than he was in. Gorgas himself seemed to agree. In 1918 when the Public Health Association put forward his name for a Nobel Prize, in his biographical essay to the committee he did not mention his tenure as surgeon general, but rather stated, "The principal works that I have accomplished have been the eradication of yellow fever from Havana, Cuba and from the Isthmus of Panama."[75] During the war, however, much of the civilian medical profession and the broader public admired Gorgas for his leadership. As Franklin Martin explained, Gorgas commanded "not by autocratic methods, but by persuasion and the example of his own industry." Nor did he allow "pride of proprietorship" to interfere with mobilizing the Medical Department and, when faced with difficult problems, he was willing to discuss all sides but then stuck by his decisions.[76] Percy Ashburn wrote that the Medical Department came through the war with "enhanced credit at home and abroad, with the Army and with the medical profession."[77] Senior War Department officials, however, resented Gorgas's political machinations, and some in the Medical Corps saw him as an aging, sick man who sat atop a chaotic Medical Department and blamed him for the department's problems.

Perhaps the most telling assessment came from the man who fired him. Newton Baker later said of Gorgas, "He remained to the last hospitable to new ideas and patient of suggestions from inexpert persons, always willing to weigh a new idea, and as little trammeled by preconceived ideas or traditions as any man I have ever known."[78] Gorgas's open mind and appreciation for expertise were crucial to fostering a modern and forward-looking Medical Department. His tenure saw many "firsts," including the creation of a program for the physical reconstruction and rehabilitation of wounded soldiers; the treatment of shell shock, or PTSD; management of the army's first chemical warfare program; aviation medicine; and the establishment of the Army School of Nursing.

Add to the list the Medical Department's magnum opus of Great War medicine, *The Medical Department in the World War*, the fifteen-volume official history, published from 1921 to 1929, covering all aspects of the Medical Department's war effort from training camp hygiene to war surgery.[79] Gorgas had long admired the "teaching value of medical war" that emerged from the Civil War and was codified in a six-volume history, *Medical and Surgical History of the War of the Rebellion*. As surgeon general he therefore followed suit and recruited scores of talented physicians and encouraged them to pursue research.[80] In 1917 his OTSG established a board to oversee the project, and when some of the initial research was published in a special issue in *Medical Clinics of North America,* Gorgas wrote the introduction. He explained that their plan was threefold: first, "continuous and liberal" publication of their clinical experience in the training camps and the battlefields; summarizing the findings in specific areas of medicine and surgery; and, finally, assimilating the work into a larger history.[81] It was Gorgas, therefore, who approved the history project, recruited many of the men who wrote it, and acquired the funds to support the research and data- and photograph-gathering. After the war, however, Ireland appointed Kean to the editorial board, and the two men put their names on every volume as it was published, materially diminishing the historical record of Gorgas's leadership.[82] Nevertheless, the official history stands as a fitting legacy to Gorgas's commitment to research. His ability to recruit talented people and let them flourish, capturing the clinical experience and science that came out of the horrible war, would thereby educate the next generation of physicians.

# CHAPTER 18

# Fighting Disease to the Last

Where will I be a year from today? If I am not teaching sanitation in Peru, I hope to be doing something equally useful in heaven. . . . What will become of the poor mosquitoes?

—William Gorgas to Ria Gorgas, October 3, 1919

Within weeks of returning from France, Gorgas was back to fighting mosquitoes. Between Christmas and New Year's, he went on a quick trip to Guatemala to investigate an outbreak of yellow fever for the PHS, but he had just had a tooth extracted and was feeling old.[1] He wrote Jessie a rather morbid letter, explaining that the end of the year often brought their mother to mind. "You were her child who was closest to her and I feel like talking to you about her," he said. Their parents had been married sixty-five years ago that day, December 29, and William realized that most of the people at the event had died and were largely forgotten. As people die, they may live on in the memories of a few descendants, but another generation or two would erase even those memories. When their mother died almost six years earlier, she had made what she liked to call the "great change," from one world to another, and "a very few [years] more and you & I will experience the same change." Then, he told his sister, "This great old world of ours will sweep along as if none of us had ever existed."[2]

Jessie would not die until 1925, but the end of William Gorgas's life was approaching. The years 1919 and 1920 would be some of the busiest of his life as he chased down yellow fever in Central and South America and made his way toward West Africa, but, driven as he was to complete his life's work, these travels would kill him.

## YELLOW FEVER COMMISSION, 1919

In the weeks after his retirement, Gorgas continued to receive honors. In January the Geographic Society of Chicago awarded him a medal for his "Service to Humanity," and the governments of Italy and France decorated him for his war service. In March the Medical Department presented a bust of his likeness to the Surgeon General's Library. After the glowing speeches, one observer wrote, "Few men have ever before heard such encomiums about themselves." Gorgas was visibly moved, and when it was his turn to speak, he invoked the memory of Walter Reed, and how Reed's work laid the basis for his own success.[3] Another kind of honor came when members of the Single Tax Party circulated Gorgas's name for president of the United States. At the party's national convention in June 1919, delegates decided to run tickets in several states in 1920, and Gorgas was among those mentioned as a candidate for president on a ticket with suffragist Carrie Chapman Catt for vice president.[4] But Gorgas was not even in the country at the time. Instead of pursuing political office, he had returned to fighting mosquitoes with the Rockefeller Foundation. "When the war is over my greatest duty is yellow fever," he had told Marie in February 1918. "I want to do all I can before I get too old and decrepit."[5]

### *Ecuador*

Gorgas gathered his team of Theo, Wrightson, and Carter, and two more scientists, W. Pareja, who was working on a yellow fever vaccine, and Israel Kligler, a Rockefeller Institute bacteriologist.[6] Marie and Lua Lyster joined the group as well, and on March 22 the IHB yellow fever commission left New York on the trusty old *Allianca* to continue the program to eliminate the key centers of yellow fever. Passing through Panama, Gorgas marveled that the jungle he had enjoyed exploring over the years was now extensive pastureland because the canal authority was running 100,000 cattle on the land to supply the US military garrisons with beef. After visiting with friends in Panama, they departed for Ecuador and were graced by smooth seas and a hawk hunting for seabirds, which entertained Gorgas during the voyage. When they arrived in Guayaquil on April 10, however, William and Marie were almost overwhelmed by the heat. Gorgas noted, "I never recollect experiencing such heat as we have in our room at this hotel."[7]

Guayaquileños were now less hostile to sanitation efforts than they had been in 1908 or 1912. The Ecuadorian government had constructed a water system, and residents could see the satisfactory results, but the city had persisted as a chief source of yellow fever infection in the world. Outbreaks had occurred every year since 1842 and averaged 259 cases annually between 1912 and 1918 with a peak of 460 in 1918.[8] The Rockefeller Foundation had assigned a scientific team to Guayaquil during the summer of 1918 to study the etiology of yellow fever, and in November, Gorgas sent Dr. Michael E. Connor, who had been with him in Panama, to work with local officials to begin mosquito mitigation. Connor's team had divided the city into districts and executed the now-familiar yellow fever campaign of isolating new cases, putting up screens, eliminating water sources where *Stegomyia* could deposit their eggs, identifying larvae predators in the lakes and streams, and draining, filling, or oiling swampland.[9] By the time Gorgas arrived, cases in Guayaquil were falling from eighty-five in January 1919 to seventeen in March and would reach zero in June.[10]

With mosquitoes and yellow fever on the run, Gorgas continued pursuing them in the other "seedbeds" or key centers in South America. The group's visit fell again into the pattern of meetings with government officials and public health officers, sanitary inspections, dinners and luncheons, and occasional outdoor adventures. Gorgas kept his travel journal but on this trip dictated his observations to Wrightson, who was typing on a new Corona typewriter that enabled them to make carbon copies to send to Aileen and the family in Tuscaloosa. From Guayaquil they visited surrounding towns that had reported yellow fever, and when they confirmed an outbreak, outlined eradication measures for it and other diseases such as plague and typhoid, including trash removal, water and sewerage systems, and mosquito mitigation. Gorgas had to repeatedly resist requests that the Rockefeller Foundation pay for local water systems, but when he found that most of the wards in the Guayaquil general hospital were unscreened for lack of funds, he paid to screen the yellow fever ward on his own account.[11] In addition to inspecting yellow fever conditions, the group practiced another form of public health diplomacy: Theo operated on patients in need of nose and throat work. His expertise in repairing cleft palates and removing infected tonsils or nasal blockages served to spread goodwill and to impress people with the power of modern science. "The rest of us are basking in reflected glory from Theo," observed Gorgas.[12]

After a week in Guayaquil, the team caught a train to Quito, where they stayed from April 18 to 27. Marie and Lua remained in Guayaquil, but the men missed not having Marie to translate. In Quito they were accompanied by Ecuadorian officials who did not speak English, so "the job is pretty hard on them," sympathized Gorgas. One evening he sat with a doctor and "in a very few minutes exhausted my Spanish," so the two men "spent two mortal hours looking at each other." He consulted his Spanish dictionary in desperation but admitted, "I have no idea to what I have committed the Foundation in this two hour conversation." They were nonetheless well entertained, Gorgas wrote, getting the "sort of attention that the circus does when it comes to one of our towns." Before they left Quito, officials held a reception and dance in their honor that lasted until dawn. But such expenditures caused Gorgas to despair, because the country was about to default on its foreign loans, and he often encountered financial roadblocks to sanitation programs. "I would much rather see them meet their obligations than spend money on entertaining us," Gorgas grumbled. "They impress me generally as being more or less irresponsible, very like children."[13]

After six weeks in Ecuador, they made their farewell rounds in Guayaquil. Marie gave a lunch for the wives of prominent officials on May 21, which was well received. They later learned that the luncheon was the first of its kind in Ecuador and that wives of two bitter political opponents had attended and given speeches, "without saying an ugly thing about the other."[14] The commission's diplomacy was rewarded when Ecuadorian officials offered Gorgas a salary of $15,000 to oversee the sanitation work for the country. Gorgas declined due to his commitments to the Rockefeller Foundation but agreed to take an honorary directorship without pay and leave Connor in charge of the yellow fever work. They had to wait, however, for the Ecuadorian government to fund the sanitation projects. "The Junta were kind enough to say that my accepting this position would insure the passage of their bill," Gorgas reported in his journal, and added less diplomatically, "Guayaquil would be permanently freed from yellow fever and then we need not give it any more thought."[15]

Some scholars have attributed the eradication of yellow fever in Ecuador to diplomatic pressure from abroad in the face of local resistance.[16] Gorgas saw it more in terms of getting the government's support and funding needed "to attain our object in dealing with yellow fever."[17] Instead of imposing the measures by fiat, public health officials had to work with the national legislature and political system to create and implement sanitation measures. Allowing those wheels to turn, Gorgas's group departed Guayaquil for the north on May 23, inspecting coastal towns along the way.

### *Colombia*

Returning to Panama, Gorgas and Theo quickly left for a trip to Colombia while the others remained behind. On the United Fruit Company's *Zacapa* to Cartagena, they had luxurious accommodations, but Gorgas was so seasick, he said, "I could feel no worse if I were in steerage." Still, the gregarious Gorgas met Americans en route to the Colombian interior "prospecting for oil," amidst a drilling boom in the jungle, and heard news of a shark biting off a man's head. Predators notwithstanding, he went for a swim in the ocean to cool off. When they arrived in Cartagena, it was so hot that Gorgas feared the "glamour of the tropics" was wearing off. "I left Panama several years ago thinking the tropics a pretty good part of the world to live in. This trip I found Guayaquil the hottest place I ever experienced, Panama hotter, and Cartagena the hottest."[18] Gorgas and Theo were not long in Colombia. Learning that there had been no yellow fever in Cartagena for three years, they advised other ports to end the quarantine against Cartagena and then returned to Panama.[19]

Gorgas loved to travel and embraced each experience as it came along. This time their vessel, the *Caribbean*, was transporting livestock and supplies to the Canal Zone, and after the ship took on five hundred cattle, Gorgas went below to see them being washed off. "They seem to enjoy it except that the flow of the water as it comes from the hose startled them," he said. "I would like to be in their stead as for being washed down is concerned." When they docked at Panama, Gorgas remained on board to watch the cattle offload. "They went out willingly enough but did not express the joy I thought they would for getting on dry land again."[20] Severe back pain dampened Gorgas's joy as well and kept him in bed until a physician named Dr. James gave him an electrical treatment. He was so much improved that he was able to dance at the Tivoli, providing "a dancing advertisement for Dr. James."[21] When Panama's President Porras loaned them his carriage, William and Marie could visit old friends, including Tranquilina at her new workplace. Gorgas observed, "She is the most important person in the laundry now and these calls from a Major General in the Army add to her prestige!"[22] He also saw a Mrs. Jesus, a friend from construction days who was supporting herself teaching French and Spanish. Gorgas credited the good influence Americans had on Panama, because "fifteen years ago no Panamanian lady could have made a living as Mrs. Jesus is now doing. She does not only not lose caste but is admired for her energy and thrift."[23]

### *Return to Ecuador and Peru*

After a quick trip to New York and Washington, the IHB yellow fever commission returned to Guayaquil while the Ecuadorian congress was in session so Gorgas could encourage officials to fund his sanitation projects. Theo and Wrightson went with him, but Marie, still ailing from her bout with influenza stayed in Washington.[24] Passing through Panama yet again, they heard that a boy from Nicaragua, the twelve-year-old son of a wealthy English mine owner, on his way to school in England, had died of yellow fever in the quarantine station. Gorgas went to Panama City to investigate and met with the boy's grieving mother, May Thomas, who spoke to him of her son and showed Gorgas some of his writings. "The child was evidently a very bright boy," wrote Gorgas, sympathizing with her loss.[25]

While in Panama they heard of 117 cases of yellow fever with twenty deaths in the town of Piura in northern Peru, so on their way to Ecuador, Gorgas wanted to investigate. The captain, however, would not enter the harbor near Piura because of the epidemic. Once in Lima, Gorgas asked President Augusto B. Leguia for help, and Leguia offered them Peru's only warship, the cruiser *Lima*, for the trip. Gorgas gladly accepted but, once on board, apologized to the captain for the trouble.[26] The captain replied that his orders were to take Gorgas anywhere he wished. When Gorgas asked if such orders would include Panama, the captain said yes, "as he would very much like to see the place." When Gorgas suggested Nicaragua, the captain said, "Even better," and when Gorgas asked about San Francisco, the captain thought that would be "the best of all," assuring Gorgas he had orders to take him anywhere he wanted. Gorgas exclaimed, "This is the greatest chance to travel I have ever had!" They could sail around the whole world! "Would it not create a commotion in Lima when it was announced that General Gorgas had run away with the whole available Peruvian navy!"[27] They did confine their itinerary to Piura, and upon return to Lima, instead of being annoyed with Gorgas's use of the ship, President Leguia asked him to be his director of sanitation, and to reorganize the health department and supervise the sanitary engineering work of Lima. Gorgas again had to decline due to other commitments, but this and the Guayaquil proposal were tempting, and he decided to talk it over with Marie.[28]

### *Central America*

Marie came down to Panama to celebrate William's sixty-fifth birthday, October 3, and in the comfort of the Tivoli Hotel, his thoughts turned again to mortality. Remembering his last birthday, when he was under fire in France, he now wondered where he would be for his next birthday, and whether he would be teaching sanitation in Peru or in heaven. A month later he even wrote to Dick, worrying about who would support their sisters when he was gone.[29]

Gorgas and the yellow fever commission spent the next two months in Central America assessing mosquito populations and yellow fever risks in Nicaragua, El Salvador, Guatemala, and Honduras. He engaged in cultural as well as public health diplomacy. While Gorgas was in El Salvador, the former president Carlos Meléndez Ramirez died, and after Gorgas spoke highly of the deceased, the family designated him a "chief mourner," seating him next to the president's brother in a funeral that went from 8:00 a.m. to 6:00 p.m. After Gorgas finally "managed to give the officials the slip at the cemetery," he vowed that "in the future, I shall have to be very careful about claiming acquaintance with deceased Presidents." In Managua, Gorgas negotiated gender politics when the government invited American and Nicaraguan women to a picnic. This was a first for the Nicaraguans. "Having ladies at an affair like this was a concession to what was supposed to be American ideas on this subject," Gorgas explained. He then upped the ante when he asked the US Marines commander's wife to dance. The Nicaraguan president followed suit, although a "Nicaraguan President had never before danced at an entertainment." Delighted, the party danced the rest of the afternoon. "We have revolutionized social customs in Nicaragua!" exclaimed Gorgas.[30]

Mexico persisted as an endemic center for yellow fever, but Gorgas decided against going there so soon after the tensions of the war. Japanese bacteriologist Hideyo Noguchi was in the country working on a vaccine, so Gorgas told the Rockefeller Foundation that as the Mexicans were going to honor Noguchi, "I think it would be of advantage to our cause to give the Mexicans full swing and not embarrass them by having an army officer of the party."[31] When relations improved, he would revisit the matter. They sailed for home on November 28 with a sense of accomplishment. The governments of Nicaragua, Salvador, Guatemala, and Honduras had all agreed to control mosquito breeding in their ports, require daily inspection of ships for *Stegomyia*, and maintain a six-day quarantine against all travelers from southern Mexico until yellow fever has been eliminated there. And, in line with Rockefeller Foundation policy, each country would pay for at least part of the cost of control.

### *South America, Again*

Once they were home, William and Marie decided he would accept the position of Peru's director of sanitation starting on January 1, 1921, after the Rockefeller Foundation mission to West Africa was complete. Until then he would leave a medical advisor and Wrightson in the country as sanitary engineers.[32] After spending the holidays with Aileen and family, the Gorgases left again for South America but got off to a bad start when their taxicab got stuck in a snowstorm, forcing them to walk with their baggage to the dock. Once on board, Gorgas sprained his ankle, which laid him up for several days. But after a short stay in Panama, Gorgas regained his stride, said goodbye to Marie, and traveled down the South American coast for the third time in a year, marking the ninth time in his life he had crossed the equator.[33]

This visit to Peru was dominated by social calls and dinners rather than sanitary inspections as he looked for housing in Lima for Aileen and William, and contemplated retirement. "This Peru work is the last job I'm going to take," he told Dick. "When I get through with it I am going to speak and write. Spend my summers in Washington and my winters in this delightful country. I have too few years left to spend them away from home."[34] He and Wrightson languished in Lima for several weeks, waiting for the Peruvian congress to pass the appropriations to make the port town of Paita a model of modern sanitation. When the legislation finally passed and included financing for water and sewage systems in thirty cities, Gorgas was gratified, writing, "I consider myself very fortunate to be able—in my old age—to supervise such a great and useful work."[35]

Gorgas then met Carter in Paita, where his colleague had been gathering the field reports to write up their findings for the Rockefeller Foundation. Carter had been troubled by Gorgas's appearance, telling his daughter that his friend appeared tired and not in "proper condition."[36] Nevertheless, they were able to report that although yellow fever continued to appear in some South American coastal areas, and West Africa remained to be investigated, they believed that they were on the cusp of eradication. Guayaquil had been free of yellow fever for eight months, work in Peru was progressing, and Mexico's last case of yellow fever was in December 1919. In Central America the disease was abating as well, and in Brazil, Rio de Janeiro had only two cases in 1919. Therefore, "the chances of complete elimination before the end of this year seemed bright."[37] Accepting the report, the Rockefeller Foundation accordingly concluded that "General Gorgas's ambition to write 'The Last Chapter of Yellow Fever' seems no Utopian dream."[38]

## THE LAST TRIP

Now the Rockefeller Commission could turn to West Africa. Despite extensive work by British scientists, physicians were still struggling to diagnose and control malaria and yellow fever in the region and could not agree on whether yellow fever even existed in West Africa. Ronald Ross, the Nobel laureate who discovered the mosquito vector for malaria, had long been frustrated by the British government's failure to wage an effective antimosquito campaign, and he hoped that Gorgas's visit might settle these questions.[39] Returning to New York in mid-April, Gorgas received a tempting invitation to attend the Australasian Medical Congress in Brisbane to explore the question of whether the permanent occupation of tropical Australia by Europeans was advisable.[40] Although it was "a subject in which I am much interested," and he was eager to see a new part of the world, Gorgas had to decline due to commitments in Peru and more immediately in West Africa.[41]

After just three weeks of preparation, the Gorgases left Washington for another demanding trip. Sailing from Quebec, they spent two nights in the historic old city before boarding the *Victoria* for London on May 8, joined by Robert Noble and his wife, Ella. Juan Guiteras would meet them in London. Their plan was to first go to Brussels for the opening day of the International Hygiene Congress, so that the king of Belgium could present Gorgas with a medal. Strong North Atlantic currents slowed the ship's crossing, however, causing them to reach Brussels too late for the medal ceremony.[42] The party then spent several days touring Brussels, where they met the queen and attended a banquet where Gorgas did receive his medal. From Brussels, William sent Jessie a check for $30 for her June "allowance," telling her that since they had arrived in Europe, they had been "in a turmoil," attending meetings, seeing the sights, and dining with friends. "Marie is well, though she tires easily. The fact is that I do the same. We are not as young as we used to be." The position in Lima was opportune: "It will not be as hard work as traveling under pressure as I have been doing for the last two years."[43] It was his last letter to his favorite sister.

On May 29 Gorgas returned to London to meet Marie at the Savoy Hotel near Covent Gardens. It was here in 1914 that the newly minted surgeon general had been feted by the British Royal Medical Society. Now Gorgas and Noble met with public health experts and officials on their West African mission, but the hard work and travel were catching up with the old sanitarian. William woke Marie at 3:00 am on May 30 to tell her that he had suffered "a slight paralytic stroke." While he did not appear to Marie to be ill, Gorgas must have self-diagnosed, because, she said, "he had not the slightest doubt of the seriousness of his experience."[44] She

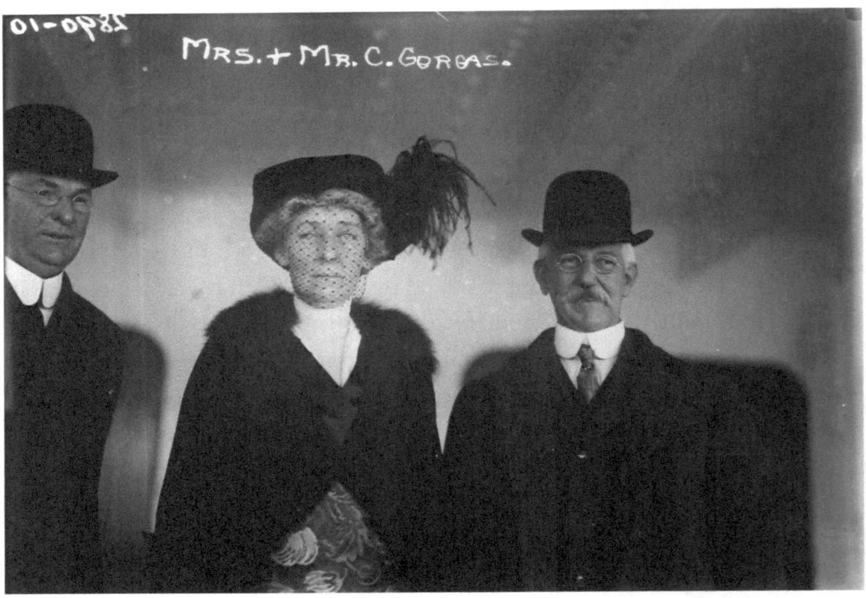


FIGURE 18.1. Marie and William Gorgas in May 1920, shortly before his fatal stroke. Library of Congress Prints and Photographs Division.

contacted Gorgas's colleague Sir John Goodwin, now in the British Army Medical Services, and he arranged for Gorgas to be admitted to the Queen Alexandra Military Hospital, a state-of-the-art general hospital during the war, and now a teaching hospital and medical school for Royal Army medical officers.[45]

Marie was at William's side for the next five weeks. They liked his cheerful room, which was supplied daily with fresh flowers and looked out on the Thames "with the passing boats and busy river life."[46] Goodwin oversaw Gorgas's care, instructing the nursing staff and advising Marie on her husband's condition. He brought in experts to consult, including the delightfully named Sir Edward Farquhar Buzzard, a baronet and specialist in neurology and reconstruction medicine at Oxford. Goodwin, however, soon faced a dilemma. Gorgas had been invited to Buckingham Palace on June 8, so King George V could decorate him for his service, but he was so weak he could not leave his hospital room. To the doctor's relief, when the king learned of Gorgas's condition, he waived protocol and came to the hospital instead.

Thus, in the last days of his life, William Gorgas had yet another extraordinary experience. "Such a wonderful event happened yesterday afternoon," Marie told Dick in a letter the next day. The king arrived at the hospital accompanied by Goodwin and several other officials, and "was as gracious and cordial as could be and talked with Will for fully five minutes," Marie wrote. He expressed distress at Gorgas's illness, wished him a speedy recovery, and thanked him for his work in tropical diseases and for sending medical officers and nurses to work with the British forces during the war. He then presented the decoration, the Most Distinguished Order of St Michael and St George, created in 1818 for service overseas or in connection with foreign or Commonwealth affairs. This gave Gorgas the title of Sir William Gorgas and put him into an elite class of several hundred individuals.[47] Marie could not hear what the king said as he handed William the decoration, but then he spoke a few words to her and left. The decoration was beautiful she told Dick, but cautioned, "We are not saying much about Will's illness—as little as possible."[48]

By mid-month, the news was out. A Florida paper reported on June 17 that the former surgeon general was in "much more serious condition than his friends have been willing heretofore to admit."[49] Get-well messages came in from around the world. Mattie, Marie's sister, sent a one-word telegram, "Love."[50] Theo Lyster—retired from the army and living in California—wrote achingly from Los Angeles. "My feeling for my uncle is too strong to make any judgement of much help. . . . Our lives have been so close for so many years that I feel this separation more than I like to admit." He would wait for news that Gorgas was better and then hoped William and Marie could come to California for him to recover. "Don't give up hope, Marie. We all see similar cases go on to complete recovery." Harking back to her own medical trials, he wrote, "You have been as sick as anyone could be and no one could believe you have been through about as much as is possible to endure and live." Theo promised to keep up the yellow fever work, but asked Marie to tell William, "I need him to guide."[51]

As days passed, however, recovery became a dream. Gorgas must have experienced additional strokes, because he became weaker and lost his appetite. He told Marie he would continue to fight, "but this time I do not believe I shall win out." He added, "If this is dying, it is very comfortable." He was also cognizant of his luck. "You know, I might have died at sea or on the way to West Africa and separated from you."[52] Farquhar Buzzard developed "profound respect and affection" for his patient. "He faced death as one hopes to face it oneself," he told Marie. "I do not suppose that anyone has heard him utter a word of complaint."[53] Charles Mayo of Rochester visited Gorgas the day before he died and told a friend, "He knew me and tried to talk, but was quite paralyzed, and he dropped off to sleep while he was talking to me."[54] That day Goodwin confided to a colleague, "I am afraid that my very dear friend Gorgas is dying."[55] Marie and Robert Noble were with him in the early hours of July 3, when he passed away at 1:35 a.m.[56] The *Washington Post* reported that Gorgas's death was "peaceful," and that the immediate cause of death was kidney failure.[57]

Condolences came to Marie from all parts of the world. One of the first was from Newton Baker. Remembering Gorgas's remarks the year before about dying on the battlefield, he wrote, "He did fall in battle, did he not? The no man's land he crossed and his object as noble as that of any war."[58] A young man from Alabama wrote that while Marie may know what her husband meant to the world, she did not know "what he meant to the young men who had the good fortune to be associated with him, I being one of them, . . . For we knew that when we wanted advice or help that General Gorgas was not only a wise advisor but a kind and loving friend."[59] Julia and Joseph Le Prince had just lost one of their fathers and now "felt for the second time in their lives the loss of a much loved and very good Father."[60] John Pershing told Marie, "The death of General Gorgas was a distinct personal loss to me, as I was proud to number him among my warmest friends." Remembering the death of his wife in a fire in the Philippines, he empathized. "None can appreciate just how severe the blow is who has not felt it."[61]

When William was courting Marie in the 1880s, he spoke of building imaginary castles with her at the center. He wrote again of castle building to his sister Minnie during Christmas in 1914, as he faced the work of surgeon general. He said that he had always felt like two people, one "occupied with the affairs of present every day life," the other occupied "with castle-building and imagery." He enjoyed building imaginary castles—images of a better world—whenever he had a leisurely moment. Those castles had been in the future, he told her, but were now images of the past, peopled with friends and family who had died. Although he was still engaged in the world, he felt his "imagery self" becoming more prominent. Death, he told Minnie, would merely be the change in which "the imagery becomes the real & the second person, which has been in the background all through this life, steps forward into the principal position."[62] William Gorgas now stepped forward to take possession of his castle.

## THE FUNERALS

In recognition of Gorgas's accomplishments and in gratitude for the American medical services' support to Britain during the war, the Crown authorized a funeral with ceremonies and pageantry befitting a three-star general in the Royal British Army. On Friday, July 9, therefore, the Stars and Stripes and the Union Jack flew at half-mast above the Queen Alexandra Military Hospital as Gorgas's flag-draped coffin adorned with lilies was brought out to rest on a gun carriage, flanked by high officials as pallbearers and followed by a riderless charger. With a thirteen-gun salute fired from Hyde Park at 11:00 a.m., the funeral procession to St. Paul's Cathedral started off to the cadence of a Coldstream Guards band with their great bearskin hats, proceeding along the Thames River and then to the Victoria embankment up New Bridge and Ludgate Hill to St. Paul's Cathedral. Bareheaded crowds lined the procession's two-mile route.[63]

The funeral party was joined at St. Paul's by other dignitaries, including representatives from the American embassy, friends Charles Mayo and Juan Guiteras, Sir John Goodwin representing the king, and a large contingent of diplomats.[64] At twelve o'clock noon, Marie entered the Cathedral on the arm of Robert Noble, with his wife and Lady Goodwin nearby. The service was almost entirely choral, with an anthem by Sir John Goss and the "Battle Hymn of the Republic."[65] Harvey Cushing watched the procession and attended the funeral with two Oxford undergraduates in tow. The traffic stopped "as by magic," he wrote, and there were "an astonishing number of distinguished people at the church." When the assemblage began singing the "Battle Hymn of the Republic," he wrote, "I could feel my young friends choking and swallowing."[66]

May Thomas, the grieving mother who had lost her talented son to yellow fever and whom Gorgas had comforted the year before in Panama, was also at the service. "Heartbroken by the death of a lovely brilliant boy of yellow fever," she explained to Marie, "I came in contact, officially, with General Gorgas in Panama, in August of last year and he spoke the most beautiful and sympathetic words to me revealing his own deep faith in God and life to come." As she sat alone in the vast cathedral, she said, "My own dark days of crushing grief and my heart flew out in sympathy to you and your irreparable loss." She wrote a poem for the occasion and sent it to Marie at the Grosvenor.

> I'd lost a lovely child, and, striving to console
> A stricken heart, he spoke to me of God, belief
> In life to come, eternal life—to ease my grief.
> And so I mourn; and grieve for you with all my heart,
> Rememb'ring well that in my grief he played the part
> Of comforter; may I not offer this to you
> My tribute to a heart so gentle, just and true?[67]

The ceremony closed with Chopin's funeral march as Gorgas's coffin was returned to the gun carriage, and then back to the hospital to await transfer to the United States. Over the next weeks, family and friends embraced Marie as she mourned and made plans to return home.[68] "No one could know how devoted & thoughtful Genl Gorgas was to you & how he loved and admired you, better than myself," wrote John Phillips's widow, Daisy.[69] William's cousin Edith Denegre wrote from New Orleans that "nothing can take from you dear Marie the knowledge of the absolute love & devotion you gave him always, which often smoothed his path & made many things possible." She added, "Thank God you were with him at the last."[70]

In early August, Marie departed England with William's casket on the *Pocahontas* to New York. Ella Noble accompanied her, but Robert Noble and the rest of the Rockefeller Yellow Fever Commission had continued on to West Africa. As the *Pocahontas* came into New York Harbor, its colors were at half-mast, and passing craft dipped their flags in tribute. Fort Jay, Governors Island, where the Gorgases once lived, saluted them with thirteen guns. They were met at the pier by colleagues from the Rockefeller Foundation, Marie's sister Hattie, Gorgas's brother Dick, and Enoch Crowder, William's old friend from Fort Brown days acting as the official representative from the War Department.[71] Aileen was on her way to Peru to join her husband, William Wrightson, and was unable to return for the funeral. Traveling by private railcar to Washington, the mourners were met with full military honors at Union Station in Washington, DC, and two companies of cavalry escorted the casket to the Church of the Epiphany at G and Fifteenth Streets, where Gorgas would lie in repose for four days.[72]

William Gorgas's funeral was the city's largest since the Great War. The service at the Church of Epiphany began at 2:30 p.m. on Monday, August 16, conducted by Reverend Doctor Percy Hall.[73] Pallbearers included Gen. John Pershing, Maj. Generals Tasker Bliss, Leonard Wood, Merritte Ireland, and Enoch Crowder, and members of the Latin American diplomatic corps; honorary pallbearers included Newton Baker and Peyton March, as well as Supreme Court justices, chairmen of the Senate and House committees on military affairs, and Rear Adm. Cary Grayson representing President Wilson.[74] Dick provided a detailed description of the ceremony for his four sisters, who for reasons unknown did not attend the funeral, and assured them that everything "passed off without a hitch & was wonderful." The hall could seat one thousand and was "packed & overflowing into the corridors." The family entered last, and Dick sat with Marie. It was "trying, of course, but we got thru it all right."[75]

A Tuscaloosa newspaper speculated that Gorgas might want to be buried alongside his parents at Tuscaloosa, but he chose the national cemetery in Arlington, Virginia.[76] After the service the mourners left the church for Arlington, passing the White House, through Georgetown, over the Potomac River, to Fort Myer, and then to Arlington, to section no. 1039, northeast of the Lee Mansion. Despite intermittent rain, people lined the Washington streets in tribute to the surgeon general and to watch the military escort of cavalry troops, a tank regiment, infantry engineer and artillery companies, motor ambulances, and three military bands. Gorgas's horse draped in black followed the flag-draped casket.[77]

At the graveside Newton Baker eloquently described watching Gorgas summon the medical profession and "organize them into a great agency to minister to young America." Others would say he was genial, gracious, courteous, considerate, Baker observed, but "I prefer to dwell upon the youthfulness of his spirit." Although Gorgas, he said, "was born in one age and lived into another, he became the adopted child of the younger age and was as elastic as any youth in it." He had an open mind and willingness to weigh new ideas to the end. Acknowledging Gorgas's wide travels, he stated, "It was appropriate that he should die on foreign soil, for he had become a citizen of the world," but added, "It is appropriate that his remains lie here, for this was his country; and in all this country there is not a fitter place to set up his final tent than Arlington, once the home of the commander under whom his father fought, now the Westminster Abbey of America's heroic military dead."[78] Gorgas, Baker declared, "fought a good fight and won the only kind of victory that counts; he added years to the length of human life; he served his generation and won a place in the lasting memory of all mankind; and withal, he was a modest gentleman—this Physician, this Soldier."[79]

At 5:00 p.m. William Gorgas was laid to rest with thirteen guns from Fort

Myer and buglers sounding "Taps." Once spurned by West Point, William Gorgas was now embraced in Arlington Cemetery, one of the most iconic military sites in the nation. His gravestone bears a phrase from the commendation that accompanied the honorary doctor of science degree Gorgas received at the University of Oxford in 1914: "William Crawford Gorgas, whose skill hath served the human lot to raise."[80]

# Epilogue

## *Remembering William C. Gorgas, 1920–2020*

THE DAY AFTER GORGAS DIED, an editorial in the *London Times* anticipated his future historical obscurity. The column noted a tendency to jealousy between scientists who make discoveries, like Walter Reed, and those who apply the new knowledge, like William Gorgas. "Gorgas did not escape the suspicion of being too ready to accept the honors of the man of science as well as those of a man of action," wrote the author. He suggested that Gorgas was so devoted to getting his "great work" done that he failed to correct his admirers on how to apportion the credit and instead accepted the praise "because it added to his momentum, and he used that momentum for the benefit of mankind."[1] This was true on occasion, but smoldering jealousy against Gorgas over his recognition and rise in the Medical Department also spurred efforts to trim his historical profile.

### HONORS AND HAGIOGRAPHY

During his lifetime, however, Gorgas achieved great recognition.[2] Congress, after all, promoted him twice outside of the Medical Corps's regular order; he held the highest office of his profession as surgeon general; seventeen colleges and universities awarded him honorary degrees; the governments of Britain, France, and Italy decorated him for his war service; and his own government gave him the Distinguished Service Medal, the highest noncombat award in the land. His death gave speakers and writers the opportunity to soar in praise. His long, even romantic history with yellow fever, his travels to distant lands to fight deadly disease, and the knighthood on his deathbed, all lent themselves to embellishment. In the North, the *New York City Telegram* called him "one of the greatest Americans that ever lived," and in the South, the *Confederate Veteran* put Gorgas on its cover for August 1920, and the *Nashville Banner* called him "easily one of the greatest men the

South has produced since the civil war." Midwest papers joined in. The *Peoria Illinois Transcript* called him "one of the most useful men of his generation" (which Gorgas would have appreciated), and the *Dayton Ohio News* observed, "His record is so incontestable that it will remain imperishable." Out west, the *Stockton California Evening Record* said, "The civilized world owes a debt of gratitude."[3] Magazine articles also hailed Gorgas as "Servant of Mankind," "Wholesale Saver of Human Lives," and "Redeemer of the Tropics."[4]

Such celebration continued into 1921, when the Southern Society of Washington held a memorial service in January and unveiled an oil portrait of Gorgas by artist Alexander R. James to hang in the OTSG library.[5] In his remarks at the unveiling, Merritte Ireland graciously said that "the name of William Crawford Gorgas will be a household name in the Western Hemisphere."[6] That seemed to be the case, as Alabama physicians had a "Gorgas Day" in 1921, and state officials named the power plant for which Gorgas had consulted after him.[7] Gorgas's alma mater, the University of the South at Sewanee, installed a stained glass window with his likeness in All Saints Chapel, in a dress frock coat and saber, holding a hypodermic needle and stethoscope, with tiny patients and a nurse at his feet.[8] Several countries issued stamps with Gorgas's image, and in 1926 Havana officials unveiled a bronze plaque with the likenesses of Finlay, Guiteras, Lazear, and Gorgas.[9] In 1928 the US Congress renamed Panama's Ancón Hospital the Gorgas Hospital, and when the American College of Surgeons commissioned Louis Tiffany to make bronze doors for its new auditorium depicting six "Important Contributors to Modern Science," it included Gorgas among the ranks of Aesculapius, Pasteur, and Osler.[10] More commercially, the pharmaceutical company E. R. Squibb & Sons used his image to sell cod liver oil and milk of magnesia with an ad in the *Ladies' Home Journal*. "The Cleansing of the Tropics" depicts a heroic Gorgas and a colleague in campaign hats consulting a pristine white map to track deadly disease in the tropics, with several West Caribbean men in the background.[11] And in England, when the London School of Hygiene and Tropical Medicine opened a new building in 1929, Gorgas's was one of twenty-three names engraved on the exterior frieze of the building, along with Koch, Pasteur, and Reed. Also adorning the stately building's first-floor balconies are ten gilded animal vectors of disease including Gorgas's nemeses, the *Aedes* and *Anopheles* mosquitoes![12]

The most well known memorial, however, was the Gorgas Memorial Institute for Tropical and Preventive Medicine in Panama (also known as the Gorgas Memorial Laboratory). Just weeks after Gorgas died, Panamanian president Porras announced the establishment of an institute to conduct research on tropical diseases and preventive medicine, and his government donated the Santo Tomás Hospital

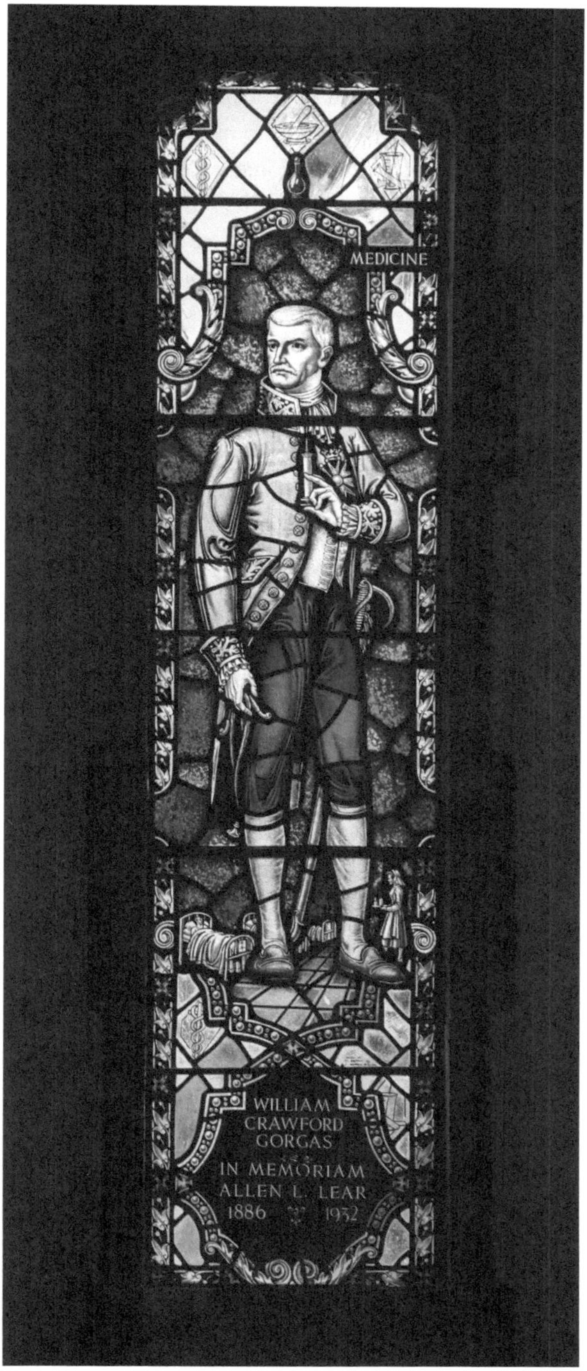


FIGURE E.1. Stained-glass window in All Saint's Chapel at the University of the South, Sewanee, Tennessee, depicting William C. Gorgas in an eighteenth-century dress frock coat with saber, wearing the Order of St Michael and St George awarded to him by King George V, and holding an upturned hypodermic needle in one hand and a stethoscope in the other, with tiny patients and a nurse at his feet. Courtesy of the University of the South, Sewanee, Tennessee.

and surrounding grounds for that purpose. Private medical organizations and individuals provided funds until Congress passed legislation in 1923 to finance the institution.[13] Opened in 1929 and graced by a replica of the bronze bust of Gorgas in the main entrance, the laboratory flourished, producing more than 630 publications on tropical diseases and parasites.[14] It also sponsored a Gorgas Essay Prize, awarded annually to the high school student who wrote the best essay on health and sanitation.[15] In cooperation with the Gorgas Memorial Laboratory, the University of Alabama at Tuscaloosa established the Gorgas School of Sanitation to train public health professionals, which exists today as the Gorgas Courses in Tropical Medicine at the University of Alabama School of Medicine in Birmingham.[16] American funding for the Gorgas Laboratory was discontinued in 1990 in anticipation of the transfer of the canal authority to Panama, but Panamanians retained the sanitarian's name in the successor organization, Instituto Conmemorativo Gorgas de Estudios de la Salud.[17]

Several proposals for a monument to Gorgas in Washington, DC, circulated, but Marie opposed the idea.[18] She preferred that the Tuscaloosa home be kept as a shrine and told his sisters, "That would please Will more than any statue."[19] The University of Alabama complied and has maintained the Gorgas House as a museum to this day.[20] Honors too numerous to mention continued. For example, in

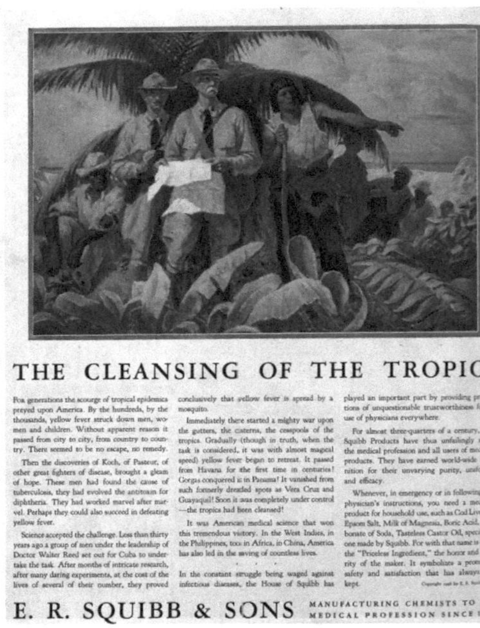


FIGURE E.2. Gorgas the Medical Hero in a Squibb Pharmaceuticals advertisement. *Ladies' Home Journal,* December 1928.

1919 the US Navy had commissioned the USS *General W. C. Gorgas*, while he was still alive, and the ship saw both civilian and military service through World War II.[21] During that war the army honored Gorgas (along with Walter Reed, George Goethals, Victor Vaughan, and others) by naming one of its 2,710 Liberty ships after him. A Texas junior college, Texas Southmost College, in Brownsville, where Gorgas served in the 1880s, established in 1947 the Gorgas Science Foundation to support conservation education.[22] New York University and the American Public Health Association named Gorgas to their Halls of Fame in the 1950s.[23] And in 1971 a little rat with big feet, discovered in 1967 and found only in northern Colombia and Venezuela, was named Gorgas's rice rat, *Oryzomys gorgasi*. As late as 2001, the army named the library in the Walter Reed Army Institute of Research the Gorgas Memorial Library.[24]

## MARIE AND THE BIOGRAPHY

Gorgas worried about money his whole life and did not die a rich man. His probated will showed an estate of $20,000 ($266,000 in 2021 dollars), with Marie and Aileen as his heirs.[25] When this became public, a Denver labor newspaper noted that Andrew Carnegie had left an estate of more than $20,000,000 when he died the previous year and asked, "Which of These Two Men Was Greatest?" Citing Gorgas's advocacy for better pay and living conditions for workers, the paper answered, "General Gorgas left comparatively little of this world's goods, but his views on poverty is [*sic*] an enduring monument."[26] In 1922 Congress approved a pension of $150 per month for Marie, and she stayed in Washington, DC, in the Adams Morgan neighborhood, living next door to Katherine Gaillard, the widow of the Panama engineer David Gaillard.[27] A visitor to her home admired the collection of old Spanish silver spoons, platters, and bowls that Marie had gathered during their Latin American travels, and noted, "Everywhere among the pieces of silver are pictures of General Gorgas, a strong purposeful face with kindly eyes."[28]

Marie's greatest project after William's death, however, was to write his biography. Just months after his death, she contacted publisher William W. Appleton of New York, who had published *Sanitation in Panama*, about a biography based on Gorgas's letters, and enlisted Burton J. Hendrick, an editor with Doubleday, to assist her.[29] Marie clearly sought to defend her husband against critics, in particular refuting the charge by Goethals that William had merely adopted mosquito-mitigation methods developed by Reed and Finlay, but she also unfortunately seemed to dismiss the work of the Reed Commission. In a preliminary chapter appearing in the monthly *World's Work* in 1924, Marie and Hendrick stated, "The story of those next few months [of yellow fever experiments] has been frequently told. It is the story of Reed and not the story of Gorgas."[30] By thus omitting the work of the Reed Commission, the excerpt implies that Gorgas had wiped out yellow fever in Havana single-handedly. Kean protested to the magazine, asserting that Gorgas had acquired enough fame: "It does not need augmentation by claiming for him what belongs to his brilliant and *unrewarded friend*, Walter Reed." The *New York Times* published Kean's critique on April 27, 1924.[31]

Kean assumed that Marie and Hendrick would modify their text in response to his comments, but when the book came out, it was the same story. The official title of *William Crawford Gorgas: His Life and Work* was tame enough, but the dust jacket spine read "The Conqueror of Yellow Fever," which again raised the question of Reed's role.[32] The language was at times grandiose, suggesting that by conquering disease in the tropics, Gorgas "added as much space to the earth's surface as Columbus himself."[33] They overstated his role with phrases such as "Gorgas cleaned up Havana" and omitted the work of others. Perhaps most annoyingly, the biography referred to him as "general" when he was in Cuba and Panama, although he was a major and colonel, respectively, and Reed died before he could be promoted to colonel.

Several reviews were positive, commenting on Gorgas's extraordinary life and accomplishments.[34] Franklin Martin wrote that it offered in layman's language "the accomplishments of scientific medicine of this quarter century which is recognized as epoch making by the medical world."[35] But Kean wrote a scathing review in the *Military Surgeon*. While he found the biography an "attractive story . . . in which no faults or imperfections appear through the shining gloss of love and hero worship," he reprised his arguments that more credit should have been given to Reed in Cuba and that Gorgas did not clean up Havana alone. "The scouring and bathing had been going on energetically for over a year before he had a chance at a scrubbing brush." Regarding Panama, Kean objected to the lack of recognition of the role of the OTSG (and Kean himself) in keeping Gorgas in his job. He also complained that Gorgas was named surgeon general even though for eighteen years he "saw no service with troops and gave but little time to military matters." Furthermore, he suggested, Gorgas spoke to Secretary of War Baker about retirement in 1917 because he had "misgivings as to his ability to handle this complex machine," and his success during the war was actually due to the efforts of previous surgeons general who had "labored to make good the errors of the Spanish War."[36] Kean sent copies of his review to a score of physicians, many of whom agreed that the book romanticized Gorgas and overstated his role.[37] He also sent copies to Hendrick and Marie, which Marie stiffly acknowledged, writing, "I regret that the biography does not meet with your approval."[38]

After the biography was published, Marie returned to Cuba and Panama to see old friends and relish her husband's successes, and lived long enough to attend the first Gorgas Essay Prize ceremony at the White House in May 1929. But later that year, having survived yellow fever and cancer, on November 9, 1929, Marie succumbed to a heart attack at her home, while spending the evening with Katherine Gaillard. She was buried next to William at Arlington National Cemetery.[39]

With Marie's death, it was largely left to Kean to tell the yellow fever story. His

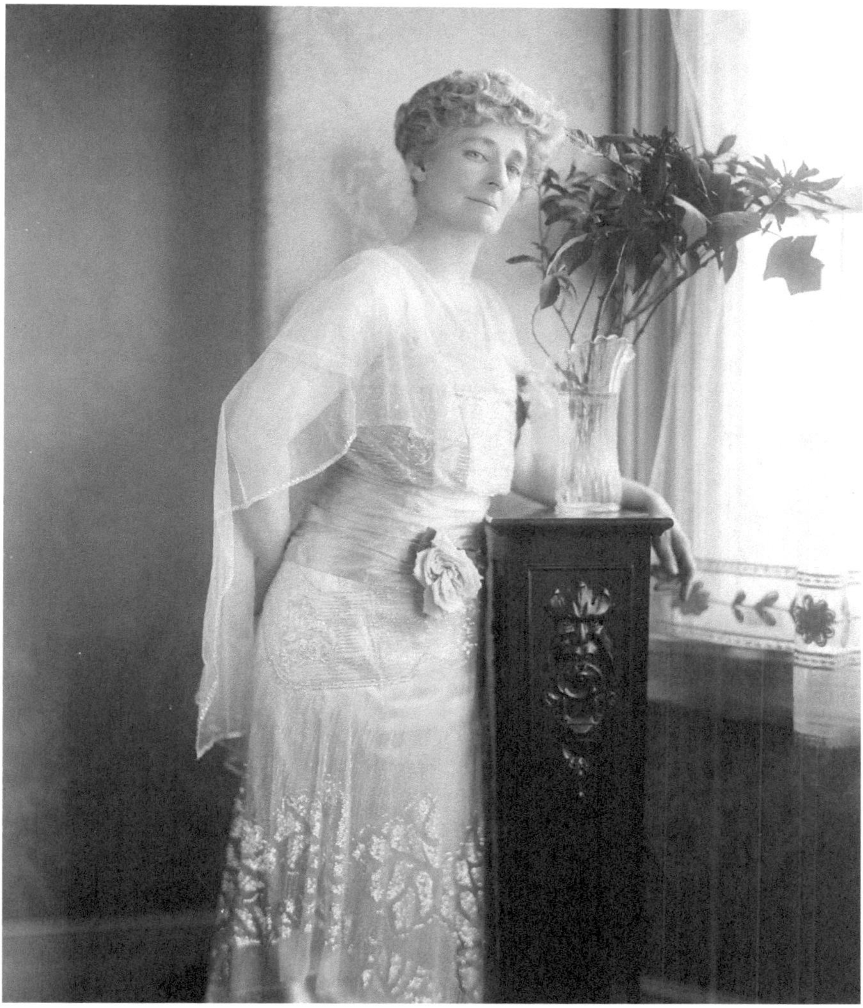

FIGURE E.3. Marie D. Gorgas, with a flower at her waist. Library of Congress Prints and Photographs Division.

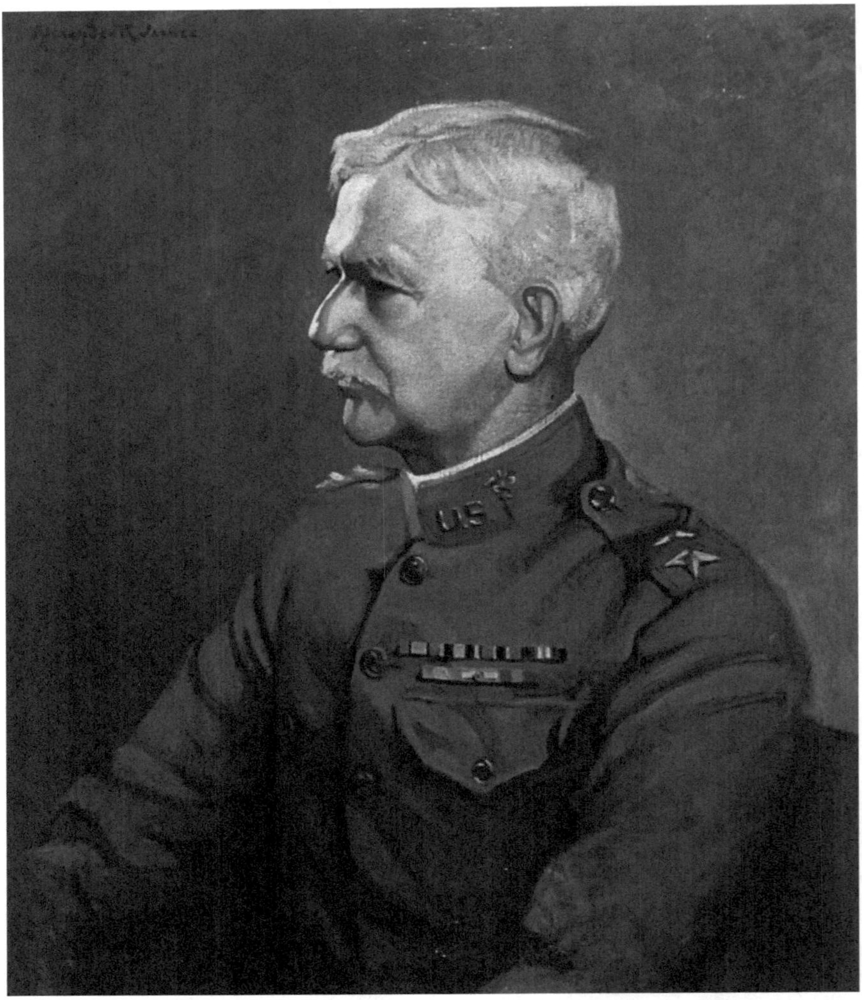

FIGURE E.4. William C. Gorgas, portrait in oil by Alexander R. James, presented to the War Department by the Southern Society of Washington, on March 3, 1921. National Library of Medicine.

critique of her biography had succeeded in dampening the book's reception. As he told one colleague, his review in the *Military Surgeon* "had a wide circulation & killed the sale of the book."[40] Few historians took up Gorgas's story. In the 1930s Robin Lampson wrote a romantic biography of Gorgas in verse, *Death Loses a Pair of Wings* (1939), which portrayed Gorgas as both an innocent and a hero.[41] Hagiographic biographies appeared as well, with titles of *Soldier Doctor*, *Tropic Fever*

*Fighter*, and *Warrior in White*.[42] When John Gibson, who worked at the Department of Public Health in Montgomery, Alabama, wrote a biography of Gorgas in the 1940s, he used much of Marie's material and produced an entertaining story, unencumbered by scholarly references, of a hero who "conquered" yellow fever.[43] Kean's campaign may have succeeded too well: so few biographies have since been written about Gorgas that Marie and Hendrick's hagiographic book still stands as an important source.

In yet another irony, Jefferson Kean was the first person to be awarded the Gorgas Medal. It had been created in 1917 by the Medical Reserve Corps Association but was never awarded. As New York physician S. A. Knopf explained to Marie when he sent her the unawarded medal in 1923, it was not presented due to the chaos of war mobilization and the reluctance of career Medical Corps officers to honor Gorgas, who they believed had shortchanged them in promotions.[44] Wyeth Laboratories, however, resurrected the Gorgas Medal in 1942, during World War II, for "distinguished work in preventive medicine," and gave the first one to Kean, now finally a general. He accepted the award in the name of "an old and valued friend," whom he called Major Gorgas (not General!) and felt the need to point out that Gorgas was skeptical of the mosquito theory "long after others accepted it" but had "lost nothing in fame or in opportunity by his scientific skepticism." Kean appreciated the honor of the medal conveyed, remarking that he had "gained something by the promptness of my conversion," and had even "obtained a place, which I hardly deserve, in Cornwell's now famous painting of the Conquerors of Yellow Fever."[45]

## THE HENCH COLLECTION

Long after William Gorgas died, another voice came to frame the story of yellow fever. Philip Hench (1896–1965) was a physician and scientist at the Mayo Clinic who became intrigued by the Reed experiments and spent his free time for more than three decades researching events in Cuba, 1900–1902. Hench met Kean in 1939, and Kean gave him more than a thousand documents, including original letters, accounts, and fever charts, many of which he annotated with his interpretation of their meaning, such as his criticism of Marie's portrayal of the Reed experiments in her biography of William.[46] Philip Hench consequently adopted Kean's position of minimizing Gorgas's role in the yellow fever work, and in his 1941 speech at the unveiling of Cornwall's *The Conquerors of Yellow Fever*, which featured fifteen men but not Gorgas, he proclaimed that it portrayed the "team who won this victory."[47] Hench's credibility was greatly enhanced after he won the 1950 Nobel Prize for Physiology and Medicine for his role in the discovery of the hormone cortisone.[48]

Kean died in 1950 at the age of ninety, and Hench died in 1965, before he could write his biography of Reed. He did, however, leave his huge archive to the University of Virginia, and today the Philip Hench Walter Reed Collection at the University of Virginia is the single most important source of information on the Reed Commission; the index alone is ninety-six pages long.[49] Thus, we complete the circle to Jefferson Randolph Kean's efforts to shape the history of the yellow fever eradication in Cuba.

## MOSQUITOES AND YELLOW FEVER ENDURE

Yellow fever and mosquitoes, meanwhile, have outlived everyone and continue to torment and kill people to this day. The wealth, reach, and expertise of the Rockefeller Foundation could not eradicate the disease, which continued to erupt in Africa, and Central and South America. Raymond Fosdick, onetime president of the Rockefeller Foundation, wrote, "On no disease in the long list of human afflictions did the Rockefeller Foundation put greater emphasis or a larger proportion of time and financial support than on yellow fever."[50] Gorgas and Carter firmly believed that the disease could be eradicated from the earth but were also aware that some scientists thought the disease could "linger for years in some unknown way in a locality without in any way being recognized, and then when conditions are favorable, develop into an epidemic Yellow Fever."[51] The mechanism, however, remained unknown until the 1930s when researchers discovered that more than one mosquito species—*Haemogogus* as well as *Aedes*—could transmit yellow fever and that some strains of the virus continued to thrive in mosquitoes and animals in the jungle such as deer and monkeys. What they called "sylvan yellow fever" could therefore escape destruction in these animal reservoirs. The foundation therefore had to abandon Gorgas and Carter's theory—and dream— that the world could be freed from yellow fever by eliminating key centers of infection.[52]

Rockefeller Foundation scientists continued to pursue a vaccine, and in that process thirty-two scientists and technicians contracted yellow fever in laboratories, and five died. The vaccine was developed in 1937 under the leadership of Max Theiler, and from 1942 to 1946 the Rockefeller Foundation helped produce and distribute 34 million vaccine doses without cost to governments, health agencies, and other official units. It then passed the responsibility for the manufacture and distribution of the vaccine on to the United States PHS and governments in other countries. For his work on the vaccine Theiler was the only scientist to receive the coveted Nobel Prize (1951) in connection with yellow fever.[53]

Although yellow fever can be prevented with the vaccine, the disease still sickens more than 100,000 people in the world annually, killing almost half of them, and remains incurable. Malaria also remains unvanquished and stands as one of the biggest killers in the world today, threatening ever larger populations as global warming and climate change expand mosquito habitat.[54] Today mosquitoes of all stripes are flourishing and resist control, evolving resistance to DDT and other pesticides.[55] Gorgas's archfoe, *Stegomyia*, has been renamed *Aedes aegypti* and now harbors even more deadly diseases. In addition to yellow fever and dengue, *Aedes* can transmit the Zika virus, first identified in Africa in the 1940s and arriving in the Western Hemisphere in the 2000s, and the chikungunya virus which prevailed in the tropics and was identified in the United States in 2013.[56] When William Gorgas wondered "what would become of the poor mosquitoes" when he died, he could not have dreamt that modern science, public health, and human civilization in the 2020s had not yet gained mastery over them.

# Notes

## *Introduction*

1. Marie D. Gorgas and Burton J. Hendrick, *William Crawford Gorgas, His Life and Works* (Garden City, NY: Doubleday, Page, 1924), 334.

2. "To Mrs. Gorgas," May Thomas to Marie Gorgas, July 12, 1920, William C. Gorgas Papers, University of Alabama Libraries Special Collections, Tuscaloosa, Alabama (hereafter cited as WCGP).

3. W. C. Gorgas, "The Conquest of the Tropics for the White Race," *JAMA* 52 (June 19, 1909): 1967–69.

4. Gorgas and Hendrick, *William Crawford Gorgas*; John M. Gibson, *Physician to the World: The Life of General William C. Gorgas* (Durham, NC: Duke University Press, 1950).

5. Donald B. Cooper, "Reviewed Works: Death by Migration by Philip Curtin and Physician to the World by John Gibson," *Hispanic American Historical Review* 71 (1991): 158–59; and John Mendinghall Gibson, *Physician to the World: The Life of General William C. Gorgas* (Whitefish, MT: Literary Licensing, 2012).

6. Jefferson Kean, "Autobiographical Sketch of Jefferson Randolph Kean," 1928, US Army Medical Department, Office of Medical History, 8, 42.

7. Public Law 858, 70th Congress, February 28, 1929; "Roll of Honor: Participants in the Yellow Fever Investigations in Cuba," *Army Register*, 1937.

8. Reed, Carroll, and Agramonte, "The Etiology of Yellow Fever—an Additional Note," *JAMA* 36 (1901): 431–40; "Informed Consent Agreement between Antonio Benigno and Walter Reed," November 26, 1900, Philip S. Hench Walter Reed Yellow Fever Collection, Claude Moore Health Sciences Library, University of Virginia Health System, Charlottesville, Virginia (hereafter cited as Hench Collection).

9. Jefferson Randolph Kean to John J. Moran, May 14, 1929, Hench Collection.

10. R. M. O'Reilly, "Yellow Fever Commission," S. doc. No. 59–10, August 30, 1906; S. doc. 61–120, April 29, 1910; and "The Yellow Fever Roll of Honor," February 16, 1928, Hench Collection.

11. After Kean's death, his wife, Cornelia, told a friend that his resentment against Gorgas had been growing for years. "Kean, McCaw, and Ireland came in time to resent the favors and publicity which followed Gorgas," she confided. Cornelia Knox Kean to Mary Standlee, May 4, 1951, Hench Collection.

12. Kean to Albert E. Truby, August 9, 1942, Hench Collection.

13. Philip Showalter Hench, "The Unveiling of Dean Cornwell's painting *Conquerors of Yellow Fever*" (speech, 1941), Hench Collection.

14. Benjamin G. Withers and Stephen C. Craig, "The Historical Impact of Preventive Medicine in War," in *Military Preventative Medicine: Mobilization and Deployment Vol. 1, Chapter 2; The Historical Impact of Preventive Medicine in War*, ed. Patrick W. Kelly (Washington, DC: Office of the Surgeon General, Borden Institute, 2003).

15. Notable Graves, "Medicine," Arlington National Cemetery website. William Gorgas is in grave 1039, Section 2 and Walter Reed in grave 1864, Section 3.

16. On the American history of yellow fever, see Molly Caldwell Crosby, *The American Plague: The Untold Story of Yellow Fever, the Epidemic That Shaped Our History* (New York: Berkley Books, 2006); John R. Pierce and James V. Writer, *Yellow Jack: How Yellow Fever Ravaged America and Walter Reed Discovered Its Deadly Secrets* (Hoboken, NJ: John Wiley and Sons, 2005); Margaret Humphreys, *Yellow Fever and the South* (New Brunswick, NJ: Rutgers University Press, 1992).

17. The naming of this insect has a long history. Gorgas and his contemporaries knew it as *Stegomyia fasciata* or *Culex fasciatus*, while the term used today is *Aedes aegypti*. In the late 1930s scientists determined that another species of mosquito, *Haemogogus*, also transmits yellow fever. See World Health Organization website, "Yellow Fever," May 7, 2019.

18. Also known as "Yellow Jack," for the yellow quarantine flag flown on ships or because of the yellow jacket that some hospitals put on patients to distinguish them from other patients.

19. Centers for Disease Control and Prevention website, "Yellow Fever," June 2, 2022.

20. Pierce and Writer, *Yellow Jack*, 10.

21. David K. Patterson, "Yellow Fever Epidemics and Mortality in the United States, 1693–1905," *Social Science and Medicine* 34 (1992): 855–65.

22. D. J. Rogers et al., "The Global Distribution of Yellow Fever and Dengue," *Advances in Parasitology* 62 (2006): 181–200; Annelies Wilder-Smith, Vernon Lee, and Duane J. Gubler, "Yellow Fever: Is Asia Prepared for an Epidemic?" *The Lancet: Infectious Diseases* 19 (March 2019): 241–42.

23. William C. Gorgas, *Sanitation in Panama* (New York: Appleton, 1915), 1–2.

24. Jefferson Kean, "William Crawford Gorgas," *Military Surgeon* (March 1925): 1–5.

25. Jean Segata writes, "Mosquito-centrism is the principal symptom of our health policies. It is as persistent as the militarization of those policies," in "Enacting Politics *with* Mosquitoes," in Marcus Hall and Dan Tamïr, eds. *Mosquitopia: The Place of Pests in a Healthy World* (London: Routledge, 2022), 174; Christian Strother, "Waging War on Mosquitoes: Scientific Research and the Formation of Mosquito Brigades in French West Africa, 1899–1920," *Journal of the History of Medicine and Allied Sciences* 71 (October 2016): 452.

## *Chapter 1*

1. Biographical information on Josiah Gorgas is drawn from Sarah Woolfolk Wiggins, *Love and Duty: Amelia and Josiah Gorgas and Their Family* (Tuscaloosa: University of Alabama Press, 2005); Frank Everson Vandiver, *Ploughshares into Swords: Josiah Gorgas and Confederate Ordnance* (Austin: University of Texas Press, 1952); Sarah Woolfolk Wiggins, "Josiah Gorgas, a Victorian Father," *Civil War History* 32 (1986): 229–46; Sarah Woolfolk Wiggins, ed., *The Journals of Josiah Gorgas, 1857–1878* (Tuscaloosa: University of

Alabama Press, 1995). The original journals may be found in the Josiah and Amelia Gorgas Family Papers.

2. Gayle served as governor (1831–1835), member of Congress (Whig Party, 1847–1849), and United States district judge of Alabama (1849–1859).

3. Gorgas and Hendrick, *William Crawford Gorgas,* 27–29.

4. Gorgas and Hendrick, *William Crawford Gorgas*, 25.

5. WCG to Mamie, January 1, 1914, Josiah Gorgas Family Papers, University of Alabama Libraries Special Collections, Tuscaloosa, Alabama (hereafter cited as JGFP).

6. Robin Lampson, *Death Loses a Pair of Wings: The Epic of William Gorgas and the Conquest of Yellow Fever: A Novel in Cadence* (New York: Charles Scribner's Sons, 1939), 18.

7. Josiah C. Nott, "Yellow Contrasted with Bilious Fever: Reasons for Believing It Is a Disease Sui Generis—Its Mode of Propagation—Remote Cause—Probable Insect or Animalcular Origin," *New Orleans Medical and Surgical Journal* 4 (1848): 563–601. Nott was also one of the southern physicians who propounded a "scientific" defense of slavery to shore up white supremacy. This pernicious view opposed the emerging theory of evolution, arguing that the races had been created separately and were therefore not of equal humanity. See Josiah Clark Nott, *An Essay on the Natural History of Mankind, Viewed in Connection with Negro Slavery Delivered before the Southern Rights Association, 14 December 1850* (Mobile, AL: Dade, Thompson, 1851).

8. Infant mortality was more than one-third for Black babies in 1859. See Michael Haines, "Fertility and Mortality in the United States," March 19, 2008, EH.Net Encyclopedia, ed. Robert Whaples.

9. When siblings Solomon and Sarah came to visit in 1857, he had not seen them for five or six years. Wiggins, *Journals of Josiah Gorgas*, September 28, 1857.

10. Wiggins, *Journals of Josiah Gorgas*, January 1, 1857.

11. Gorgas and Hendrick, *William Crawford Gorgas*, 30.

12. Wiggins, *Journals of Josiah Gorgas,* January 28, 1857.

13. Gorgas and Hendrick, *William Crawford Gorgas*, 31.

14. JG to AGG, August 4, 1858, JGFP, emphasis in original.

15. Gorgas and Hendrick, *William Crawford Gorgas*, 32; Lampson, *Death Loses a Pair of Wings*, 38–41.

16. WCG to Helen Longstreet, November 26, 1910, William Crawford Gorgas Papers, Library of Congress, Washington, DC (hereafter cited as Gorgas Papers, LoC). The Confederate Memorial in Arlington National Cemetery, unveiled by President Woodrow Wilson in 1914, has the figure of a Black mammy holding a child for the white father to kiss as he goes off to war.

17. Wiggins, *Love and Duty*, 31–50.

18. Wiggins, *Journals of Josiah Gorgas*, April 24, 1857.

19. Lampson, *Death Loses a Pair of Wings*, 34.

20. Wiggins, *Journals of Josiah Gorgas*, February 9, 1858.

21. Wiggins, *Journals of Josiah Gorgas*, April 12, 1858.

22. AGG to JG, July 4, 1858, JGFP.

23. Wiggins, *Journals of Josiah Gorgas*, April 30, 1858.

24. Wiggins, *Journals of Josiah Gorgas*, June 7, 1857, emphasis in the original.

25. Wiggins, *Journals of Josiah Gorgas*, April 3, 1860.

26. Wiggins, *Journals of Josiah Gorgas*, June 3, 1860, emphasis in the original.

27. Wiggins, *Journals of Josiah Gorgas*, March 31, 1861.

28. Lampson, *Death Loses a Pair of Wings*, 43.

29. Wiggins, *Journals of Josiah Gorgas*, March 31, 1861.

30. Gorgas and Hendrick, *William Crawford Gorgas*, 34.

31. James M. McPherson, *Battle Cry of Freedom: The Civil War Era: Oxford History of the United States* (New York: Oxford University Press, 1988), 319–20; Frank Everson Vandiver, *Ploughshares into Swords: Josiah Gorgas and Confederate Ordnance* (Austin: University of Texas Press, 1952); Frank E. Vandiver, ed., *The Civil War Diary of General Josiah Gorgas* (Tuscaloosa: University of Alabama Press, 1947); Ezra J. Warner, *Generals in Gray: Lives of the Confederate Commanders* (Baton Rouge: Louisiana State University Press, 1959).

32. Lampson, *Death Loses a Pair of Wings*, 45.

33. David Walker to WCG, July 20, 1917, WCGP.

34. Wiggins, *Journals of Josiah Gorgas*, March 13, 1864, and August 10, 1864.

35. Henry St. George Tucker, *Gorgas Memorial Laboratory*, House of Representatives, Committee on Foreign Affairs, 70th Cong., 1st sess., January 20, 1928, 103.

36. Gibson, *Physician to the World*, 22.

37. WCG to Helen Longstreet, November 26, 1910, Gorgas Papers, LoC.

38. Wiggins, *Journals of Josiah Gorgas*, July 27, 1862.

39. Wiggins, *Journals of Josiah Gorgas*, February 21, 1864.

40. Wiggins, *Journals of Josiah Gorgas*, May 13, 1863.

41. Wiggins, *Journals of Josiah Gorgas*, April 1, 1864.

42. Wiggins, *Journals of Josiah Gorgas*, November 3, 1864.

43. Anne Kelly Knowles, "Labor, Race, and Technology in the Confederate Iron Industry," *Technology and Culture* 42 (2001): 1–26.

44. Wiggins, *Journals of Josiah Gorgas*, April 26, 1864.

45. Gorgas and Hendrick, *William Crawford Gorgas*, 38.

46. Wiggins, *Journals of Josiah Gorgas*, May 15, 1865.

47. Quoted in Gibson, *Physician to the World*, 25.

48. Wiggins, *Journals of Josiah Gorgas*, February 23, 1865.

49. Wiggins, *Journals of Josiah Gorgas*, April 30, 1865.

50. "The Evacuation of Richmond," *Confederate Veteran* 25 (March 1917): 110.

51. Gorgas and Hendrick, *William Crawford Gorgas*, 40. This story is also told in an editorial in the *News Leader*, Richmond, VA: November 10, 1914, WCGP.

52. Wiggins, *Journals of Josiah Gorgas*, April 9, 1867, reflecting on the event two years later.

53. Elizabeth R. Varor, *Appomattox: Victory, Defeat, and Freedom at the End of the Civil War* (New York: Oxford University Press, 2015), 1–2.

54. Drew Gilpin Faust, *Mothers of Invention: Women of the Slaveholding South* (Chapel Hill: University of North Carolina Press, 2000); Laura F. Edwards, *Scarlett Doesn't Live Here Anymore: Southern Women in the Civil War Era* (Urbana: University of Illinois Press, 2000).

55. Gorgas and Hendrick, *William Crawford Gorgas*, 26.

56. Wiggins, *Love and Duty: Amelia and Josiah Gorgas and Their Family*, 37.

57. Gibson, *Physician to the World*, 24.

58. Wiggins, *Journals of Josiah Gorgas*, xxiii; and JG to AGG, circa July 1865, JGFP.

59. AGG to JG, July 29, 1865, JGFP.

60. JG to AGG, circa June 14, 1865, JGFP.

61. AGG to JG, August 14, 1865, JGFP.

62. JG to AGG, September 11, 1865, JGFP.

63. Congress restored Robert E. Lee's citizenship in 1975 and Jefferson Davis's citizenship in 1978.

64. AGG to JG, June 26, 1865, JGFP.

65. JG to AGG, July 7, 1865; and AGG to JG, July 29, 1865, JGFP.

66. AGG to JG, August 23, 1865, JGFP.

67. AGG to JG, August 23, 1865, JGFP.

68. WCG to JG, August 23, 1865, JGFP.

69. WCG to AGG, February 1870, JGFP.

70. Gorgas and Hendrick, *William Crawford Gorgas*, 46.

71. Wiggins, *Journals of Josiah Gorgas*, November 4, 1865, emphasis in the original.

72. AGG to JG, March 10, 1866, JGFP.

73. Gorgas and Hendrick, *William Crawford Gorgas*, 41.

74. JG to AGG, February 11, 1866, JGFP.

75. See Letter from WCG to E. D. Gayle, September 18, 1915, WCGP.

76. Wiggins, *Journals of Josiah Gorgas*, January 27, 1867, emphasis in the original.

77. Wiggins, *Journals of Josiah Gorgas*, October 10, 1867.

78. Wiggins, *Journals of Josiah Gorgas*, January 6, 1867.

79. WCG to RHG, August 31, 1879, WCGP.

80. Gibson, *Physician to the World*, 27–28.

81. Knowles, "Labor, Race, and Technology in the Confederate Iron Industry."

82. Wiggins, *Journals of Josiah Gorgas*, January 6, 1867.

83. Wiggins, *Journals of Josiah Gorgas*, January 3, 1868.

84. JG to WCG, February 25, 1868, JGFP.

85. Report cards, William Crawford Gorgas, Marshall School, New Orleans, Louisiana, February and April 1868, JGFP.

86. Eric Foner, *Reconstruction: America's Unfinished Revolution, 1863–1877* (New York: Harper and Rowe, 1988, 2014).

87. AGG to WCG, April 19, 1868, JGFP.

88. Wiggins, *Journals of Josiah Gorgas*, November 5, 1869; Ian Webster, "CPI Inflation Calculator," Official Inflation Data, Alioth Finance, November 21, 2022.

89. Charles Reagan Wilson, *Baptized in Blood: The Religion of the Lost Cause, 1865–1920* (Athens: University of Georgia Press, 1980, 2009), 145–51. Also on the Lost Cause, see Karen L. Cox, *Dixie's Daughters: The United Daughters of the Confederacy and the Preservation of Confederate Culture* (Tallahassee: University Press of Florida, 2019).

90. Steven Deyle, *Carry Me Back: The Domestic Slave Trade in American Life* (Oxford: Oxford University Press, 2013), 205; David Paulsen, "Sewanee Seeks Untold Story of University's Ties to Slavery, Segregation in Reconciliation Project," *Episcopal News Service*, posted online March 6, 2018.

91. JG to AGG, February 17, 1870, WCG to Mother, 1869, JGFP.

92. Wilson, *Baptized in Blood*, 145–51.

93. Gibson, *Physician to the World*, 35; Gorgas and Hendrick, *William Crawford Gorgas*, 45.

94. Wiggins, *Journals of Josiah Gorgas*, August 20, 1871.

95. Gorgas and Hendrick, *William Crawford Gorgas*; A. F. Kilpatrick to WCG, April 24, 1915, WCGP.

96. WCG to Jessie, October 1, 1871, JGFP.

97. Equal Justice Initiative website, "Reconstruction in America: Racial Violence after the Civil War, 1865–1876," 2020.

98. William Crawford Gorgas, "Address Delivered at the University of the South," Sewanee, Tennessee, June 13, 1912, WCGP.

99. Wilson, *Baptized in Blood*, 15.

## *Chapter 2*

1. WCG to Frank Polk, June 26, 1918, WCGP. This officer was William Mecklenburg Polk, a graduate of the Virginia Military Institute, who, after working at the ironworks, went to medical school and later became Marie Gorgas's surgeon.

2. Wiggins, *Journals of Josiah Gorgas*, June 3, 1860.

3. AGG to WCG, n.d., JGFP.

4. AGG to WCG, n.d., JGFP.

5. Gibson, *Physician to the World*, 39.

6. AGG to WCG, February 11, 1876, JGFP.

7. JG to AGG, February 4, 1876, JGFP.

8. Marie made this point in Gorgas and Hendrick, *William Crawford Gorgas*, 48.

9. David Oshinsky, *Bellevue: Three Centuries of Medicine and Mayhem at America's Most Storied Hospital* (New York: Doubleday, 2016); Lampson, *Death Loses a Pair of Wings*, 119–20.

10. Wiggins, *Journals of Josiah Gorgas*, October 29, 1876.

11. WCG to Jessie, November 19, 1876, WCGP.

12. David Adams, "Internal Military Intervention in the United States," *Journal of Peace Research* 32 (1995): 197–211.

13. The uncle was David Wyatt Aiken (D-SC). WCG to Jessie, November 19, 1876, WCGP.

14. Rosemary Stevens, *American Medicine and the Public Interest* (New Haven: Yale University Press, 1971), chapter 3; Kenneth M. Ludmerer, *Learning to Heal: The Development of Medical Education* (New York: Basic Books, 1985).

15. Table 15, "Life expectancy at birth, at age 65, and at age 75, by sex, race, and Hispanic origin: United States, selected years 1900–2015, in National Center for Health Statistics, *Health, United States, 2019,* (Hyattsville, MD, 2021); Elizabeth Arias, Betzaida Tejada-Vera, Farida Ahmad, and Kenneth D. Kochanek, "Provisional Life Expectancy Estimates for 2020," *Vital Statistics Rapid Release* 15 (July 2021): 1–12.

16. Simon Flexner and James Thomas Flexner, *William Henry Welch and the Heroic Age of American Medicine* (Baltimore: Johns Hopkins University Press, 1941, 1993).

17. Notably, William Welch and William Halstead. Oshinsky, *Bellevue*, 148–51.

18. Oshinsky, *Bellevue*, 117.

19. Austin Flint, *Clinical Medicine: A Systematic Treatise on the Diagnosis and Treatment of Diseases: Designed for the Use of Students and Practitioners of Medicine* (Philadelphia: H. C. Lea, 1879); Flexner and Flexner, *William Henry Welch.*

20. WCG to AGG, October 3, 1884, WCGP.

21. Benjamin J. Baldwin to MG, January 1, 1921, WCGP; Gibson, *Physician to the World*, 42–44.

22. James D. Stanley, to WCG, June 5, 1917, WCGP.

23. Benjamin J. Baldwin to MG, January 1, 1921, and Anecdotes on Life of W. C. Gorgas, chapter II, Early Years, circa 1925, WCGP.

24. Account book, WCG, 1877, WCGP.

25. Gorgas and Hendrick, *William Crawford Gorgas*, 50.

26. Lampson, *Death Loses a Pair of Wings*, 134.

27. WCG to RHG, August 22, 1881, WCGP.

28. "A Day of Fierce Heat," *New York Tribune*, July 19, 1878; "No Relief from Heat," *New York Tribune*, July 20, 1878.

29. "The Hot Wave's Approach," *NYT*, July 19, 1878; Lampson, *Death Loses a Pair of Wings*, 145.

30. On the 1878 epidemic, see Jeanette Keith, *Fever Season: The Story of a Terrifying Epidemic and the People Who Saved the City* (New York: Bloomsbury Press, 2012); Khaled J. Bloom, *The Mississippi Valley's Great Yellow Fever Epidemic of 1878* (Baton Rouge: Louisiana State University Press, 1993); Deanne Stephens Nuwer, *Plague among the Magnolias: The 1878 Yellow Fever Epidemic in Mississippi* (Tuscaloosa: University of Alabama Press, 2009); Crosby, *American Plague.*

31. Nuwer, *Plague among the Magnolias*, 114, 118.

32. Nuwer, *Plague among the Magnolias*, 126–28; Pierce and Writer, *Yellow Jack*, 69.

33. Flint, *Clinical Medicine*, 733–35.

34. Lampson, *Death Loses a Pair of Wings*, 161–238.

35. Benjamin J. Baldwin to MG, January 1, 1921, WCGP.

36. JG to AGG, September 15, 1878, JGFP. Josiah's biographer speculates that he had a brain tumor, because his condition continued to worsen. See Vandiver, *Ploughshares into Swords,* 314.

37. JG to AGG, October 23, 1878, JGFP.

38. JG to AGG, December 5, 1878, JGFP.

39. JG to WCG, December 8, 1878, JGFP.

40. AGG to WCG, December 8, 1878, JGFP.

41. AGG to WCG, February 27, 1879, JGFP.

42. AGG to WCG, March 8, 1879, JGFP.

43. Transcribed newspaper article, *Tuscaloosa Gazette*, October 9, 1879, JGFP.

44. WCG to Jessie, June 1, 1879, WCGP.

45. Gibson, *Physician to the World*, 45

46. Lampson, *Death Loses a Pair of Wings,* 225–28.

47. Benjamin Baldwin to MG, January 1, 1921, WCGP.

48. Nellie Bly, "Ten Days in a Mad-House or Nellie Bly's Experience on Blackwell's Island," in *Miscellaneous Sketches: Trying to Be a Servant* (New York: Ian L. Munro, 1887).

49. AGG to WCG, April 4, 1880, WCGP.

50. Ruth Gordon, "William Crawford Gorgas: A Modern Pioneer," typescript, 1935, 24, WCGP.

51. Roy E. Gandy et al., "The Statesmanship of William Crawford Gorgas, M.D., Surgeon General, Medical Corps, United States Army," *American Surgeon* 83 (March 2017): 223–25; Gillett, *Army Medical Department, 1865–1917,* 13–18; Jack McCallum, *Leonard Wood: Rough Rider, Surgeon, Architect of American Imperialism* (New York: New York University Press, 2006), 15.

52. Ian Webster, "CPI Inflation Calculator," Official Inflation Data, Alioth Finance, November 21, 2022.

53. Gillett, *Army Medical Department, 1865–1917,* 27; Miles Wyndam, *A History of the National Library of Medicine* (Bethesda, MD: Department of Health and Human Services, PHS, National Institutes of Health, National Library of Medicine (hereafter cited as NLM), Bethesda, MD, 1982).

54. WCG to RHG, November 8, 1880, WCGP.

55. Edward M. Coffman, *The Old Army: A Portrait of the American Army in Peacetime, 1784–1898* (New York: Oxford University Press, 1986), 348.

56. Charles A. Byler, "Civil-Military Relations on the Frontier and Beyond, 1865–1917," in *In War and in Peace: U.S. Civil-Military Relations,* ed. David S. and Jeanne T. Heidler (Westport, CT: Praeger Security International, 2006); Peter D. Olch, "Medicine in the Indian-Fighting Army, 1866–1890," *Journal of the West* 21 (1982): 32–48; and Kevin Adams, *Class and Race in the Frontier Army: Military Life in the West, 1870–1890* (Norman: University of Oklahoma Press, 2009).

57. WCG to RHG, August 22, 1881, WCGP.

58. WCG to RHG, November 8, 1880, WCGP.

59. V. H. Bridgman to MG, December 28, 1920, WCGP.

60. WCG to RHG, August 22, 1881, WCGP.

61. "Anecdotes on the Life of W. C. Gorgas, General Sherman and the Mint Julep," circa 1925, WCGP.

62. WCG to RHG, December 7, 1879, WCGP.

## *Chapter 3*

1. Aileen Lyster, "Anecdotes on Life of WC Gorgas, Life in Matamoros in Brownsville," circa 1920, WCGP.

2. Quoted in Gorgas and Hendrick, *William Crawford Gorgas,* 4.

3. Harriet N. Dunn and Eveline Guthrie Dunn, *Records of the Guthrie Family, of Pennsylvania, Connecticut, and Virginia, with Ancestry of Those Who Have Intermarried with the Family* (Chicago: H. N. and S. L. Dunn, 1898), 135–60, has the Doughty family genealogy.

4. "Mrs. William C. Gorgas Tells of Life in Panama during Work on Canal," newspaper clipping, circa 1915, WCGP.

5. Gorgas and Hendrick, *William Crawford Gorgas,* 2.

6. WCG to Jessie, August 14, 1882, WCGP.

7. Medical Log for Fort Brown, Record Group 94, Records of the Adjutant General's Office, NARA, (hereafter cited as RG 94), Entry 547.

8. Thus began a lifelong friendship between Crowder, who served as provost general during World War I, and Gorgas, the army surgeon general during the war.

9. Gorgas and Hendrick, *William Crawford Gorgas*, 8–9.

10. WCG to MG, January 10, 1884, WCGP. She referred to Lyster as "Colonel," which was his rank when she wrote the story, but he was a captain at the time.

11. Gorgas and Hendrick, *William Crawford Gorgas*, 10.

12. "List of Patients Suffering from Epidemic Yellow Fever, Fort Brown, Texas, 1882," RG 94, Entry 620, Box 5, NARA.

13. T. C. Lyster, "Memories of WC Gorgas," circa 1915, WCGP.

14. E. Mellou, telegram, October 4, 1882, RG 94, Entry 561, Box 225; and Medical Log for Fort Brown, RG 94, Entry 547, NARA.

15. Gorgas and Hendrick, *William Crawford Gorgas*, 11.

16. "Report on Epidemic of Yellow Fever at Fort Brown, Texas during the Summer of 1882," RG 94, Entry 620, Box 5, NARA; and C. C. Hewitt, "Nineteenth Regiment of Infantry," in *The Army of the US Historical Sketches of Staff and Line with Portraits of Generals-In-Chief*, ed. Theophilus Francis Rodenbough and William L. Haskin (New York: Maynard, Merrill, 1896), 664–65.

17. The young woman was Dora E. Reynolds, who had died September 29. See "List of Patients Suffering from Epidemic Yellow Fever, Fort Brown, Texas, 1882," RG 94, Entry 620, Box 5, NARA.

18. "Social and Personal," *Washington Post*, September 4, 1905.

19. Gorgas and Hendrick, *William Crawford Gorgas*, 13.

20. Gorgas and Hendrick, *William Crawford Gorgas*, 43.

21. Gorgas and Hendrick, *William Crawford Gorgas*, 14.

22. Gorgas and Hendrick, *William Crawford Gorgas*, 16.

23. AGG to WCG, April 26, 1885, WCGP.

24. AGG to WCG, May 20, 1884, WCGP

25. WCG to OTSG, June 1, 1883, RG 94, Entry 561, Box 225, NARA.

26. Gorgas and Hendrick, *William Crawford Gorgas*, 16–17.

27. WCG to MG, May 8,1883, WCGP.

28. WCG to MG, August 11, 1883, WCGP.

29. Marie, "Anecdotes on the Life of W. C. Gorgas, Chapter II, Early Years, circa 1925," WCGP.

30. WCG to Jessie, February 26, 1883, WCGP.

31. Account Book, WCG, 1879, WCGP. The book has notations for the years 1878 to 1883.

32. WCG to MG, January 16, 1884, WCGP.

33. Medical Log for Fort Brown, RG 94, Entry 547, NARA; AGG to WCG, August 6, 1884, WCGP.

34. J. H. Woodward to Mary [Marie] Doughty, May 26, 1884, Woodward Family Papers, University of Alabama Special Collections, Tuscaloosa, Alabama; AGG to WCG, August 6, 1884, WCGP.

35. WCG to Surgeon General Murray, July 1, 1884, RG 94, Entry 620, Box 5, NARA.

36. WCG to AGG, October 3, 1884, WCGP.

37. AGG to WCG, April 26, 1885, WCGP.

38. WCG to Jessie, May 18, 1885, WCGP.

39. WCG to Ria, July 6, 1885, WCGP.

40. "Partial letter from Marie Gorgas," circa 1920 (probably earlier), WCGP.

41. Gorgas and Hendrick, *William Crawford Gorgas*, 17–18.

42. WCG to AGG, October 11, 1885, WCGP.

43. Fort Sill was known as Camp Oklahoma, Indian Territory, at the time. Records of Gorgas's duty reports can be found in RG 94, Entry 561, Box 225, NARA.

44. Brenda K. Jackson, "Holding Down the Fort: A History of Dakota Territory's Fort Randall," *South Dakota History* 32 (2002): 1–28.

45. WCG to C. E. Anderson, December 26, 1917, and WCG to Colonel, August 14, 1891, WCGP. Thanks to Peter H. Wood for bringing to my attention the Lee connection to Traveler's name.

46. WCG to Colonel, August 14, 1891, WCGP.

47. Gorgas and Hendrick, *William Crawford Gorgas*, 56–57.

48. Coffman, *Old Army*, 370–78.

49. Gorgas and Hendrick, *William Crawford Gorgas*, 55.

50. The journal is now *Military Medicine*. See Editorial, *Military Medicine* 116 (January 1955): 58–59. Lampson says that Gorgas was an inaugural subscriber to the journal; see *Death Loses a Pair of Wings*, 313.

51. Peter D. Olch, "Medicine in the Indian-Fighting Army, 1866–1890," *Journal of the West* 21 (July 1982): 36.

52. Fort Randall Medical Log, RG 94, Entry 547, vol. 85, NARA.

53. *War Department Annual Report, 1893*, 439 (hereafter cited as *WDAR*).

54. "Medical History of Patients Treated by W. C. Gorgas," and five booklets of patient records, "Physician's Visiting List 1894," beginning 1891, Gorgas Papers, Box 38, LoC. On frontier medicine, see Anton Paul Sohn, *A Saw, Pocket Instruments, and Two Ounces of Whiskey: Frontier Military Medicine in the Great Basin* (Spokane, WA: Arthur H. Clarke, 1998).

55. "Medical History of Patients Treated by W. C. Gorgas," January 28, 1897, Gorgas Papers, Box 32, LoC.

56. Quoted in Hyson et al., *A History of Dentistry in the US Army to World War II*, (Washington, DC: Borden Institute, 2008), 102; W. C. Gorgas, "Consideration of Some of the Important Changes That Have Been Made in the Medical Department of the United States Army during the past Four Years," *Journal of the National Dental Association* 5 (1918):1154–55.

57. Gorgas and Hendrick, *William Crawford Gorgas*, 59–60.

58. WCG, bound journal with records of patient cases, Gorgas Papers, Box 33, LoC.

59. Gorgas and Hendrick, *William Crawford Gorgas*, 53.

60. "Anecdotes on Life of W. C. Gorgas, Characteristics and Anecdote," circa 1925, WCGP.

61. "Medical History of Patients Treated by W. C. Gorgas," Gorgas Papers, Box 32, LoC.

62. WCG to AGG, September 10, 1893; and WCG to AGG, October 8, 1901, WCGP.

63. Lampson, *Death Loses a Pair of Wings,* 314, 323–24.

64. MG to Mattie, September 28, 1889, WCGP.

65. Robert J. Kamish, "Doctor William Crawford Gorgas—1854–1920," *American Journal of Surgery* 108 (1964): 921–28.

66. William C. Gorgas, "Nine Cases of Wounds of the Abdomen," *Proceedings of the Florida Medical Association* 2 (1891): 56–62.

67. *WDAR, 1894,* 360.

68. John P. Kelly to MG, March 7, 1921, WCGP.

69. WCG to Col. H. D. Snyder, November 7, 1914, WCGP.

70. John P. Kelly to MG, March 7, 1921, WCGP. The Index of OTSG Document Files, 1894–1917, also has an entry under Gorgas's name, "Special Report, Double Amputation, 1897," file 34813, Record Group 112, Records of the Office of the Surgeon General, NARA (hereafter cited as RG 112), Entry 23.

71. Marie wrote this in dialect: "Suttenly it's more! 'Tain't everybody whut can git washing done by a pusson what has two wooden legs!" Gorgas and Hendrick, *William Crawford Gorgas,* 63.

72. V. H. Bridgman to MG, December 28, 1920, WCGP.

73. "Letter from Champe McCulloch, Fort Sheridan, Illinois, to Mrs. Gorgas, Washington, D.C.," August 13, 1921, WCGP.

74. The following discussion is from the records of RG 112, Entry 26, Box 33, NARA. Also see George F. Pearce, "Torment of Pestilence: Yellow Fever Epidemics in Pensacola," *Florida Historical Quarterly* 56 (1978): 448–72.

75. W. C. Gorgas, "A Short Account of the Yellow Fever Epidemic of 1897, and More Particularly Its Relations to the Garrisons of the Regular Army," *Proceedings of the Eighth Annual Meeting of the Association of Military Surgeons* (Columbus: Berlin Printing, 1900): 282–89; and *WDAR, 1898,* 626.

76. Junius W. MacMurray to adjutant general, December 8, 1897, RG 112, Entry 26, Box 33, NARA.

77. Champe McCulloch to MG, August 13, 1921, WCGP.

78. Gorgas to Surgeon General, November 1894, RG 112, Entry 26, Box 33, NARA.

79. WCG to Mamie, December 17, 1897, WCGP.

## *Chapter 4*

1. Louis A. Pérez Jr., *The War of 1898: The United States and Cuba in History and Historiography* (Chapel Hill: University of North Carolina Press, 1998); Nancy Stepan, "The Interplay between Socio-Economic Factors and Medical Science: Yellow Fever Research, Cuba and the United States," *Social Studies of Science* 8 (1978): 397–423; Mariola Espinosa, *Epidemic Invasions: Yellow Fever and the Limits of Cuban Independence, 1878–1930* (Chicago: University of Chicago Press, 2009).

2. On depopulation of the Americas, see Noble David Cook, *Born to Die: Disease and New World Conquest, 1492–1650* (Cambridge: Cambridge University Press, 1998); J. R. McNeill, *Mosquito Empires: Ecology and War in the Greater Caribbean, 1620–1914.* (Cambridge: Cambridge University Press, 2010); Alfred W. Crosby Jr., *The Columbian Exchange: Biological and Cultural Consequences of 1492* (Westport, CT: Greenwood Press, 1972).

3. Quoted in Cook, *Born to Die*, 63.

4. Cook, *Born to Die*, 205.

5. Pierce and Writer, *Yellow Jack*, 9–13; Cook, *Born to Die*, 178–82.

6. Gorgas, "A Short Account of the Yellow Fever Epidemic of 1897," 282–89.

7. John Lawrence Tone, *War and Genocide in Cuba*, 1895–1898 (Chapel Hill: University of North Carolina Press, 2008); Pérez Jr., *War of 1898*.

8. Espinosa, *Epidemic Invasions*; Mariola Espinosa, "The Threat from Havana: Southern Public Health, Yellow Fever, and the U.S. Intervention in the Cuban Struggle for Independence, 1878–1898," *Journal of Southern History* 72 (2006): 541–68; Stepan, "The Interplay between Socio-Economic Factors and Medical Science," 397–423; Randall M. Packard, *A History of Global Health: Interventions into the Lives of Other Peoples* (Baltimore: Johns Hopkins University Press, 2016).

9. H. G. Rickover, *How the Battleship Maine Was Destroyed* (Annapolis: Naval Institute Press, 1995), 321–22; Thomas B. Allen, "A Special Report: What Really Sank the Maine?" *Naval History* 12 (1998): 30–44.

10. Gregory Weeks, *U.S. and Latin American Relations* (New York: Pearson, 2008), 56.

11. Paul A. Kramer, *The Blood of Government: Race, Empire, the United States, & the Philippines* (Chapel Hill: University of North Carolina Press, 2006), 91–96.

12. Stephen C. Craig, *In the Interest of Truth: The Life and Science of Surgeon General George Miller Sternberg* (Fort Sam Houston, TX: Borden Institute, 2013); John Gibson, *George Sternberg—Soldier in White: The Life of General George Miller Sternberg* (Durham, NC: Duke University Press, 1958); Martha Sternberg, *George Miller Sternberg: A Biography* (Chicago: American Medical Association, 1920).

13. George M. Sternberg, *A Manual of Bacteriology* (New York: W. Wood, 1893).

14. George M. Sternberg, "Dr. Finlay's Mosquito Inoculations," *American Journal of Medical Sciences* 102 (1891): 627–30.

15. WCG to Jessie, June 3, 1893; and WCG to RHG, June 9, 1893, WCGP.

16. George Sternberg to Secretary of War, March 25, 1898, Hench Collection; *WDAR, 1899*, 490–94.

17. McNeill, *Mosquito Empires*, 302.

18. *WDAR, 1898*, 602.

19. Pierce and Writer, *Yellow Jack*, 102–3; *WDAR, 1899*, 495–97.

20. Other hospital ships were the *Solace*, the *Missouri*, and the *Olivette*.

21. Nicholas Senn, *War Correspondence (Hispano-American War): Letters from Dr. Nicholas Senn* (Chicago: American Medical Association Press, 1899), 52. See Gillett, *Army Medical Department, 1865–1917*, 173–228, on medical support during the war.

22. WCG to AGG, May 30, 1898, WCGP.

23. Ester V. Hasson, "The First Trip of the Army Hospital Ship *Relief*," RG 112, Entry 230, Box 1, NARA.

24. WCG to Theo, April 6, 1898, WCGP.

25. Louis La Garde testimony, *Report of the Commission Appointed by the President to Investigate the Conduct of the War Department in the War with Spain* (hereafter cited as Dodge Commission Report), S. doc. 221, vol. 5, US 56th Cong., 1st sess. (Washington, DC: GPO), 1829.

26. Dodge Commission Report, vol. 5, 1919.

27. "Journal, William Crawford Gorgas, partial," July 1898, WCGP.

28. Hasson, "The First Trip of the Army Hospital Ship *Relief*."

29. "Major General Merritte W. Ireland," Medical Memoir, 1931, US Army, Office of Medical History website (hereafter cited as Merritte Ireland memoir).

30. On the history of nursing, see Susan M. Reverby, *Ordered to Care: The Dilemma of American Nursing: 1850–1945* (Cambridge: Cambridge University Press, 1987); Mary Sarnecky, *History of the Army Nurse Corps* (Philadelphia: University of Pennsylvania Press, 1999); Philip A. Kalisch and Beatrice J. Kalisch, *American Nursing: A History*, 4th ed. (Lippincott Williams & Wilkins, 2003); Patricia D'Antonio, *American Nursing: A History of Knowledge, Authority, and the Meaning of Work* (Baltimore: Johns Hopkins University Press, 2010).

31. Gorgas and Hendrick, *William Crawford Gorgas*, 51.

32. *WDAR, 1899*, 375.

33. Until 1943 the Army Nurse Corps did not allow nurses to marry and would not admit Black women until 1947. Men were not enlisted in the Army Nurse Corps until the Korean War. See Sarnecky, *History of the Army Nurse Corps*; "Rules Governing Army Nurse Corps," in *WDAR*, 1899, 378–82; Anita Newcome McGee, "The Status of the Army Nurse of 1898," *Trained Nurse and Hospital Review* 39 (August/September, 1907): 1–8.

34. Dodge Commission Report, vol. 1, 370.

35. La Garde testimony, Dodge Commission Report, vol. 5, 1829; WCG to OTSG, July 15, 1898, RG 94, Entry 561, Box 225, NARA.

36. La Garde testimony, Dodge Commission Report, vol. 5, 1839.

37. *WDAR, 1898*, 784; Maj. Charles Greenleaf's report on Dept. of Santiago, *WDAR, 1898*, 732–33; Greenleaf, "Memorandum for Sanitary Precautions," July 15, 1898, in Dodge Commission Report, vol. 2, 614–15.

38. "Personal Recollections of General Gorgas by Victor C. Vaughan," included with a letter from Burton J. Hendrick to MG, December 3, 1923, WCGP.

39. W. C. Gorgas, "General Directions as to the Treatment of Yellow Fever," handwritten, 1898, WCGP.

40. "Personal Recollections of General Gorgas by Victor C. Vaughan," WCGP.

41. Pierce and Writer, *Yellow Jack*, 108.

42. WCG to James Bowles, December 29, 1910, Gorgas Papers, Box 9, LoC.

43. La Garde testimony, Dodge Commission Report, vol. 5, 1835; *WDAR, 1900*, 737.

44. All quotes from "Journal, William Crawford Gorgas, partial," July 1898, WCGP.

45. *WDAR, 1899*, vol. 1, pt. 2, 522

46. WCG to Home, August 6, 1898, WCGP.

47. Mariola Espinosa, "The Question of Racial Immunity to Yellow Fever in History and Historiography." *Social Science History* 38 (2014): 437–53.

48. Roger D. Cunningham, "The Black 'Immune' Regiments in the Spanish-American War," the National Museum of the United States Army website, 2015.

49. WCG to MG, August 4, 1898, WCGP.

50. WCG to MG, August 26, 1898, WCGP.

51. WCG to Home, August 19, 1898, WCGP.

52. WCG to MG, August 3, 1898, WCGP.

53. WCG to Home, August 19, 1898, WCGP.

54. Theodore Roosevelt, *The Roughriders* (New York: Da Capo Press, 1990), Appendix A, 281–82. Originally published 1902.

55. *NYT*, August 5, 1898, and *Chicago Daily Tribune*, August 28, 1898, quoted in Mark A. Youngren, "A Sickly Little War: Epidemic Disease, Military Campaigns, and the Spanish-American War," PhD diss., (Michigan State University, 2016), 521–22.

56. WCG to MG, August 9, 1898, WCGP

57. WCG to MG, August 12, 1898, WCGP.

58. WCG to MG, August 15, 1898, WCGP.

59. WCG to MG, August 16, 1898, WCGP

60. WCG to MG, August 21, 1898, WCGP.

61. WCG to MG, August 26, 1898, WCGP.

62. Carolina M. Anthony to WCG, January 5, 1905, Gorgas Papers, Box 7, LoC.

63. Vincent J. Cirillo, *Bullets and Bacilli: The Spanish-American War and Military Medicine* (New Brunswick, NJ: Rutgers University Press, 2004).

64. Craig, *In the Interest of Truth*, 242–43.

65. "Typhoid," World Health Organization website, March 2018.

66. *WDAR, 1899*, 525; La Garde testimony, Dodge Commission Report, vol. 5, 1840.

67. WCG to MG, August 26, 1898, WCGP. The letter is dated the twenty-sixth, but he wrote it over several days.

68. WCG to Dearest, August 30, 1898, WCGP.

69. WCG to MG, August 31 and September 1–2, 1898, WCGP.

70. William H. Arthur to WCG, April 2, 1915, WCGP.

71. WCG to William H. Arthur, March 25, 1915, WCGP.

72. Sternberg, Dodge Commission Report, vol. 5, 1922.

73. "Memorial of the Late Dr. George McCreery," *New York Medical Journal* 69 (January 1899): 136–37; Dodge Commission Report, 1833 and 2021; Merritte Ireland memoir.

74. "Note signed by Dr. Andrew K. Smith, concerning Mrs. Mary D. Gorgas' health," handwritten on letterhead, September 12, 1898, WCGP.

75. "Patient record, The Presbyterian Hospital," and WCG to OTSG, September 30, 1898, RG 94, Entry 561, Box 225, NARA; Lampson, *Death Loses a Pair of Wings*, 375–76.

76. Cirillo, *Bullets and Bacilli*.

77. Leonard Porter Ayres, *The War with Germany: A Statistical Summary* (Washington, DC: GPO, 1919), 124.

78. Walter Reed, Victor C. Vaughan, and E. O. Shakespeare, *Reports on the Origin and Spread of Typhoid Fever in the U.S. Military Camps during the Spanish War of 1898*, 2 vols. (Washington, DC: GPO, 1904). The commission published three different reports; the one commonly cited is the final report of 1904.

79. The formal name was The Commission Appointed by the President to Investigate the Conduct of the War Department in the War with Spain.

80. Sternberg, Dodge Commission Report, vol. 5, 1925.

81. Dodge Commission Report, passim; Gillett, *Army Medical Department, 1865–1917*, chapter 7; Vincent J. Cirillo, "Fever and Reform: The Typhoid Epidemic and the

Spanish-American War," *Journal of the History of Medicine* 55 (October 2000): 363–97; Stanhope Bayne-Jones, *The Evolution of Preventive Medicine in the U.S. Army, 1607–1939* (Washington, DC: Office of the Surgeon General of the Army, 1968), 123–46.

82. Dodge Commission Report, vol. 1 (Appendices), 188–89.

## *Chapter 5*

1. The following discussion is drawn from William Crawford Gorgas, "Diary, February 1899–August 1899," Box 4, and "Yellow Fever Cases, 1899," Gorgas Papers, Box 25, LoC.

2. MG to AGG, January 2, 1899, WCGP.

3. MG to Mother, February 3, 1899, WCGP.

4. Gorgas and Hendrick, *William Crawford Gorgas*, 82.

5. On the US occupation of Cuba, see Marial Iglesias Utset, *A Cultural History of Cuba during the U.S. Occupation, 1898–1902*, trans. Russ Davidson (Chapel Hill: University of North Carolina Press, 2011); Louis A. Pérez Jr. "Insurrection, Intervention, and the Transformation of Land Tenure Systems in Cuba, 1895–1902," *Hispanic American Historical Review* 65 (1985): 229–54; Howard Gillette, "Military Occupation of Cuba, 1899–1902: Workshop for American Progressivism," *American Quarterly* 2 (October 1973): 410–25; Graham A. Cosmas, "Securing the Fruits of Victory: The U.S. Army Occupies Cuba, 1898–1899," *Military Affairs* 38 (October 1974): 90; McCallum, *Leonard Wood*, chapter 7; Leonard Wood, "Military Government of Cuba," *Annals of the American Academy of Political and Social Science* 21 (March 1903): 153–82.

6. Pérez Jr., "Insurrection, Intervention, and the Transformation of Land Tenure Systems in Cuba," 229–54.

7. Cosmas, "Securing the Fruits of Victory," 90.

8. Wood, "Military Government of Cuba," 153–54.

9. McCallum, *Leonard Wood*, chapter 7.

10. Utset, *Cultural History of Cuba during the U.S. Occupation*, 122–24; McCallum, *Leonard Wood*, 124, 148.

11. WCG to Carlos Finlay, June 16, 1906; Kean to WCG, October 8, 1907, WCGP.

12. Gorgas and Hendrick, *William Crawford Gorgas*, 82–83.

13. G. C. Cook, "Ronald Ross (1857–1932): 100 Years since the Demonstration of Mosquito Transmission of *Plasmodium* spp.—on 20 August 1897," *Transactions of the Royal Society of Tropical Medicine and Hygiene* 91 (July–August 1997):487–88; Wood, "Military Government of Cuba," 15–17.

14. Craig, *In the Interest of Truth*, 248.

15. Hugh Lenox Scott, *Some Memories of a Soldier* (New York: Century, 1928), 239; Leonard Wood in *WDAR, 1900*, 262.

16. Mariola Espinosa, "A Fever for Empire: U.S. Disease Eradication in Cuba as Colonial Public Health," National Library of Medicine, Digital Collections, recorded lecture, Bethesda, MD, 2007.

17. Scott, *Some Memories of a Soldier*, 239.

18. Caldwell, *American Plague*, 89.

19. Scott, *Some Memories of a Soldier*, 236.

20. WCG to AGG, August 5, 1899, WCGP. Date on transcript is September 15, 1899.

21. "Yellow Fever Cases, 1899," Gorgas Papers, Box 25, LoC.

22. W. C. Gorgas, "Notes on the Treatment of Yellow Fever at Las Animas Hospital, the Hospital of the Sanitary Department, during the Epidemic of 1900 at Havana, Cuba," *Military Surgeon* (1903): 1–7.

23. Aspirin was a recent invention and may have been administered, but it may have also aggravated internal bleeding. The FDA banned phenacetin in 1983 for its carcinogenic and kidney-damaging properties.

24. Osler, *Principles and Practice of Medicine* (New York: D. Appleton, 1912), 362–63; Gorgas, "Notes on the Treatment of Yellow Fever at Las Animas Hospital."

25. "Stories from Nurses," Anita Newcomb McGee Files, RG 112, Entry 230, Box 1, NARA.

26. "Hospitals of Cuba," *New York Medical Journal* (November 2, 1901), 855.

27. WCG to MG, November 21, 1899, Gorgas Papers, Box 2, LoC.

28. WCG to John Ross, December 30, 1899, Box 3, John Ross Papers.

29. WCG to MG, September 15, 1900, WCGP.

30. W. C. Gorgas, *Report of Vital Statistics of Havana, April 1900* (Havana, Cuba: Office of Adjutant General, War Department, April 1900).

31. Utset, *Cultural History of Cuba during the U.S. Occupation*, 23.

32. "Cuba: Yellow-Fever Mortality in Havana, 1884–1900—Statistics and Deductions," *PHR* 15 (July 20, 1900): 1840–54.

33. William C. Gorgas, "Cuba. Vital Statistics of Havana for September, 1900," *PHR* 15 (1900): 2644–49.

34. *WDAR* 1900, "Revenues and Expenditures in Cuba," 221.

35. WCG to MG, September 6, 1900, WCGP.

36. "Letter from Will Gorgas, Havana Cuba," typewritten letter, May 8, 1900, WCGP.

37. WCG to MG, September 5, 1899, WCGP.

38. AGG to WCG, n.d. (probably April 1901), JGFP. On the Southern Cross of Honor, see Spencer C. Tucker, *American Civil War: The Definitive Encyclopedia and Document Collection* (Santa Barbara, CA: ABC-CLIO, 2013), 2202.

39. WCG to AGG, May 3, 1901, WCGP; emphasis in the original.

40. WCG to AGG, August 20, 1899, transcript, and AGG to WCG, July 1, 1900, WCGP.

41. Juan F. Vizcaino, "Carlos J. Finlay, Gloria Americana," *Journal of Inter-American Studies* 7 (1965): 497.

42. Gorgas, *Sanitation in Panama*, 6–7.

43. WCG to RHG, August 16, 1900, WCGP.

44. Craig, *In the Interest of Truth*, 265.

45. WCG to MG, September 4, 1900, WCGP.

46. *PHR* 16 (1901): 2589; "Officials Get Yellow Fever?" *NYT*, October 12, 1900.

47. "Flags of Morro Castle Lowered at Half Mast," *Cincinnati Times*, October 19, 1900; "Devoted Wife," *Boston Daily Globe,* October 19, 1900; "Dual Tragedy in Havana; Major Peterson Dies of Yellow Fever and His Wife Kills Herself," *NYT*, October 19, 1900.

48. William B. Bean, *Walter Reed: A Biography* (Charlottesville: University of Virginia Press, 1982), 123.

49. "Less Yellow Fever in Cuba," *NYT*, October 21, 1900.

50. "A Commotion in Cuba," *New York Evening Post*, November 2, 1900.

## *Chapter 6*

1. Although such ad hoc investigatory bodies were technically army boards, they were also called commissions. Walter Reed, for example, signed documents "On the Part of the Commission." See the informed consent agreement between Antonio Benigno and Walter Reed, November 26, 1900, Hench Collection.

For a discussion of the myth that no one died in the experiments, see D. Hachenburg, "Deaths Associated with Yellow Fever Experiments," *JAMA* 249 (1983): 1150–51. Even Hachenburg ignores the Spanish men who died in the vaccine trials.

2. Bert Hansen, "Medical History for the Masses: How American Comic Books Celebrated Heroes of Medicine in the 1940s," *Bulletin of the History of Medicine* 78 (2004): 148–91.

3. Guiseppe Sanarelli, "A Lecture on Yellow Fever, with a Description of the *Bacillus Icteroides*," *British Medical Journal* (July 3, 1897): 7–11; Walter Reed and James Carroll, "A Comparative Study of the Biological Characters and Pathogenesis of *Bacillus X* (Sternberg), *Bacillus Icteroides* (Sanarelli), and the Hog-Cholera Bacillus (Salmon and Smith)," *Journal of Experimental Medicine* 5 (1900): 215–70. On early efforts to find the yellow fever pathogen, see Margaret Warner, "Hunting the Yellow Fever Germ: The Principle and Practice of Etiological Proof in Late Nineteenth-Century America," *Bulletin of the History of Medicine* 59 (1985): 361–82.

4. William B. Bean, *Walter Reed: A Biography* (Charlottesville: University of Virginia Press, 1982); Laura Wood Roper, *Walter Reed, Doctor in Uniform* (New York: J. Messner, 1996). Originally published 1961.

5. John A. Garraty and Mark C. Carnes, eds., *American National Biography*, vol. 4 (New York: Oxford University Press, 1999), 459–61.

6. Headquarters of the Army, Special Order No. 122, "Military Orders Regarding the Appointment of a Board to Study Infectious Diseases in Cuba," May 24, 1900, Hench Collection.

7. Kean, "Autobiographical Sketch," 1928, US Army Medical Department, Office of Medical History.

8. "Military Orders for William Crawford Gorgas and Jefferson Randolph Kean," April 9, 1900, Hench Collection.

9. Theo Lyster to Mother, May 25, 1900, WCGP.

10. Enrique Chaves-Carballo, "Carlos Finlay and Yellow Fever: Triumph over Adversity," *Military Medicine* 170 (2005); Juan F. Vizcaino, "Carlos J. Finlay, Gloria Americana," *Journal of Inter-American Studies* 7 (1965): 493–502.

11. Carlos J. Finlay, "El mosquito hipoteticamento considerado como agente de transmision de la fiebre amarilla" (The Mosquito Hypothetically Considered as the Agent of Transmission of Yellow Fever), *Anales de Academia de Sciencia Medica de la Habana* 18 (1881): 147–69.

12. John Lawrence Tone, "How the Mosquito (Man) Liberated Cuba," *History and Technology* 18 (2002): 277–308.

13. Gorgas, *Sanitation in Panama*, 15.

14. Reed and Carroll, "Comparative Study of the Biological Characters and Pathogenesis of Bacillus X," 215–70.

15. Randall M. Packard, *The Making of a Tropical Disease: A Short History of Malaria* (Baltimore: Johns Hopkins University Press, 2007), 115–17. Ross was awarded the Nobel Prize in Medicine in 1902, and Laveran in 1907.

16. Aristides Agramonte to Kean, July 3, 1908, Hench Collection.

17. *WDAR, 1900*, 683.

18. "Inquiry into Yellow Fever Outbreak," *Washington Post*, August 12, 1900.

19. Walter Reed, "The Propagation of Yellow Fever—Observations Based on Recent Researches," in *Medical and Chirurgical Faculty of the State of Maryland* (Baltimore, 1901).

20. Henry R. Carter, "A Note on the Interval between Infecting and Secondary Cases of Yellow Fever from the Records of the Yellow Fever at Orwood and Taylor, Miss., 1898," *New Orleans Medical and Surgical Journal* 52 (1900): 617–36. Alan N. Clements and Ralph E. Harbach single out Carter for credit in "History of the Discovery of the Mode of Transmission of Yellow Fever Virus," *Journal of Vector Ecology* (December 2017): 208–22.

21. Walter Reed, "Recent Researches concerning the Etiology, Propagation, and Prevention of Yellow Fever, by the United States Army Commission (Three Charts)," *Journal of Hygiene* 2 (April 1902):101–19.

22. "Address by Doctor Antonio Albertini," translation [from Spanish] of speech by Antonio D. Albertini, September 28, 1936, Hench Collection.

23. W. C. Gorgas, "Personal Reports," RG 94, Entry 561, Box 225, NARA; "Albert E. Truby's Answers for a Questionnaire from Philip Showalter Hench concerning Truby's Book," February 1947, Hench Collection. Thanks to Daniel Cavanaugh of the Claude Moore Health Sciences Library, University of Virginia, for background information on Rafael Lillo.

24. Walter Reed to George M. Sternberg, July 24, 1900, Hench Collection

25. Carroll was confined to bed until September 13, 1900. Jefferson Kean, "Chronology of the Yellow Fever Work in Cuba 1899 and 1900 and Personal Experiences," June 1, 1929, Hench Collection; Senate Report no. 6009, *James Carroll*, February 2, 1907, 60th Cong., 1st sess.

26. "Statement by Aristides Agramonte concerning the Work of the U.S. Yellow Fever Commission," August 31, 1908: Hench Collection.

27. WCG to MG, September 6, 1900, WCGP.

28. Walter Reed's biographer believes that it was an accident. William B. Bean, *Walter Reed: A Biography* (Charlottesville: University of Virginia Press, 1982), 134–37. Crosby suggests Reed and others believed it to be experimental but presented his infection as accidental because his life insurance company would not pay his widow for a self-inflicted death, in *American Plague*, 165–66.

29. WCG to Mabel Lazear, April 4, 1903, Hench Collection.

30. Jefferson Kean, "Autobiographical Sketch," 1928, US Army Medical Department, Office of Medical History; Bean, *Walter Reed*, 139.

31. Walter Reed, James Carroll, Aristides Agramonte, and Jesse Lazear, "The Etiology of Yellow Fever: A Preliminary Note," *Proceedings of the Annual Meeting of the American Public Health Association* (October 23, 1900): 37–53.

32. "Military Orders to Commanding Officers," Chief Surgeon's Office, Headquarters Department of Western Cuba, Circular No. 8, October 15, 1900, Hench Collection.

33. Aristides Agramonte to Kean, July 3, 1908, Hench Collection.

34. Sternberg to Reed, November 17, 1900; "Informed Consent Agreement [in Spanish] for Antonio Benigno," November 26, 1900, Hench Collection.

35. Walter Reed, James Carroll, and Aristides Agramonte, "The Etiology of Yellow Fever—an Additional Note," *JAMA* 36 (1901): 431–40.

36. Quoted in Crosby, *American Plague*, 178.

37. Albert E. Truby, *Memoir of Walter Reed: The Yellow Fever Episode* (New York: Hoeber, 1943), 142.

38. John J. Moran to MG, February 22, 1924, WCGP.

39. Telegram from Reed to War Department, December 15, 1900, Hench Collection.

40. Jefferson Kean, "Chronology of the Yellow Fever Work in Cuba 1899 and 1900 and Personal Experiences, by Jefferson Kean, June 1, 1929;" Kean to John Moran, April 12, 1938, Hench Collection.

41. "General Orders No. 6, Havana," December 21, 1900, Hench Collection.

42. Reed, Carroll, and Agramonte, "Etiology of Yellow Fever–an Additional Note," 431–40.

43. William Crawford Gorgas, "Solving the Health Problem at Panama," *Review of Reviews* 30 (1904): 52–56.

44. L. O. Howard, "An Experiment against Mosquitoes," *Insect Life* 5 (September 1892): 12–14.

45. Gorgas, *Sanitation in Panama*, 61.

46. Gorgas and Hendrick, *William Crawford Gorgas*, 128.

47. Gorgas, *Sanitation in Panama*, 57.

48. William C. Gorgas, "Cuba: Vital Statistics of Havana, Guanabacoa, Regla, and Marianao for July, 1901," *PHR* 16 (1901): 2006–8; William Crawford Gorgas, "The Work of the Sanitary Department of Havana; with Special Reference to the Repression of Yellow Fever," *Medical Record* 60 (September 1901): 1–15.

49. Gorgas, *Sanitation in Panama*, 88.

50. WCG to Walter Reed, August 26, 1901, in Gorgas, *Sanitation in Panama*, 94.

51. Walter Reed to WCG, June 27, 1901, WCGP.

52. Walter Reed to WCG, June 5, 1901, WCGP.

53. WCG to Walter Reed, June 13, 1901, WCGP.

54. Walter Reed to WCG, July 29, 1901, WCGP.

55. Walter Reed to WCG, January 31, 1902, WCGP.

56. WCG to Walter Reed, February 6, 1902, Hench Collection.

57. Reed et al., "Etiology of Yellow Fever—a Preliminary Note." Regarding credit for the mosquito theory and the Cuban partisans, see Ellen Griffith Spears and Rosa López-Oceguera, "Carlos Juan Finlay, William Gorgas, Walter Reed and the U.S. Army Yellow Fever Controversy: Competing Historical Memories," *Alabama Review* 74 (January 2021): 62–76; C. E. Finlay, "Carlos Finlay and Yellow Fever," *Journal of Parasitology* 28 (1942): 172–74; Carlos Martinez Duran et al., "125th Anniversary of the Birth of Carlos J. Finlay," *Revista de la Sociedad Cubana de Historia de la Medicina* 1 (1958): 6–52; C. Corbitt

Duvon, "Carlos J. Finlay, Cuban Physician," *Hispanic American Historical Review* 45 (1965): 439–41; Ines Pinto Alicea, "Conquerors of Yellow Fever: Dr. Carlos Juan Finlay, Unsung Hero," *Hispanic Outlook in Higher Education* 12 (2002): 24.

58. WCG to Henry Rose Carter, December 13, 1900, Hench Collection.

59. Marie made this point in Gorgas and Hendrick, *William Crawford Gorgas*, 109.

60. "Headquarters Department of Cuba, Circular No. 5, April 27, 1901, Hench Collection.

61. William C. Gorgas, "Results in Havana during the Year 1901 of Disinfection for Yellow Fever," *The Lancet* 160 (September 6, 1902): 669.

62. W. C. Gorgas, "Letter to the editor," *Philadelphia Medical Journal*, December 17, 1901, WCGP.

63. WCG to Walter Reed, August 26, 1901, WCGP.

64. WCG to Walter Reed, June 13, 1901, WCGP; William Crawford Gorgas, "Methods of Quarantine against Yellow Fever Adopted in Havana, Cuba, during the Year 1901," *Medical Record* 62 (January 17, 1903).

65. W. C. Gorgas, "Cuba: Vital Statistics of Havana during November, 1901," *PHR* 16 (1901): 3060–61.

66. *WDAR, 1901*, 667.

67. WCG to Henry Carter, August 31, 1901, Gorgas Papers, Box 3, LoC.

68. William C. Gorgas, "Period of the Disease in Man during Which Yellow Fever Can Be Transmitted to the Mosquito," *PHR* 29 (1903): 65–7.

69. Quoted in William B. Bean, *Walter Reed: A Biography* (Charlottesville: University of Virginia Press, 1982), 168.

70. "American Success in Havana," *Chicago Daily Tribune*, March 14, 1902; "Havana Purged of Fever: Major Gorgas Regards 'Yellow Jack' as a Back Number—the Anti-Mosquito Plan's Success," *NYT*, February 16, 1902; "Yellow Fever Stamped Out: Dr. Gorgas Says Mosquito Crusade Has Eradicated Disease in Havana," *Washington Post*, February 16, 1902; "Havana Is Now Healthy," *Jacksonville Metropolis*, April 15, 1901.

71. Henry Romeike, 110 Fifth Ave., New York, Newspaper Cutting Bureau.

72. WCG to H. L Scott, March 29, 1902, RG 140, Entry 3, Box 241, NARA.

73. "Mosquitoes and Yellow Fever in Havana," *The Lancet* 12 (April 1902): 1045–46; William C. Gorgas, "Cuba: Vital Statistics of Havana for August, 1900," *PHR* 15 (1900): 2402–6; William Crawford Gorgas, "The Work of the Sanitary Department of Havana; with Special Reference to the Repression of Yellow Fever," *Medical Record* (September 7, 1901): 361–65.

74. "Havana's Health," *Los Angeles Times*, March 27, 1901; "Havana Healthy City," *Boston Daily Globe*, March 18, 1901.

75. "A Prophet in Havana!" *Washington Post*, April 6, 1901.

76. WCG to George Sternberg, February 25, 1901, RG 112, Entry 26, Box 218, NARA; Craig, *In the Interest of Truth*, 280.

77. John Guiteras, "Experimental Yellow Fever at the Inoculation Station of the Sanitary Department of Havana with a View to Producing Immunization," *American Medicine* (November 23, 1901): 809–17; Enrique Chaves-Carballo, "Clara Maass, Yellow Fever and Human Experimentation," *Military Medicine* 178 (2013): 557–62; Ingrid Gessner, "Heroines

of Health: Examining the Other Side of the 'Splendid Little War,'" Special issue: Women in the USA, *European Journal of American Studies* 10, no. 1 (2015).

78. "Fatal Experiments," *New York Daily Standard*, August 22, 1901; "Mosquitoes Kill This Trained Nurse," *New York Evening Journal*, August 26, 1901, clippings found in Gorgas Papers, Box 29a, LoC.

79. Guiteras, "Experimental Yellow Fever at the Inoculation Station of the Sanitary Department of Havana with a View to Producing Immunization."

80. "Fatal Experiments," *New York Daily Standard*, August 22, 1901.

81. WCG to Walter Reed, August 26, 1901, Hench Collection.

82. Walter Reed and James Carroll, "The Prevention of Yellow Fever," *Public Health Papers and Reports* 27 (1901): 113–29; William C. Gorgas, "The Results of Yellow Fever Sanitation in Havana, Cuba, for the Year 1901 up to September 1st, Carried on upon the Basis That the Stegomyia Mosquito Is the Sole Means of Its Transmission," *Public Health Papers and Reports* 27 (1901): 130–33.

83. WCG to Henry Carter, October 8, 1901, Gorgas Papers, Box 3, LoC.

84. James Carroll, "The Transmission of Yellow Fever," *JAMA* (May 23, 1903); James Carroll, "Yellow Fever: A Popular Lecture," *American Medicine* 9 (June 3, 1903): 907–15; J. A. del Regato, "James Carroll: A Biography," *Annals of Diagnostic Pathology* 5 (October 1998): 335–49.

85. James H. Hitchman, "Unfinished Business: Public Works in Cuba, 1898–1902," *The Americas* 31 (1975): 335–59.

86. Section V of the Platt amendment. "For the sanitation of the cities of the island, to the end that a recurrence of epidemic and infectious diseases may be prevented, thereby ensuring protection to the people and commerce of Cuba, as well as to the commerce of the southern ports of the United States and the people residing in them." Most of the Platt amendment's provisions were repealed in the 1934 treaty with the United States under Franklin Roosevelt's "Good Neighbor Policy," and in 1940 the Cuban constitutional convention eliminated the amendment language from the new constitution.

87. J. H. Hitchman, "The American Touch in Imperial Administration: Leonard Wood in Cuba, 1898–1902," *The Americas* 24 (1968): 394–403.

88. "Letter from Will Gorgas, Havana, Cuba," n.d., WCGP.

89. WCG to AGG, July 3, 1903, WCGP.

90. McCallum, *Leonard Wood*, 196.

91. *WDAR, 1902*, 99.

## *Chapter 7*

1. Jefferson Kean, *The Scientific Work and Discoveries of the Late Maj. Walter Reed; and Major William Crawford Gorgas*, February 6, 1903, S. Rep. 2878, 57th Cong., 2nd sess.

2. Gorgas, *Sanitation in Panama*, 138.

3. WCG to AGG, July 3, 1902, WCGP.

4. Reed, "Recent Researches concerning the Etiology, Propagation, and Prevention of Yellow Fever"; Walter Reed and James Carroll, "The Etiology of Yellow Fever—a Supplemental Note," *American Medicine* 3 (February 22, 1902): 301–5.

5. *WDAR, 1904*, 129.

6. "The Kerosene Can and the Mosquito," *Cincinnati Lancet and Clinic* 47 (1901): 325.

7. William Osler, *Principles and Practice of Medicine*, 4th ed. (New York: D. Appleton, 1902), 361–62.

8. WCG to Surgeon General, June 28, 1902, Gorgas Papers, Box 12, LoC; Gorgas, *Sanitation in Panama*, 138.

9. "A Lesson in Sanitation," *Medical News* 81 (November 15, 1902): 941.

10. "In the Cuban Capital: No Friction over Naval Situations–Major Gorgas's Departure," *NYT*, September 29, 1902.

11. WCG to RHG, December 1, 1902, WCGP.

12. Mary W. Standlee, *Borden's Dream: The Walter Reed Army Medical Center in Washington, D.C.* (Washington, DC: Borden Institute, 2009), originally published 1952.

13. WCG to AGG, November 26, 1902, WCGP.

14. Emilie Lawrence Reed, "Emilie Lawrence Reed's Description of Walter Reed's Final Illness for Howard A. Kelly," 1922, Hench Collection.

15. WCG to AGG, December 11, 1902, WCGP.

16. Gorgas, *Sanitation in Panama*, 139–41; WCG to Carter, August 22, 1903, WCGP.

17. Aileen Gorgas to John W. Ross, February 21, 1903, Box 3, John Ross Papers.

18. WCG to Family, January 17, 1903, WCGP.

19. WCG to AGG, February 7, 1903, WCGP.

20. O'Reilly statement in *Major William Crawford Gorgas*, February 6, 1903, S. Rep. 2878, 57th Cong., 2nd sess.

21. "Statement concerning Army Promotion of Doctor WC Gorgas, 1902," WCGP.

22. WCG to Theo, March 13, 1903, WCGP.

23. Consideration of S. 6895, legislation to promote William C. Gorgas, *Congressional Record*, House of Representatives, March 2, 1903, 2328.

24. Joseph Ohl, "Southern Man Goes up Higher," *Atlanta Constitution*, February 21, 1903.

25. WCG to AGG, March 7, 1903, WCGP.

26. Jessica Adler, "The Founding of Walter Reed General Hospital and the Beginning of Modern Institutional Army Medical Care in the United States," *Journal of the History of Medicine and Allied Sciences* 69 (October 2014): 521–53; Standlee, *Borden's Dream*.

27. "Yellow Fever Stamped Out: Dr. Gorgas Says Mosquito Crusade Has Eradicated Disease in Havana," *Washington Post*, February 16, 1902.

28. On the history of Panama, see Aims McGuinness, *Path of Empire: Panama and the California Gold Rush* (Ithaca: Cornell University Press, 2008); Matthew Parker, *Panama Fever: The Epic Story of One of the Greatest Human Achievements of All Time—The Building of the Panama Canal*, 1st US ed. (New York: Doubleday, 2007).

29. Noel Maurer and Carlos Yu, *The Big Ditch: How America Took, Built, Ran, and Ultimately Gave Away the Panama Canal* (Princeton, NJ: Princeton University Press, 2011), 10.

30. Walter LaFeber, *The Panama Canal: The Crisis in Historical Perspective* (New York: Oxford University Press, 1989).

31. WCG to AGG, April 6, 1903, WCGP.

32. O'Reilly to Taft, February 2, 1903, WCGP.

33. WCG to La Garde, June 4, 1903, WCGP.

34. La Garde to WCG, November 17, 1903, WCGP; "The Panama Canal Commission's Sanitation Problem," *JAMA* 42 (March 5, 1904): 655; "Sanitation and the Panama Canal," *JAMA* 42 (April 2, 1904); "The Panama Canal Commission and Medical Service on the Isthmus," *JAMA* 42 (May 1904): 1082.

35. Kean to WCG, April 3, 1903, RG 112, Entry 26, B659, NARA.

36. John Walker to WCG, June 26, 1903, WCGP.

37. WCG to Henry Carter, April 29, 1904, WCGP.

38. WCG to John Ross, September 24, 1903, WCGP.

39. W. C. Gorgas, "Results in Havana during the Year 1901 of Disinfection for Yellow Fever," *The Lancet* 160 (1902): 667–70; William C. Gorgas, "The Method of Transmission of Yellow Fever from Man to Man," *PHR* 28 (1902): 238–46; William Crawford Gorgas, *A Short Account of the Results of Mosquito Work in Havana, Cuba* (Carlisle, PA: 1903); William Crawford Gorgas, "Recent Experiences of the United States Army with Regard to Sanitation of Yellow Fever in the Tropics," *The Lancet* (March 28, 1903): 880–83; William C. Gorgas, "Period of the Disease in Man during Which Yellow Fever Can Be Transmitted to the Mosquito," *PHR* 29 (1903): 65–67; William C. Gorgas, "The Practical Mosquito Work Done at Havana, Cuba, Which Resulted in the Disappearance of Yellow Fever from That Locality," *Washington Medical Annals* 2 (1903): 170–80.

40. La Garde to WCG, June 12, 1903, WCGP.

41. O'Reilly to WCG, August 8, 1903, WCGP. On the Panama Canal Treaty, see David McCullough, *The Path between the Seas: The Creation of the Panama Canal, 1870–1914* (New York: Touchstone, 1977); Parker, *Panama Fever*, 241–49.

42. William C. Gorgas, "International Sanitary Convention: Appendix C.: Remarks on Yellow Fever," (Washington, DC: U.S. Army, 1903), 82–85.

43. WCG to MG, November 14, 1903, WCGP.

44. Convention for the Construction of the Ship Canal (Hay-Bunau-Varilla Treaty), November 18, 1903.

45. McGuinness, *Path of the Empire*, 31.

46. WCG to the Secretary of State (through the surgeon general), December 7, 1903, RG 185, Records of the Panama Canal, Entry 30, Box 767, NARA.

47. O'Reilly to WCG, December 9, 1903, WCGP.

48. O'Reilly to WCG, January 13, 1904, WCGP. The resulting pamphlet was William Crawford Gorgas, *A Few General Directions with Regard to Destroying Mosquitoes, Particularly the Yellow Fever Mosquito*, 1904, H. doc. 756, 58th Cong., 2nd sess.

49. WCG to John Ross, January 29, 1904, WCGP.

50. John Walker to WCG, telegram, March 12, 1904, WCGP.

51. Alexander Lambert to WCG, January 19, 1904, WCGP.

52. Lambert to WCG, March 15, 1904; WCG to Lambert, March 17, 1904, WCGP.

53. WCG to AGG, May 27, 1901, WCGP.

54. WCG to AGG, June 2, 1903, WCGP.

55. MG to John Ross, April 18, 1904, Box 3, John Ross Papers. Letters between Marie and William during this month have not survived.

56. WCG to AGG, April 3, 1904, WCGP.

57. Gorgas, *Sanitation in Panama*, 144.

58. "Colon Not Safe Enough," *New York Tribune*, April 28, 1904.

59. W. C. Gorgas, "Report on the Isthmian Canal," *Engineering Record* (1904): 7.

60. "Panama Sanitation," *New York Tribune*, May 2, 1904.

61. William Crawford Gorgas, "Solving the Health Problem at Panama," *Review of Reviews* 30 (1904): 52–56; Gorgas, "Report on the Isthmian Canal," *Engineering Record*.

62. "To Fight Malaria along Canal Route," *NYT*, May 15, 1904.

63. John Ross to WCG, May 17, 1904, WCGP.

64. John Walker to WCG, May 26, 1904, WCGP.

65. United States War Department, Special Order No. 125, May 27, 1904.

66. Surgeon General R. M. O'Reilly to Secretary of War Taft, June 14, 1904, WCGP.

67. WCG to La Garde, June 14, 1904, WCGP.

68. WCG to Lambert, June 9, 1904, WCGP.

69. WCG to La Garde, June 4 and 14, 1904, WCGP; "Dr. Gorgas Choses His Panama Staff," *Birmingham Ledger*, June 14, 1904.

70. La Garde to WCG, June 7, 1904, WCGP.

71. WCG to O'Reilly, June 23, 1904, WCGP.

72. "300 Doctors for Panama," *NYT*, June 19, 1904.

73. "Housecleaning on the Isthmus," *Washington Post*, July 5, 1904, 6.

## *Chapter 8*

1. Henry Carter, quoted in Mayme Ober Peak, "Pioneering in Panama, Authority on Yellow Fever Tells How They Conquered the Foe in the Tropics," Hench Collection.

2. Enrique Chaves-Carballo suggests this in "Ancon Hospital: An American Hospital during the Construction of the Panama Canal, 1904–1914," *Military Medicine* 164 (1999): 725–30.

3. Carter, quoted in Peak, "Pioneering in Panama."

4. Gorgas and Hendrick, *William Crawford Gorgas*, 141.

5. Gorgas, *Sanitation in Panama*, 149–50, 283.

6. Lloyd Noland, "The Panama Adventure," *Annals of Surgery* 125 (May 1939): 645.

7. One of his colleagues wrote of his admiration for this policy: A. J. Ornstein, South Africa, to WCG, May 23, 1919, WCGP. For an analysis of Gorgas's management style, see Faisal H. Aboul-Enein, "Dr. William Gorgas and His Style of Management against Yellow Fever during the Construction of the Panama Canal: A Historical Case Study," DrPH dissertation, University of Texas Health Science Center, ProQuest, 2009.

8. WCG, "Sanitation of the Panama Canal Zone," *Smithsonian Institution Annual Report of the Board of Regents* (1904): 745–49.

9. Gorgas and Hendrick, *William Crawford Gorgas*, 170.

10. Gorgas, *Sanitation in Panama*, 149.

11. Carter quoted in Peak, "Pioneering in Panama."

12. Gorgas, *Sanitation in Panama*, 148.

13. Gorgas, *Sanitation in Panama*, 273; and Alexandra Minna Stern, "The Public Health Service in the Panama Canal: A Forgotten Chapter of U.S. Public Health," *PHR* 120 (2005): 675–79.

14. Gorgas and Hendrick, *William Crawford Gorgas*, 164–65.

15. WCG to Gen. George Davis, August 8, 1904, WCGP.

16. Gibson provides a litany of these refusals in *Physician to the World*, 119–23.

17. McCullough, *Path between the Seas*, 420.

18. Gorgas and Hendrick, *William Crawford Gorgas*, 170.

19. WCG, "Illustrating Some of the Difficulties of Construction" (speech draft, 1905), WCGP.

20. Joseph Albert Augustin Le Prince, "The Achievements of William Crawford Gorgas," reprint from *Health Officer* 2 (March 1938): 563–70.

21. Peak, "Pioneering in Panama"; "Ancon Yellow Fever Log Book, 1904," Clendening History of Medicine Library and Museum, University of Kansas Medical Center, Kansas City, Kansas. Courtesy of Enrique Chavez-Carballo; "Yellow Fever in Canal Zone: T. C. Cunningham, of New-York, Dies from the Disease," *New York Tribune*, July 17, 1904; "First Yellow Fever Victim," *Great Falls Daily Tribune* [Great Falls, Montana], July 18, 1904.

22. WCG to John Walker, July 26, 1904, WCGP.

23. McCullough, *Path between the Seas*, 422.

24. Gorgas, *Sanitation in Panama*, 152, 158.

25. I am indebted to Dr. Elene Mooney for her careful reading and interpretation of Marie's medical records and experience.

26. WCG to Ria Gorgas, August 15, 1904, WCGP.

27. WCG to Kean, September 24, 1904, Hench Collection.

28. After tuberculosis, respiratory diseases, diarrheal ailments, heart and renal diseases, and accidents. See Rebecca Tippett, "Mortality and Cause of Death, 1900 v. 2010," University of North Carolina, Carolina Population Center website, July 30, 2019. Today, cancer ranks second in cause of death behind heart disease. See "Leading Causes of Death," Centers for Disease Control website, September 6, 2022.

29. Barron H. Lerner, *The Breast Cancer Wars: Fear, Hope, and the Pursuit of a Cure in Twentieth-Century America* (New York: Oxford University Press, 2001); Robert A. Aronowitz, *Unnatural History: Breast Cancer and American Society* (New York: Cambridge University Press, 2007).

30. Thomas Bryant, "An Analysis of Forty-Six Cases of Cancer of the Breast Which Have Been Operated upon and Survived the Operation from 5 to 32 Years," *British Medical Journal* 20 (May 17, 1902): 1200–1203.

31. William Osler, "Medical Aspects of Carcinoma of the Breast," *British Medical Journal* 24 (January 6, 1906): 4.

32. Lerner, *Breast Cancer Wars*, 21.

33. William Stewart Halstead, "The Results of Radical Operations for the Cure of Carcinoma of the Breast," *Annals of Surgery* 46 (July 1907): 1–19.

34. Charles Morton, "The Results of Operation in Fifty-Four Cases of Cancer of the Breast," *British Medical Journal* 20 (December 20, 1902): 305–15; Bryant, "Analysis of Forty-Six Cases of Cancer of the Breast."

35. H. T. Butlin, "Oophorectomy in the Treatment of Cancer of the Breast," *British Medical Journal* 20 (January 4, 1902): 10–13.

36. Lerner, *Breast Cancer Wars*, 34; Aronowitz, *Unnatural History*, 138; Bryant, "Analysis of Forty-Six Cases of Cancer of the Breast."

37. James R. Riddell, "The 'X' Rays in Treatment," *British Medical Journal* (April 29, 1911): 987.

38. The ultraviolet light treatment was developed by Danish scientist Niels Finsen, for which he received the 1903 Nobel Prize in Medicine. See Kirsten Iversen Møller et al., "How Finsen's Light Cured Lupus Vulgaris," *Photodermatology, Photoimmunology, and Photomedicine* 21, no. 3 (June 2005): 118–24; Gunver S. Kienle, "Fever in Cancer Treatment: Coley's Therapy and Epidemiologic Observations," *Global Advances in Health and Medicine* 1 (2012): 92–100. Methods similar to Coley's are still being used today. See Robert D. Carlson et al., "Talkin' Toxins: From Coley's to Modern Cancer Immunotherapy," *Toxins* 12 (April 9, 2020): 241.

39. "Journal, William Crawford Gorgas, January–March 1905," transcript used by Marie Gorgas to write *William C. Gorgas, His Life and Work*, WCGP (hereafter cited as Gorgas Journal, 1905).

40. "Ancon Yellow Fever Log," Clendening History of Medicine Library and Museum.

41. Connie L. Lester, "John Walton Ross," *Tennessee Encyclopedia*, Tennessee Historical Society, online edition, 2017.

42. Gorgas Journal, 1905, 160, WCGP.

43. Keen to WCG, December 1904, Gorgas Papers, Box 15, LoC.

44. Keen to WCG, September 30, 1904, Gorgas Papers, Box 12, LoC.

45. Keen to WCG, October 6, 1904, Gorgas Papers, Box 12, LoC.

46. Gorgas Journal, 1905, 160, WCGP.

47. WCG to RHG, January 16, 1905, WCGP.

48. Carter quoted in Peak, "Pioneering in Panama"; Gorgas Journal, 1905, WCGP; "Fever Seizes Officers," *NYT*, January 27, 1905.

49. Gorgas Journal, 1905, WCGP.

50. WCG to R. M. O'Reilly, January 3, 1905, Hench Collection.

51. WCG to RHG, January 16, 1905, WCGP.

52. William W. Keen, "Amputation of the Female Breast," *Cleveland Medical Gazette* (1894): 1–16.

53. Keen to WCG, February 2, 1905, Gorgas Papers, Box 12, LoC.

54. Gorgas Journal, 1905, WCGP.

55. Keen to WCG, March 6, 1905, Gorgas Papers, Box 12, LoC.

56. This is not now believed to be true.

57. Keen to WCG, March 6, 1905; and Keen to WCG, March 30, 1905, Gorgas Papers, Box 12, LoC.

58. MG to Keen, January 12, 1914, William W. Keen Papers, MS-1U-K2, John Hay Library, Brown University, Providence, Rhode Island.

59. Gorgas sent this letter and related correspondence to Henry Carter. See Henry Rose Carter Papers, MS-10, Claude Moore Health Sciences Library, University of Virginia, Charlottesville, Virginia.

60. WCG to Charles A. L. Reed, February 17, 1905, Hench Collection.

61. "The Panama Canal Management: Report to the Government by Dr. Charles A. L. Reed, Showing How the Commission Makes Efficient Sanitation Impossible," *JAMA* 44 (March 11, 1905): 812–18.

62. Reed, "Panama Canal Management Report," 812–18.

63. Gorgas Journal, 1905, WCGP.

64. Kean to WCG, March 13, 1905, WCGP.

65. Gorgas and Hendrick, *William Crawford Gorgas*, 194.

66. Henry F. Pringle, *The Life and Times of William Howard Taft*, vol. 1 (Hamden, CT: Archon Books, 1964), 283.

67. WCG to Taft, April 1, 1905, Hench Collection; WCG to Taft, May 16, 1905, WCGP.

68. WCG to Lambert, April 1, 1905; WCG to O'Reilly, April 1, 1905, WCGP. See also "Theodore Roosevelt in Colorado," *Colorado Magazine* 35 (October 1958): 259–60.

69. Lambert to WCG, April 22, 1905, WCGP.

70. WCG to RHG, March 13, 1905, WCGP.

71. Gorgas Journal, 1905, March 14, WCGP.

72. The patients were Father Pablo Arcardio, Girgliano Fulinio, and Giuseppe Giantollo. See "Ancon Yellow Fever Log Book, 1904," Clendening History of Medicine Library and Museum.

73. Gorgas Journal, 1905, March 22, WCGP.

74. Mary Price to MG, September 8, 1920, WCGP.

75. Gorgas Journal, 1905, March 28, WCGP.

76. Verbatim transcript of the letter from Kean, March 13, 1905, in Gorgas Journal, 1905, WCGP.

77. Kean to WCG, April 10, 1905, WCGP.

78. Gorgas Journal, 1905, WCGP.

79. WCG to Kean, April 20, 1905, Hench Collection; emphasis in original.

80. Harry E. Bovay to MG, January 14, 1924, WCGP.

81. Joseph A. Le Prince, A. J. Orenstein, and L. O. Howard, *Mosquito Control in Panama: The Eradication of Malaria and Yellow Fever in Cuba and Panama* (New York: G. P. Putnam's Sons, 1916), 282.

82. In line with contemporary decorum, Gorgas addressed the letter to the chief engineer John Findley Wallace so he could send it to the young woman. WCG to Wallace, May 3, 1905, WCGP.

83. WCG to Charles Reed, May 5, 1905, WCGP.

84. WCG to Charles Magoon, April 20, 1905, WCGP.

85. WCG to O'Reilly, May 5, 1905, Hench Collection.

86. "Letter to the editor," *NYT*, June 6, 1905.

87. J. F. Stevens, "Momentous Hour at Panama," *Science* 71 (1930): 550–52.

88. Charles A. L. Reed to WCG, July 4, 1905, WCGP. See, for example, "The Sanitary Problem of Panama," *JAMA* 45 (September 9, 1905): 794–95; "Improved Conditions on the Isthmus of Panama," *JAMA* 45 (1905): 1328–29.

89. Lambert to MG, May 20, 1922, WCGP.

90. Gorgas and Hendrick, *William Crawford Gorgas*, 211.

91. Jefferson Randolph Kean, unpublished autobiography, 95, MS C14, Jefferson R. Kean Papers, NLM.

92. J. F. Stevens, "Momentous Hour at Panama," *Science* 71 (1930): 550–52.

93. Congressional Research Service, "Salaries of Members of Congress: Recent Actions and Historical Tables," August 8, 2022. This would be more than $300,000 in 2021 dollars. See Ian Webster, "CPI Inflation Calculator," Official Inflation Data, Alioth Finance, November 21, 2022.

94. Taft to WCG, April 25, 1905, and Magoon to WCG, June 1, 1905, Hench Collection.

95. WCG to John Ross, May 12, 1905, WCGP, emphasis in original.

96. WCG to Kean, June 29, 1905, Hench Collection.

## *Chapter 9*

1. AGG to MG, July 25, 1905, WCGP.

2. Marixa Lasso, *Erased: The Untold Story of the Panama Canal* (Cambridge: Harvard University Press, 2019), 96. See also Julie Greene, *The Canal Builders: Making America's Empire at the Panama Canal* (New York: Penguin Press, 2009): 1; Sarah J. Moore, *Empire on Display: San Francisco's Panama-Pacific International Exposition of 1915* (Norman: University of Oklahoma Press, 2013).

3. McCullough, *Path between the Seas*, 466.

4. Main sources for this discussion are Gorgas, *Sanitation in Panama*; Le Prince et al., *Mosquito Control in Panama*; William C. Gorgas, "Sanitation of the Tropics with Special Reference to Malaria and Yellow Fever," *JAMA* 52 (April 3, 1909): 1075–77.

5. Le Prince et al., *Mosquito Control in Panama*, 273; "New Zone Building Laws," *Canal Record* (September 25, 1907): 4.

6. Le Prince et al., *Mosquito Control in Panama*, 286.

7. Gorgas, *Sanitation in Panama*, 141.

8. William C. Gorgas, "Etiology and Prophylaxis of Yellow Fever," paper for the Fifteenth International Congress of Medicine, held at Lisbon, Portugal, April 1906, WCGP.

9. Excerpt from Laura Carter's diary in Peak, "Pioneering in Panama."

10. Mary A. Chatfield, *Light on Dark Places at Panama: By an Isthmian Stenographer* (New York: Broadway, 1908), 70.

11. Fania de Obarrio to Le Prince, August 31, 1905; and Fania de Obarrio to WCG, September 1, 1905, WCGP.

12. "New Zone Building Laws," *Canal Record* (September 25, 1907): 4.

13. Henry S. Wellcome, "Observations on the Medical and Sanitary Department of the Panama Canal Commission during My Visits to the Isthmus the First Week in March and at the End of April and the Beginning of May, 1910," *Military Surgeon* 27 (1910): 7.

14. Gustavo A. Mellander and Nelly Maldonado Mellander, *Charles Edward Magoon: The Panama Years* (Rio Piedras, Puerto Rico: Editorial Plaza Mayor, 1999), 22.

15. Gorgas and Hendrick, *William Crawford Gorgas*, 243–44.

16. WCG to Kean, April 20, 1905, Hench Collection, italics added by author.

17. A Panamanian official quoted by A. J. Orenstein to MG, March 30, 1921, WCGP.

18. William C. Gorgas, "Purified Panama: An Entire Republic under Sanitary Law," *Sunday Magazine*, February 4, 1906.

19. WCG to AGG, October 17, 1905, WCGP.

20. *ICC Annual Report, 1905* (Washington, DC: GPO), 33.

21. WCG Journal, August 1905, Gorgas Papers, Box 31, LoC.

22. *ICC Annual Report, 1905*, 33.

23. "Taft Pleased in Panama," *NYT*, November 5, 1905.

24. "Colonel Gorgas says Health of the Isthmus Is Excellent," November 24, 1905, *New York Tribune*.

25. W. C. Gorgas, "A Short Account of the Sanitary Department of the Isthmian Canal Commission," *PHR* 32 (1906): 52–57.

26. See, for example, *WDAR, 1919*, vol. 1, pt. 2, 1448–49, 1463–64.

27. Department of Sanitation, ICC, monthly report, March 1906.

28. Gorgas, *Sanitation in Panama*, 213–15; *ICC Annual Report*, 1909.

29. World Monuments Fund website, "Mount Hope Cemetery, Colón, Panama," July 2010.

30. Chaves-Carballo, "Ancon Hospital," 55–56; Eugenie Hibbard, "Isthmus of Panama: A Sketch," Canal Zone Library–Museum Papers, Box 22, LoC.

31. Chaves-Carballo, "Ancon Hospital," 725–30.

32. Gorgas, *Sanitation in Panama*, 211.

33. Chaves-Carballo, "Ancon Hospital," 727.

34. Gorgas, *Sanitation in Panama*, 214.

35. For a discussion of the various diseases and injuries physicians encountered in Panama, see C. L. Overlander, "Medical Practice in the Canal Zone," *JAMA* 60 (March 15, 1913): 806–10.

36. "Notice: Bubonic Plague," *Canal Record* (April 29, 1908); Department of Sanitation, *ICC Annual Report*, 1908, 62–64.

37. WCG to Governor of Canal Zone, August 17, 1906, RG 112, Entry 26, Box 654; Department of Sanitation, ICC, monthly report, July 1906, 3.

38. WCG to Kean, April 20, 1905, Hench Collection.

39. Gorgas, *Sanitation in Panama*, 208.

40. Charles Morrow Wilson, *Ambassadors in White: The Story of American Tropical Medicine* (New York: Henry Holt, 1942), 165–66.

41. *ICC Annual Report*, 1905, 107; and "Death of Dr. John H. Purnell," *Canal Record* (1908): 75.

42. WCG to Furbush, June 6, 1904, WCGP.

43. WCG to Furbush, February 3, 1905, WCGP.

44. Samuel Darling to MG, March 2, 1922, WCGP.

45. "Anecdotes on Life of WC Gorgas, Reminiscences of Construction Days," circa 1925, WCGP.

46. John J. Moran to MG, February 22, 1924, WCGP.

47. Greene, *Canal Builders*, 111–14.

48. "Anecdotes on Life of WC Gorgas, Reminiscences of Construction Days," WCGP.

49. E. B. Williston to WCG, c. 1904, WCGP.

50. WCG to E. B. Williston, December 15, 1904, WCGP; "Doctor Weds Nurse in Fever-Stricken Canal Zone," newspaper clipping, no publication name, July 5, 1905, WCGP.

51. On Roosevelt's visit, see Greene, *Canal Builders*, 235–36.

52. Gorgas, *Sanitation in Panama*, 236.

53. WCG to George Davis, November 23, 1906, WCGP.

54. Theodore Roosevelt to WCG, November 27, 1906, WCGP.

55. Gorgas and Hendrick, *William Crawford Gorgas*, 208–9.

56. Theodore Roosevelt, "Special Message concerning the Panama Canal," *Congressional Record*, 60th Cong., 2nd sess., December 17, 1906, 458.

57. Gibson, *Physician to the World*, 159.

58. Theodore Roosevelt to WCG, April 1, 1907, WCGP.

59. Notation by Aileen Gorgas Wrightson on letter from Roosevelt to WCG, April 19, 1907, WCGP.

60. Theodore Roosevelt speech, 1906, in "Men Dug the Canal—But Women Played a Vital Role," *Panama Canal Review* (Spring 1976), published on Canal Zone Brats website, July 15, 1998.

61. "Men Dug the Canal—But Women Played a Vital Role."

62. Newspaper clipping, "Mrs. William C. Gorgas Tells of Life in Panama during Work on Canal," circa 1915, WCGP. On Panama during the construction period, see Ralph Emmett Avery, *America's Triumph at Panama* (Chicago: Reagan Printing House, 1913); Forbes Lindsay, *Panama and the Canal Today* (Boston: L. C. Page, 1912); John Owen Collins, *The Panama Guide* (Mount Hope, Canal Zone: I.C.C. Press, 1912).

63. "Anecdotes on Life of W. C. Gorgas, a Silhouette," circa 1925, WCGP.

64. Gorgas and Hendrick, *William Crawford Gorgas*, 240.

65. Gorgas Journal, 1905, WCGP.

66. Greene, *Canal Builders*, 107–16; Reverby, *Ordered to Care*, 39–59; D'Antonio, *American Nursing*, chapter 2.

67. Greene, *Canal Builders*, 207–23.

68. Newspaper clipping, "Mrs. William C. Gorgas Tells of Life in Panama during Work on Canal," circa 1915, WCGP.

69. "Activities of the Young Men's Christian Association: Corozal," *Canal Record*, 1911.

70. D. L. Wilkinson to WCG, June 7, 1910, WCGP.

71. Mrs. Ernst Ulrich von Munchow, ed., *The American Woman on the Panama Canal, 1905–1916* (Panama: Star and Herald, 1916), 39.

72. WCG to Rev. A. W. Knight, April 4, 1910, WCGP.

73. Theodore Roosevelt, "National Duties," address at Minnesota State Fair, September 2, 1901, in *The Strenuous Life* (New York: Century, 1902), 241. See also Emily Rosenberg, *Spreading the American Dream: American Economic and Cultural Expansion, 1890–1945* (New York: Hill and Wang, 1982); Gretchen Murphy, *Shadowing White Man's Burden: U.S. Imperialism and the Problem of the Color Line* (New York: New York University Press, 2010).

74. G. Anguizola, "Negroes in the Building of the Panama Canal," *Phylon* 29 (1968): 351–59.

75. ICC, "Invitation for Proposal to Furnish Chinese Labor to Be Used, under Direction of the Isthmian Canal Commission," August 20, 1906, RG 112, Entry 26, Box 659, NARA.

76. Michael L. Conniff, *Black Labor on a White Canal: Panama, 1904–1981* (Pittsburgh: University of Pittsburgh Press, 1985).

77. *ICC Annual Report*, 1911, 5; Greene, *Canal Builders*, Appendix.

78. "Journal, William Crawford Gorgas" (Partial typescript copy), February 4, 1920, WCGP.

79. Minutes of the ICC, 1696.

80. Conniff, *Black Labor on a White Canal*, 34; John Lindsay-Poland, "The Great White Canal," *Peacework*, no. 287 (July/Aug 1998): 11.

81. See *ICC Annual Report*, 1910.

82. Avery, *America's Triumph*, 122.

83. "Precautions to Be Observed for Avoiding Diseases Incident to the Isthmus," *Canal Record* (September 18, 1907): 21.

84. *ICC Annual Report*, 1906, 5. On Goethals's racism, see Rory McGovern, *George W. Goethals and the Army: Change and Continuity in the Gilded Age and Progressive Era* (Lawrence: University of Kansas Press, 2019), 125–26.

85. WCG to AGG, April 3, 1905, WCGP.

86. WCG to Sen. Morgan, August 8, 1906, WCGP.

87. H. Pilgrim Wilkins to MG, September 26, 1922, WCGP.

88. "Hospital and Sanitation Work on the Isthmus of Panama," newspaper clipping, October 20, 1910, Gorgas Papers, LoC.

89. Kean to WCG, August 16, 1907, WCGP.

90. Gorgas Ledger, c. 1899 to 1910, 184, Gorgas Papers, Box 31, LoC. Amelia mentioned this to Minnie in AGG to Minnie Gorgas, June 1906, WCGP.

## *Chapter 10*

1. WCG to AGG, June 19, 1906, WCGP.

2. Stevens to Roosevelt, January 30, 1907, quoted in McCullough, *Path between the Seas*, 503–4.

3. See David McCullough, "A Man, a Plan, a Canal, Panama!" *American Heritage* 22 (June 1971).

4. McGovern, *George W. Goethals and the Army*, 93.

5. Quoted in Harry E. Bovay to MG, January 23, 1924, WCGP.

6. "Panama Items," *Steam Shovel and Dredge*," 3 (1909): 832. On engineering during construction, see Jon T. Hoffman et al., *The Panama Canal: An Army's Enterprise* (Washington, DC: United States Army Center for Military History, 2019), originally published 2009; Henry Petroski, "Engineering: The Panama Canal," *American Scientist* 81 (1993): 13–18.

7. George Goethals, "The Building of the Canal in Panama: The Human Element in Administration," *Scribner's Magazine* 57 (June 1915): 720–34.

8. Gorgas and Hendrick, *William Crawford Gorgas*, 214–15.

9. Both quotes in McGovern, *George W. Goethals and the Army*, 111, 112.

10. William L. Sibert to MG, May 30, 1921, WCGP.

11. McCullough, *Path between the Seas*, 571–72.

12. "Portrait," *Columbia University Quarterly* 15 (1913): 341.

13. For more on this rivalry, see McCullough, *Path between the Seas*, 571–73; Gillett, *Army Medical Department, 1865–1917*, 276–77.

14. Gorgas and Hendrick, *William Crawford Gorgas*, 221.

15. Gorgas and Hendrick, *William Crawford Gorgas*, 216–20.

16. William C. Gorgas, "Malaria in the Tropics," *JAMA* 46 (May 12, 1906): 1416. On malaria, see Margaret Humphreys, *Malaria: Poverty, Race, and Public Health in the United States* (Baltimore: Johns Hopkins University Press, 2001); Randall M. Packard, *The Making of a Tropical Disease: A Short History of Malaria* (Baltimore: Johns Hopkins University Press, 2007); Frank M. Snowden, *The Conquest of Malaria: Italy, 1900–1962* (New Haven: Yale University Press, 2006).

17. Chaves-Carballo, *American Medicine and the Panama Canal*, 70.

18. Gorgas and Hendrick, *William Crawford Gorgas*, 226.

19. E. Chaves-Carballo, *American Medicine and the Panama Canal: Proceedings of the Medical Association of the Isthmian Canal Zone* (Morgan Hill, CA: Bookstand, 2014); E. Chaves-Carballo, *The Tropical World of Samuel Taylor Darling: Parasites, Pathology and Philanthropy* (Portland, OR: Sussex Academic Press, 2007).

20. See, for example, Arthur I. Kendall, "Malarial Infection in Certain Native Villages of the Canal Zone," *JAMA* 46 (April 21, 1906): 1151–54 and (April 28, 1906): 1266–73; Samuel T. Darling, "Transmission of Malarial Fever in the Canal Zone by *Anopheles* Mosquitoes," *JAMA* 53 (December 18, 1909): 2051–53; Le Prince et al., *Mosquito Control in Panama*. See also L. J. Bruce-Chwatt, "Ronald Ross, William Gorgas, and Malaria Eradication," *American Journal of Tropical Medical Hygiene* 26 Suppl. (1977): 1071–79. On mosquitoes, see Hall and Tamïr, *Mosquitopia*.

21. Gorgas, *Sanitation in Panama*, 184.

22. Gorgas, *Sanitation in Panama*, 192–94.

23. Adele Steiner Burleson to MG, February 17, 1923, WCGP.

24. Quinine is still used to treat some forms of malaria. See Centers for Disease Control website, "Treatment of Malaria: Guidelines for Clinicians."

25. Gorgas, "Malaria in the Tropics," 1417.

26. Gorgas, *Sanitation in Panama*, 220–21.

27. Gorgas, "Conquest of the Tropics for the White Race," 1968.

28. Gorgas, *Sanitation in Panama*, 222–23.

29. Ronald Ross, *The Prevention of Malaria* (London: Dutton, 1910), 136; Chaves-Carballo, *Tropical World of Samuel Taylor Darling*.

30. Le Prince et al., *Mosquito Control in Panama*, 113. Scientists are continuing to study this phenomenon. See, for example, Diego Girando et al., "Human Scent Guides Mosquito Thermotaxis and Host Selection under Naturalistic Conditions," *Current Biology* 33 (June 19, 2023): 2367–82.

31. Le Prince et al., *Mosquito Control in Panama*, 297.

32. Gorgas, *Sanitation in Panama*, 197.

33. Le Prince et al., *Mosquito Control in Panama*, passim.

34. Department of Sanitation, *ICC Annual Report*, 1908, 62–64.

35. Gorgas, *Sanitation in Panama*, 187.

36. Gorgas, *Sanitation in Panama*, 233–34.

37. See Lasso, *Erased*; Ashley Carse et al., "Panama Canal Forum: From the Conquest of Nature to the Construction of New Ecologies," *Environmental History* 21 (April 2016): 206–87; Paul Sutter, "Nature's Agents or Agents of Empire? Entomological Workers and Environmental Change during the Construction of the Panama Canal," *Isis* 98 (2007):

724–54; Guillermo H. Castro, "Isthmus in the World: Elements for an Environmental History of Panama," *Global Environment* 1 (2008): 10–55.

38. Hall and Tamïr, *Mosquitopia*.

39. Chaves-Carballo, *Tropical World of Samuel Taylor Darling*; *ICC Annual Report*, 1910; H. R. Carter, "Notes on the Sanitation of Yellow Fever and Malaria from Isthmian Experience," *Medical Record* (July 10, 1909); Chaves-Carballo, *American Medicine and the Panama Canal*.

40. Samuel T. Darling, "Transmission of Malarial Fever in the Canal Zone by *Anopheles* Mosquitoes," *JAMA* 53 (1909): 2051–53; Gorgas, *Sanitation in Panama*, 238.

41. Le Prince, *Mosquito Control in Panama*, 226.

42. "A Steam Shovel Man's View," *Canal Record* (September 18, 1907): 23.

43. WCG to Goethals, September 3, 1907, Goethals Papers, Box 5, LoC; Le Prince to MG, January 9, 1924, WCGP.

44. Kean, autobiographical sketch, 124.

45. WCG to Torney, May 13, 1909, WCGP.

46. WCG to Goethals, August 7, 1908, Gorgas Papers, Box 24, LoC.

47. Torney to WCG, March 30, 1909, WCGP.

48. WCG to William Merry, April 3, 1908, Gorgas Papers, Box 17; and WCG to F. M. Sandwith, April 28, 1910, Gorgas Papers, Box 9, LoC.

49. WCG to Goethals, August 16, 1907, Gorgas Papers, Box 23, LoC.

50. "The First Pan-American Scientific Congress, Held in Santiago, Chile, December 25, 1908–January 6, 1909," *Science* 29 (March 19, 1909): 441–48; WCG, "Sanitation of the Tropics with Special Reference to Malaria and Yellow Fever," December 25, 1908, Gorgas Papers, Box 16, LoC; *Report of the Delegates of the United States to the Pan-American Scientific Congress*, S. doc. 64, 61st Cong., 1st sess., May 29, 1909.

51. Gorgas and Hendrick, *William Crawford Gorgas*, 212.

52. WCG to O'Reilly, July 21, 1908, Hench Collection; Harry E. Bovay to MG, January 23, 1924, WCGP.

53. See McCullough, *Path between the Seas*, 571, for a profile of Effie Goethals.

54. "The Women's Movement," *Canal Record* (October 1917): 2.

55. "Officers' Wives Are Waging War," *Washington Star*, December 25, 1909; "Women's Social Feud Hits Canal Commission: May Disrupt Isthmian Board, and Mean Retirement of an Officer," *Minneapolis Morning Tribune*, December 26, 1909.

56. Newspaper clipping "Who Is Social Queen at the Isthmus?" *The World*, December 25, 1909, WCGP.

57. Dillard to MG, January 17, 1910, WCGP.

58. George Goethals, "The Building of the Panama Canal: Organization of the Force," *Scribner's* (March 1915): 545.

59. WCG to Goethals, July 21, 1908, Gorgas Papers, Box 24, LoC.

60. WCG to Goethals, July 25, 1908, Gorgas Papers, Box 24, LoC.

61. *ICC Annual Report* for 1908, 28.

62. William C. Gorgas, "The Part Sanitation Is Playing in the Construction of the Panama Canal," *JAMA* 53 (August 21, 1909): 597–99.

63. WCG to C. A. Devol, November 4, 1908, Gorgas Papers, Box 24, LoC.

64. WCG to Torney, May 13, 1909, WCGP.

65. William L. Sibert to MG, May 30, 1921, WCGP.

66. *ICC Annual Report*, 1910, 419, 422.

67. WCG to Kean, December 14, 1910, WCGP.

68. "Memorandum to Col. John L. Phillips, March 29, 1911; and John L. Phillips to Goethals, August 22, 1911, Gorgas Papers, Box 24, LoC.

69. On the screening debate, see Lasso, *Erased*, 125–34.

70. Gillett, *Army Medical Department, 1865–1917*, 277.

71. Arthur Bullard, *Panama: The Canal, the Country, and the People* (New York: Macmillan, 1914), 523–24.

72. WCG to W. W. Keen, April 16, 1908, WCGP.

73. WCG to Dr. J. R. Broome, July 26, 1909, WCGP.

74. WCG to Mamie, October 27, 1909, WCGP.

75. WCG to Jessie, February 2, 1911, WCGP.

76. WCG to AGG, November 9, 1909, WCGP.

## *Chapter 11*

1. WCG to AGG, August 20, 1899, WCGP.

2. Eric Hobsbawm, *The Age of Empire, 1875–1914* (New York: Vintage Books, 1989), 251. On tropical medicine and imperialism, see José Amador, *Medicine and Nation Building in the Americas, 1890–1940* (Nashville: Vanderbilt University Press, 2015); Gillett, *Medical Department of the Army, 1917–1941*, 201–306; Warwick Anderson, "Immunities of Empire: Race, Disease, and the New Tropical Medicine, 1900–1920," *Bulletin of the History of Medicine* 70 (Spring 1996): 94–118; Marcos Cueto, "Sanitation from Above: Yellow Fever and Foreign Intervention in Peru, 1919–1922," *Hispanic American Historical Review* 72 (1992): 1–22; Marcos Cueto and Steven Palmer, *Medicine and Public Health in Latin America: A History* (New York: Cambridge University Press, 2015).

3. Gorgas, "Conquest of the Tropics for the White Race," 1969.

4. "Gorgas's Conquest of Disease," *NYT*, September 22, 1912. Also *New England Journal of Medicine* 160 (1909): 765–67; and *Boston Medical and Surgical Journal* 101 (June 19, 1909): 663.

5. "Conquest of the Tropics for the White Race," *Youth's Companion* 83 (July 29, 1909): 366.

6. Warwick Anderson, *Colonial Pathologies: American Tropical Medicine, Race, and Hygiene in the Philippines* (Durham, NC: Duke University Press, 2006); McNeill, *Mosquito Empires*; Jonathan B. T. Herron, James Alexander, and Thomas Dunbar, "The British Army's Contribution to Tropical Medicine," *Clinical Medicine* 18 (2018): 380–83.

7. Equal Justice Initiative, *Lynching in America: Confronting the Legacy of Racial Terror*, 3rd ed. (Montgomery: Equal Justice Initiative, 2017); Douglas O. Linder, "Lynching in America: Statistics, Information, Images," in Famous Trials website, University of Missouri, Kansas City, 2022.

8. *ICC Annual Report*, 1910, 409–11.

9. "Report of Hearing in Sen. Blackburn's Office, July 17, 1909," transcript; Goethals to WCG, July 21, 1909, WCGP.

10. John T. Morgan to WCG, May 30, 1905, WCGP.

11. WCG to John T. Morgan, August 8, 1906, WCGP.

12. WCG to Kean, August 4, 1906, WCGP.

13. Department of Sanitation, ICC, monthly report, April 1906.

14. US Congress, "Hearings concerning Construction of the Isthmian Canal," November 12, 1907, 810–11.

15. "Report of H. R. Carter to W. C. Gorgas, 28 August 1907," RG 185, Entry 30, Box 795, NARA; "Hearings concerning Construction of the Isthmian Canal," November 12, 1907, 810–11.

16. William C. Gorgas, "Economic Causes of Disease," speech to Business Men's Club, Cincinnati, Ohio, September 28, 1914, published in "Two Papers on Public Sanitation and the Single Tax" (Cincinnati: Joseph Fels Fund of America, 1915), 9–13; and "Relation between Wages and Health," speech before Consumers' League of Washington, April 3, 1916, WCGP.

17. WCG to Charles F. Adams, November 7, 1912, WCGP.

18. "Concerning the Estimates for Construction of the Isthmian Canal for FY12," Hearings before the House Committee on Appropriations, in Culebra, Panama, November 22, 24–25, 1910, 194.

19. WCG to Charles F. Adams, November 7, 1912, WCGP.

20. Department of Sanitation, *ICC Annual Report*, 1914.

21. *Canal Record*, September 9, 1908, 10.

22. "Fatal Explosions of Dynamite," *Canal Record*, October 14, 1908.

23. "Premature Explosion" *Canal Record*, December 16, 1908.

24. "Money Flows Like Apples," Canal Zone-Library Museum Papers, Box 33, LoC. Transcribed into English.

25. "Memorial Window Unveiling," *Canal Record*, October 25, 1910; and Joseph Bucklin Bishop, "An Address at the Unveiling and Dedication of the Memorial Windows at St. Luke's Church, Ancon Hospital," May 8, 1910 (Ancón: Executive Committee of St. Luke's Church, 1910).

26. Department of Sanitation, *ICC Annual Report*, 1910; William R. Scott, *The Americans in Panama* (New York: Statler, 1913).

27. *Estimates for Construction of the Isthmian Canal for FY 12*, 196–97.

28. *ICC Annual Report*, 1910, 434.

29. William C. Gorgas, "The Expenses Necessary for Sanitation in the Tropics," *Journal of the Southern Medical Association* 17 (1910): 1–7.

30. For example, W. C. Gorgas, "Sanitation on the Canal Zone," *JAMA* 60 (March 29, 1913): 955.

31. E. Chaves-Carballo, "The Cost of Running American City Hospitals: The Gorgas 1910 Survey," *Southern Medical Journal* 93 (February 2000): 191–4; and E. Chaves-Carballo, "Ancon Hospital," 729.

32. Gorgas, *Sanitation in Panama*, 241–47.

33. William C. Gorgas, "The Part Sanitation Is Playing in the Construction of the Panama Canal," *JAMA* 53 (August 21, 1909): 597–99.

34. Gorgas, "Expenses Necessary for Sanitation in the Tropics," 7.

35. William C. Gorgas, "Sanitation at Panama," *JAMA* 58 (March 20, 1912): 907–9.

36. See WCG to Edgar Jadwin, August 15, 1910, Gorgas Papers, Box 14, LoC; Gorgas, "Expenses Necessary for Sanitation in the Tropics."

37. WCG to Sen. Bankhead, August 10, 1910, Gorgas Papers, Box 7, LoC.

38. William C. Gorgas, "Sanitation in the Tropics with Special Reference to Malaria and Yellow Fever," *JAMA* 52 (April 3, 1909): 1075–77.

39. "Health Report for September," *Canal Record*, 1907.

40. See, for example, "Sensible Sanitary Measures on the Isthmus," *JAMA* 46 (1906): 366; "Health of White Men in the Canal Zone," *JAMA* 53 (August 27, 1909): 783; "Sanitation in Panama," *JAMA* 54 (April 9, 1910): 1214; "Improved Outlook for Canal Sanitation," *JAMA* 56 (January 20, 1911): 380; "Panama an Object-Lesson to Civilization," *JAMA* 56 (June 10, 1911): 1728; "Medical Importance of Panama," *JAMA* 59 (1912): 1725; "A Clean Record in the Canal Zone," *JAMA* 61 (October 25, 1913): 1544; "Another Clean Record in the Canal Zone," *JAMA* 62 (May 9, 1914): 1481.

41. Kean to WCG, March 9, 1910, WCGP.

42. "Memorandum, "Appropriations and Expenditures of the Sanitary Department," April 25, 1911, Gorgas Papers, Box 24, LoC.

43. WCG to Jessie, February 20, 1911, WCGP.

44. Account Book, WCG, 1910–1914, WCGP.

45. WCG to AGG, October 27, 1909, WCGP.

46. WCG to Mamie, October 27, 1912, WCGP.

47. "Anecdote," WCGP. A version of this conversation appeared in the press, but Goethals denied such a conversation ever occurred.

48. Account Book, WCG, 1910–1914, 66, WCGP.

49. Adele Steiner Burleson to MG, February 17, 1923, WCGP.

50. Le Prince to MG, March 23, 1921, WCGP.

51. Le Prince to MG, March 23, 1921, WCGP; Gorgas and Hendrick, *William Crawford Gorgas*, 254–58.

52. Account Book, WCG, 1915–1916, WCGP, has an inventory of the books.

53. WCG to AGG, December 29, 1911, WCGP.

54. Dixon was the author of *The Clansman* (1905), the book on which the film *Birth of a Nation* was based.

55. Wilson, *Baptized in Blood*, 34; WCG to S. A. Cunningham, *Confederate Veteran*, February 16, 1912, Gorgas Papers, Box 10, LoC.

56. WCG to AAAS, June 22, 1908, Gorgas Papers, Box 7, LoC.

57. WCG to Mamie, October 27, 1912, WCGP. Original typescript of Josiah's war diary is in the Library of Congress, "Josiah Gorgas Journal 1857–1877," Gorgas Papers, Box 35, LoC.

58. Blake Scott, "From Disease to Desire: The Rise of Tourism at the Panama Canal," *Environmental History* 21 (April 2016): 270–77.

59. A. Bienkowski, "Souvenir of the Canal Zone," 1906, WCGP.

60. "The Canal Zone an Ideal Health Resort," *JAMA* 57 (December 23, 1911): 2090–91; "Panama as a Resort," *NYT*, September 22, 1912.

61. "Gorgas's Conquest of Disease," *NYT*, September 22, 1912.

62. John Owen Collins, *The Panama Guide* (Mount Hope, Canal Zone: I.C.C. Press, 1912).

63. Quoted in Anderson, *Colonial Pathologies*, 215.

64. MG, "Memory Jogs," WCGP.

65. OTSG to WCG, February 10, 1910, WCGP; Henry S. Wellcome, "Observations on the Medical and Sanitary Department of the Panama Canal Commission," *Military Surgeon* 27 (1910): 1–33.

66. Hiram Bingham to WCG, January 10, 1910, Gorgas Papers, Box 9, LoC; James Bryce to WCG, August 10, 1910, WCGP; WCG to Goethals, September 7, 1910, Goethals Papers, Box 11, LoC.

67. Account Book, WCG, 1910–1914, WCGP.

68. WCG to Jessie, February 20, 1911, WCGP.

69. WCG to AGG, August 14, 1911, WCGP.

70. Account Book, WCG, 1910–1914, WCGP.

71. *Operation of Panama Canal, Etc., Hearings before the House Committee on Interstate and Foreign Affairs*, June 7, 1911, 62nd Cong., 1st sess., 23. For a discussion of this debate, see Lasso, *Erased*, 136–53.

72. William C. Gorgas, "Address Delivered at the Commencement of the Johns Hopkins University," Baltimore, June 11, 1912, WCGP. See also WCG, "Sanitation in Its Relations to Race Betterment," circa 1915, delivered to Philadelphia County Medical Society, WCGP; William Crawford Gorgas, "The Relation That Modern Tropical Sanitation Will Probably Have on the Future Movements of Populations," *Southern Medical Journal* (1916): 131–34.

## *Chapter 12*

1. *Dr. William Gorgas*, film, Theodore Roosevelt Association Collection, LoC.

2. *Estimates for Construction of the Isthmian Canal for FY12*, 194.

3. W.C. Gorgas, "The Effect that the Completion of the Panama Canal Will Have upon the Probable Extension of Yellow Fever to Asia," in *The History of Yellow Fever*, edited by George Augustin (New Orleans: Searcy and Pfaff, 1909), 135–45.

4. Elihu Root to WCG, June 1, 1906, WCGP.

5. Ronn F. Pineo, "Misery and Death in the Pearl of the Pacific: Health Care in Guayaquil, Ecuador, 1870–1925," *Hispanic American Historical Review* 70 (1990): 609–34; Department of Commerce, Bureau of The Census, "Mortality Statistics 1912" (Washington, DC: GPO, 1913), 9.

6. Pineo, "Misery and Death in the Pearl of the Pacific," 637.

7. O'Reilly to WCG, March 9, 1907, WCGP.

8. B. J. Lloyd to WCG, June 4, 1908, Gorgas Papers, Box 13, LoC; and US Department of State, "Historical Summary Prepared in the Division of Latin American Affairs of the Department of State," Papers Relating to the Foreign Relations of the United States (Washington, DC: GPO, 1920), 513–16.

9. Lois F. Parks and Gustave A. Nuremberger, "The Sanitation of Guayaquil," *Hispanic American Historical Review* 23 (1943): 203.

10. Gorgas, "The Effect That the Completion of the Panama Canal Will Have," 137.

11. "United States Will Take Hold: Insists on Better Sanitation at Guayaquil," *Los Angeles Times*, January 25, 1912; "American Officer a Yellow Fever Victim," *Hartford Courant*, January 25, 1912.

12. Taft to WCG, July 13, 1910, WCGP.

13. "Memorandum of Proposed Convention between the Governments of the United States and Ecuador regarding the Sanitation of Guayaquil," n.d., Gorgas Papers, Box 13, LoC.

14. A Joint resolution to permit Col. William C. Gorgas and certain other officers of the Medical Corps and of the Engineer Corps of the Army to accept service under the Republic of Ecuador, H. J. Res. 365, House Report No. 1286, "Sanitation of Republic of Ecuador," January 10, 1913; *Congressional Record*, 62nd Cong., 3rd sess., February 17, 1913, 3282–84; Parks and Nuremberger, "Sanitation of Guayaquil;" Pineo, "Misery and Death in the Pearl of the Pacific," 609–37.

15. "The Pest Hole of the Pacific: Yellow Fever, Smallpox, Leprosy and Bubonic Plague Stalk Unhampered through the Streets of Guayaquil, Ecuador," *Courier-Journal*, April 7, 1912; "Find a Menace in Guayaquil: United States Will Order the City to Clean Up . . . If Ecuador Doesn't Act Uncle Sam Will," *Los Angeles Times*, February 5, 1912; Scott, *Americans in Panama*, chapter 2.

16. Account Book, WCG, 1910–1914, December 9, 1912, WCGP.

17. WCG, "Speech, Sanitation, Address Delivered at the Canadian Club Meeting," Ottawa, Canada, January 15, 1916, WCGP.

18. Photograph of the car in "Colonel Gorgas's Tour in Ecuador Recounted by One Who Made Trip," *Christian Science Monitor*, January 21, 1913.

19. "Sanitation of Guayaquil, a Report by Colonel Wm. C. Gorgas, Medical Corps, U.S.A., January 9, 1913," submitted to the Hon. Secretary of State, Washington, D.C., Gorgas Papers, Box 25, LoC; "Gorgas to Report: Will Tell of Sanitary Conditions in Guayaquil," *Arizona Republican*, January 21, 1913.

20. Newspaper clipping, "Las cuentas del Coronel Gorgas," *La Prensa*, May 17, 1913, WCGP; Translation of editorial appearing in *El Telégrafo* of Guayaquil, Ecuador, April 16, 1913; "El fondeadero de los vapores," "The Anchorage of Steamers," *El Telégrafo*, n.d., Gorgas Papers, Box 13 LoC. Although Congress approved a delegation of six, Gorgas took a party of four and used only half of the $8,000 Ecuador had authorized for the trip, returning the remainder of the funds. US Department of State, *Papers Relating to the Foreign Relations of the United States*, "Sanitation of Guayaquil," 505–7.

21. Translation of editorial from *El comercio de Quito*, April 26, 1913, Gorgas Papers, Box 13, LoC.

22. Walter V. Scholes and Marie V. Scholes, "The United States and Ecuador, 1909–1913," *The Americas* 19 (1963): 276–90.

23. WCG to RHG, January 4, 1913, WCGP.

24. As recounted in Account Book, WCG, 1915–1916, 3, WCGP.

25. Account Book, WCG, 1915–1916, 176, WCGP. This is the only entry on this page. He also copied in his account book important family birthdays, anniversaries, and the dates of his parents' deaths.

26. WCG to Jessie, April 4, 1913, WCGP. The portrait still hangs in the Amelia Gayle Gorgas Library, University of Alabama, Tuscaloosa.

27. WCG to Mamie, October 27, 1912, WCGP.

28. Wrightson to WCG, c. 1912, Gorgas Papers, Box 23, LoC.

29. WCG to Jessie, April 4, 1913, WCGP.

30. "Account of Wrightson-Gorgas Wedding from Issue May 10, 1913," source unknown, WCGP.

31. Account Book, WCG, 1910–1914, WCGP.

32. WCG to Mamie, October 27, 1912, WCGP.

33. WCG to Dick, September 20, 1913, WCGP.

34. Frank G. Carpenter, "Goethals tells about the Canal: Dictator of Zone Explains How Some Difficult Problems Were Met," *Chicago Daily Tribune,* April 21, 1912. Also, McGovern, *George W. Goethals and the Army*, passim.

35. Account Book, WCG, 1910–1914, WCGP.

36. Department of Sanitation, *ICC Annual Report*, 1913.

37. Gorgas, *Sanitation in Panama*, 292.

38. Chaves-Carballo, "Ancon Hospital," 729.

39. "William Crawford Gorgas," *American Journal of Public Health* 3 (1913).

40. WCG to Dick, September 20, 1913, WCGP.

41. "Paper by S. Evans," RG 185, Entry 30, Box 795, NARA; WCG to Sec., Chamber of Mines, Johannesburg, August 18,1913, and WCG to Samuel Evans, August 16, 1913, WCGP,

42. WCG to Dick, September 20, 1913, WCGP.

43. WCG to Mamie, August 27, 1913, WCGP.

44. "Colonel Gorgas and Assistants to Investigate Sanitary Conditions in South Africa," *Canal Record*, October 15, 1913.

45. McGovern, *George W. Goethals and the Army*, 115.

46. WCG to Dick, November 4, 1913, WCGP.

47. "Letter from Dr. Gorgas to His Sister, Courtesy of Mrs. William D. Wrightson," November 26, 1913, Gorgas Papers, LoC.

48. "In the Cause of Health," *South Africa*, November 15, 1913, in WCGP.

49. WCG to Dick, November 4, 1913, and WCG to Marie, November 25, 1914, WCGP.

50. WCG to Dick, November 4, 1913, WCGP. Haggard was an English novelist known for African adventure stories.

51. "Transcript of letters from W. C. Gorgas, onboard the *Briton*, to Dearest, November–December 1913," WCGP.

52. W.C. Gorgas, "Recommendation as to Sanitation concerning Employees of the Mines on the Rand Made to the Transvaal Chamber of Mines," *JAMA* 62 (June 13, 1914): 1855–56.

53. "A Sanitary Visit to South Africa," address before the Alumni Association of Bellevue Hospital, NYC, February 3, 1915, WCGP.

54. Gorgas, "Recommendation as to Sanitation concerning Employees of the Mines on the Rand," 1863.

55. WCG to MG, December 4, 1913, WCGP.

56. *Canal Record*, January 21, 1914; Account Book, WCG, 1910–1914, in WCGP.

57. "Le Roi Est Mort; Vive le Roi," *Military Surgeon* 34 (February 1914): 156–57.

58. WCG to Edward Munson, June 27, 1912, Gorgas Papers, Box 17, LoC.

59. Account Book, WCG, 1910–1914, January 10, 1914, WCGP.

60. Account Book, WCG, 1910–1914, January 18, 1914, WCGP.

61. "Honor to Col. Gorgas: Named Army Surgeon General for Cleaning up Panama," *Washington Post*, January 18, 1914.

62. ZimFieldGuide.com, "Historic, Cultural and Wildlife Information for Zimbabwe," 2022.

63. William C. Gorgas, "Surgeon-General Gorgas' Report on Malaria and Blackwater Fever in Southern Rhodesia," *Southern Medical Journal* 7 (September 1914): 687–93.

64. Helen Williams to MG, January 11, 1921, WCGP; and S. T. Darling, "Proceedings of the Medical Association of the Isthmian Canal Zone, April 1914 to October 1914," in Chaves-Carballo, *American Medicine and the Panama Canal.*

65. Account Book, WCG, 1910–1914, *WCGP*; Gorgas and Hendrick, *William Crawford Gorgas*, 278–90.

66. Editorial, "Sanitation on the Isthmus of Panama and on the Rand," *JAMA* 62 (June 13, 1914): 1892–93; "South Africa: Sanitation of the Mines: Report of Surgeon-General Gorgas," *The Lancet* (May 2, 1914): 1281–82.

67. WCG to William Keen, March 3, 1914, William W. Keen Papers, John Hay Library, Brown University.

68. WCG quoted in Arthur B. Krock, "Surgeon-General William C. Gorgas," *Technical World* 21 (1914): 820; Philip D. Curtin, "The End of the 'White Man's Grave'? Nineteenth-Century Mortality in West Africa," *Journal of Interdisciplinary History* 21 (1990): 63–88.

69. "A Chat with General Gorgas," *South Africa*, March 21, 1914.

70. W. C. Gorgas, "Anti-mosquito Work at Panama," *Proceedings of the Royal Society of Medicine* 7 (April 1, 1914): 31–40.

71. Menu, bound and autographed, from dinner honoring W. C. Gorgas given by the Medical Profession, London, England, March 23, 1914, WCGP.

72. Newspaper clipping, "Surgeon-General Gorgas, Tribute by the Medical Profession," *London Times*, March 24, 1914; "Surgeon-General Gorgas," *British Medical Journal* (March 28, 1914): 723–24; "Surgeon-General Gorgas and the Panama Canal," *The Lancet* (March 28, 1914): 912–14.

73. Quoted in W. L. Craddock, "The Achievements of William Crawford Gorgas," *Military Medicine* 162 (May 1997): 325–27.

74. John L. Phillips to WCG, February 18, 1914, and March 24, 1914, WCGP.

75. Tranquilina Gustamante File, Gorgas Papers, Box 13, LoC.

## *Chapter 13*

1. WCG to Jessie, December 24, 1914, WCGP.

2. Kean, "Autobiographical Sketch," 159; and Kean to Gen. Henry McCain, September, 1914, WCGP.

3. Kean to WCG, March 17, 1914, WCGP.

4. Editorial, "Surgeon General Gorgas and the Nation's Greatest Need," *Southern Medical Journal* 7 (September 1914): 751–54.

5. WCG to John Ross, September 18, 1914, WCGP.

6. See Greene, *Canal Builders.*

7. Congress gave no recognition or reward to the hundreds of enlisted American personnel who served in Panama, or to the thousands of Caribbean workers who had done the hard labor. Public Law No. 316, "An Act to Provide for Recognizing the Services of Certain Officers of the Army, Navy and Public Health Service for Their Services in Connection with the Construction of the Panama Canal," March 4, 1915.

8. Kean to WCG, March 10, 1915, WCGP.

9. Account Book, WCG, 1910–1914, WCGP; House Committee on Military Affairs, H. Report 1022, *Recognition of Services of Members of Isthmian Canal Commission and Recognition of Services of Certain Officers of the Army and Navy*, July 27, 1914.

10. "Presentation of Gold Medal to Surgeon General Gorgas," *JAMA* 62 (July 4, 1914).

11. John L. Phillips to WCG, May 2, 1914, WCGP.

12. "Report of the Surgeon General, OTSG Priorities, FY 1915," September 1, 1914, *WDAR*, 1914, 335–37; Gillett, *Army Medical Department, 1865–1917*, 313–46.

13. WCG to John Ross, September 18, 1914, WCGP.

14. T. C. Lyster pamphlet, "Report of Department of Health of Veracruz Mexico, for month of August, 1914," WCGP.

15. Gillett, *Army Medical Department, 1865–1917*, 395.

16. WCG to Turtle, August 14, 1914, WCGP. [Note, letter mislabeled "Samuel Evans, July 25, 1914."]

17. "A Bearer of White Man's Burden," *Munsey's Magazine* (December 1915): 413–15.

18. Henry George, *Progress and Poverty: An Inquiry into the Cause of Industrial Depressions and of Increase of Want with Increase of Wealth*, 50th anniversary ed. (New York: Robert Schalkenbach Foundation, 1942).

19. As Dominic Candeloro writes, "The Single Tax movement indicates that the movement was rich in ideas and inspiration but short on organization and tangible accomplishments . . . middle-class, altruistic, and attractive, but not very effective." See "The Single Tax Movement and Progressivism, 1880–1920," *American Journal of Economics and Sociology* 38 (April 1979): 126. Libertarians' interest in George and the Single Tax has endured into the twenty-first century. See Annika Neklason, "The 140-Year-Old Dream of Government without Taxation," *The Atlantic* (April 15, 2019); "The Time May be Right for Land-Value Taxes," *The Economist*, August 9, 2018; *The Gilded Age*, digital short *Henry George: From Poverty to Politics*, dir. Sarah Colt, written by Mark Zwonitzer, PBS, The American Experience, 2018.

20. Henry George, *Progress and Poverty*, 47, 248.

21. Gorgas and Hendricks, *William Crawford Gorgas*, 14; V. H. Bridgman to MG, December 28, 1920, WCGP; Lawrence M. Lipin, "Nature, the City, and the Family Circle: Domesticity and the Urban Home in Henry George's Thought," *Journal of the Gilded Age and Progressive Era* 13 (July 2014): 305–35.

22. WCG to Miss M. B. Ely, October 24, 1914, WCGP.

23. Joseph Miller, *Single Tax Review*, February 1912 and 1913, Gorgas Papers, Box 20, LoC. Gorgas subscribed to *Single Tax Review* from at least 1908 to 1913.

24. "Notables on Henry George," Earth Rights Institute website, accessed March 2022.

25. Robert C. Macauley, "The Single Tax Party in 1920," *Single Tax Review* (September–October 1920).

26. For example, when one writer noted that President Wilson appointed Single Taxers to his administration, he cited Louis F. Post, assistant secretary in the Department of Labor, and others, but not Gorgas, who was speaking around the country in favor of the single tax. Dominic Candeloro, "The Single Tax Movement and Progressivism, 1880–1920," *American Journal of Economics and Sociology* 38 (April 1979): 113–27.

27. "Address Delivered Before the Women's Single Tax Club," February 8, 1915, WCGP.

28. Gorgas, "Economic Causes of Disease."

29. W. C. Gorgas, "Sanitation and Morality," *Constructive Quarterly* 4 (1916): 320–28.

30. "Two Papers on Public Sanitation and the Single Tax" (Cincinnati: Joseph Fels Fund of America, 1915); "Surgeon-General Gorgas Appeals to Christians to Help Increase Wages," *Constructive Quarterly*, c. 1916, 337.

31. Chris Bishop, *The Lion and the Journalist: The Unlikely Friendship of Theodore Roosevelt and Joseph Bucklin Bishop* (Guilford, CT: Lyons Press, 2012), 173.

32. "Announcement," *Canal Record* 1 (September 4, 1907): 1.

33. Joseph Bucklin Bishop, "A Benevolent Despot," *Scribner's Magazine* 53 (March 1913): 303–19. Mark Sullivan's voluminous history *Our Times, 1900–1925*, vol. 1 (New York: Scribner's Sons, 1971), 167–75, reported on the Gorgas-Goethals controversy.

34. Joseph Bucklin Bishop, "Sanitation of the Isthmus," *Scribner's Magazine* (February 1913): 234–51.

35. Joseph Bucklin Bishop, *The Panama Gateway* (New York: Scribner's Sons, 1913).

36. Ralph Emmett Avery, *America's Triumph at Panama* (Chicago: Reagan Printing House, 1913).

37. M. H. Thatcher to WCG, April 29, 1915, WCGP. The articles were Joseph Bucklin Bishop, "Personality of Colonel Goethals," *Scribner's Magazine* 57 (February 1915): 129–52; and George W. Goethals, "The Building of the Panama Canal," Parts I–IV (March–June 1915): 265–82; 395–418; 531–48; 720–34. Bishop's subsequent hagiographic biography, *Goethals—Genius of the Panama Canal* (New York: Harpers and Brothers, 1930), was completed after his death in 1928 by son Farnham Bishop.

38. "Speech, Address at the Commencement of the Washington University, W. C. Gorgas, St. Louis, Missouri, April 30, 1915," WCGP.

39. "Failure to Eliminate Malaria," *Cincinnati Enquirer*, May 1, 1915; "Gorgas, Who Cleaned Up Havana, Holds Chairman of Panama Commission Responsible for Failure to Eradicate Malaria from Canal Zone," *St. Louis Post Dispatch*, April 30, 1915, WCGP.

40. Kean, "Autobiographical Sketch," 133–34.

41. WCG to William L. Sibert, September 17, 1914, WCGP. The three volumes were William L. Sibert and John F. Stevens, *The Construction of the Panama Canal* (New York, D. Appleton, 1915); Emory Richard Johnson, *The Panama Canal and Commerce* (New York, D. Appleton, 1916); and Gorgas, *Sanitation in Panama*, 1915.

Goethals (and Bishop) produced two books on Panama: George Washington Goethals,

*Government of the Canal Zone* (Princeton: Princeton University Press, 1915); and George W. Goethals, *The Panama Canal: An Engineering Treatise* (New York: McGraw Hill, 1916).

42. See Account Book, WCG, 1910–1914, WCGP.

43. Gorgas, *Sanitation in Panama*, 239–40.

44. WCG to Theodore Roosevelt, December 21, 1914, and Le Prince to WCG, January 26, 1915, WCGP. Le Prince published the dye work in "*Annals of the Entomological Society of America* 6 (1913).

45. Gorgas, *Sanitation in Panama*, 286, 288.

46. Gorgas, *Sanitation in Panama*, 291–92.

47. Robert M. Brown, "Eradication of Yellow Fever in Panama," *Geographical Review* 9 (February 1920): 147.

48. Emory R. Johnson, "Reviews," *Annals of the American Academy of Political and Social Science* (November 1915): 301–4.

49. "Book Notices," *JAMA* 65 (July 17, 1915): 273.

50. WCG to Emory Johnson, July 8, 1915, WCGP.

51. WCG to Mamie, November 7, 1914, WCGP.

52. WCG to George Crile, August 24, 1915, cited in E. I. Rutkow and I. M. Rutkow, "George Crile, Harvey Cushing, and the Ambulance Americaine: Military Medical Preparedness in World War I," *Archives of Surgery* 139 (2004): 678–85.

53. WCG to Cushing, September 25, 1915, and Cushing to MG, September 23, 1923, WCGP; John H. Fulton, *Harvey Cushing: A Biography* (Springfield, IL: Charles C. Thomas, 1946), 419; *A History of United States Army Base Hospital No. 19, American Expeditionary Forces, Vichy, France, A.P.O. 781* (Rochester, NY: Wegman-Walsh Press, 1922), 3.

54. WCG to President A. Lawrence Lowell, Harvard University, October 7, 1915, and WCG to Cushing, November 24, 1915, WCGP.

55. Kean, "Autobiographical Sketch," 178; and Julia C. Stimson, *History and Manual of the Army Nurse Corps* (Carlisle Barracks Medical Field Service School, 1937), 19.

56. Jefferson Kean, "The New Role of the American Red Cross," *Military Surgeon* (May 1916): 539.

57. These six hospitals were: Base Hospital No. 2, from Presbyterian Hospital, NY; No. 4 from Lakeside in Cleveland; No. 5 from Harvard; No. 10 from Pennsylvania Hospital in Philadelphia; No. 12 from N.W. Hospital in Chicago; and No. 21 from Washington University in St. Louis.

58. Percy M. Ashburn, *A History of the Medical Department of the U.S. Army* (Boston: Houghton Mifflin, 1929), 256–57.

59. "Career of Gorgas Lauded by Nations: Memorial Services at Pan-American Building Honor Conqueror of Yellow Fever," *Washington Post*, January 17, 1921.

60. WCG to Jerome D. Greene, Rockefeller Foundation, April 16, 1915, WCGP.

61. "Extracts from Minutes of the Rockefeller Foundation, April 4, 1915," Rockefeller Foundation Records, International Health Board, Rockefeller Archive Center, New York (hereafter cited as RF, IHB, RG 5 [FA115]). For more on the Rockefeller Foundation, see chapter 14.

62. Account Book, WCG, 1915–1916, WCGP.

63. Wickliffe Rose to Lindley M. Garrison, March 31, 1915, and Woodrow Wilson to Lindley M. Garrison, April 2, 1915, WCGP.

64. "Rockefeller Foundation and General Gorgas," *Science* 41 (1915): 572.

65. WCG to Jerome D. Greene, Rockefeller Foundation, April 14, 1915, WCGP.

66. WCG to Jacob Dickinson, April 16, 1915, and WCG to W. W. Keen, April 14, 1915, WCGP.

67. Sen. Duncan Fletcher to WCG, April 12, 1915, WCGP.

68. WCG to Jerome D. Greene, April 26, 1915, WCGP.

69. WCG to Jessie, March 17, 1915, WCGP. The Red Cross in coordination with the Rockefeller Foundation and other groups did send an American mission to Serbia that helped contain the outbreak by the end of 1915, but not before almost 150,000 people died. See "Rockefeller Foundation Annual Report, 1915" (New York: The Foundation, 1915), Rockefeller Foundation website; Gaines M. Foster, "Typhus Disaster in the Wake of War," *Bulletin of the History of Medicine* 55 (1981): 221–32.

70. Account Book, WCG, 1915–1916, WCGP.

71. WCG to Henry D Snyder, November 14, 1915, and Account Book, WCG, 1915–1916, WCGP.

72. U.S. Bureau of Labor Statistics, CPI Inflation Calculator website.

73. Account Book, WCG, 1910–1914, April 1914, WCGP.

74. Account Book, WCG, 1915–1916, WCGP.

75. William Sibert to WCG, May 17, 1915, and Account Book, WCG, 1915-1916, WCGP; Standlee, *Borden's Dream*, 105–6.

76. William C. Gorgas, "Dr. Carlos Finlay," *American Journal of Public Health* 5 (November 1915): 1176–78. Finlay received numerous awards during his lifetime but never the Nobel Prize, although he was nominated by Gorgas and others several times. WCG to Ronald Ross, August 9, 1905, Hench Collection.

77. WCG to E. D. Gayle, September 18, 1915, WCGP.

78. "Panama Hat for Any Occasion," *Ladies' Home Journal*, circa 1916, in WCGP.

79. "Her Life Never Dull," *Semi-Weekly Tribune*, North Platte, Nebraska, March 26, 1915.

80. Newspaper clipping, "Mrs. William C. Gorgas Tells of Life in Panama during Work on Canal," n.p., n.d., circa 1915, WCGP.

## *Chapter 14*

1. On preparedness, see John Whiteclay Chambers, *To Raise an Army: The Draft Comes to Modern America* (New York: Free Press, 1987).

2. Osler to WCG, January 30, 1916, WCGP.

3. Carol R. Byerly, *Fever of War: The Influenza Epidemic in the United States Army during World War I* (New York: New York University Press, 2005), chapters 1 and 2.

4. H. C. Fisher, "Preparedness of the Medical Department for War," *Military Surgeon* 38 (February 1915): 123–30.

5. Gillett, *Army Medical Department, 1865–1917*, 348–49. An effort in 1904 to immunize soldiers in the army failed. See W. D. Tigertt, "The Initial Effort to Immunize American Soldier Volunteers with Typhoid Vaccine," *Military Medicine* 124 (1959): 342–49.

6. "Report of the Surgeon General U.S. Army, 1917" (Washington, DC: GPO, 1917); William Sanders Marble, "Medical Support for Pershing's Punitive Expedition in Mexico, 1916 –1917," *Military Medicine* 73 (March 2008): 287–92.

7. Edward Marshall, "Sanitary Lessons from the War," *NYT*, June 27, 1915.

8. *Preparedness for National Defense, Hearings before the Senate Committee on Military Affairs*, 64th Cong., 2nd sess., Gorgas testimony, January 31, 1916, 687–705.

9. Gorgas testimony, *Preparedness for National Defense*, 699. Gorgas's testimony included Exhibit A, letters of support for earlier legislation from Taft and Root; Exhibit B, Dodge Commission on needs of Medical Department; Exhibits C and D, on British war emergency in medical services and editorial support in medical journals; and Exhibit E, number of medical students in the United States.

10. "Vast Body of Surgeons Needed When Army of Million Is Raised, Gorgas Says," *Cincinnati Enquirer*, February 8, 1916.

11. The National Defense Act was approved June 3, 1916 (39 Stat. L., 166); William O. Owen, *A Chronological Arrangement of Congressional Legislation Relating to the Medical Corps of the United States Army from 1785 to 1917* (Chicago: AMA, 1918), 49–59; James A. Tobey, *The Medical Department of the Army: Its History, Activities, and Organization* (Baltimore: Johns Hopkins University Press, 1927), 34–36.

12. Stephen C. Craig, "The Life of Brigadier General Theodore C. Lyster," *Aviation, Space, and Environmental Medicine* 65 (1994): 1047–53.

13. *WDAR, 1916*, 470.

14. See Franklin H. Martin, *Digest of the Proceedings of the Council of National Defense during the World War* (Washington, DC: GPO, 1934).

15. Franklin H. Martin, *Fifty Years of Medicine and Surgery* (Chicago: Surgical Publishing Company of Chicago, 1934), 33–35.

16. Martin, *Fifty Years of Medicine and Surgery*, 33.

17. *Military Appropriations, FY 1917, Hearings before the House Committee on Military Affairs*, Gorgas testimony, April 11, 1916, 859, 876.

18. *WDAR*, 1916, 656; William C. Gorgas, "Yellow Fever and Its Eradication," *Proceedings of the Second American Scientific Congress, 1915–1916* (Washington, DC: GPO, 1917), 7–9.

19. WCG Speech, "Yellow Fever," Address delivered at the Meeting of the American Medical Association, San Francisco, June 1916, WCGP.

20. WCG, unpublished essay, "The Two Greatest Events of 1915," January 1, 1915, WCGP.

21. "The Rockefeller Institute for Medical Research," *Science* 40 (July 3, 1914): 20–21.

22. R. B. Fosdick, *The Story of the Rockefeller Foundation* (New York: Harper, 1952), 15.

23. John Farley makes this point in *To Cast Out Disease: A History of the International Health Division of the Rockefeller Foundation, 1913–1951* (Oxford: Oxford University Press, 2004).

24. Farley, *To Cast Out Disease*, 88–106; R. B. Fosdick, *Story of the Rockefeller Foundation* (New York: Harper, 1952), 58.

25. Wickliffe Rose memo, "Yellow Fever," April 6, 1916, Rockefeller Foundation, IHB, RG 5 (FA115), Box 14.

26. Gorgas, "Yellow Fever and Its Eradication," 7–9.

27. WCG Speech, "Yellow Fever," Address delivered at the Meeting of the American Medical Association, San Francisco, June 1916, WCGP.

28. Quoted in R. B. Fosdick, *Story of the Rockefeller Foundation* (New York: Harper, 1952), 59.

29. For example, Espinosa, *Epidemic Invasions*; Cueto and Palmer, *Medicine and Public Health in Latin America: A History*.

30. Quoted in Gorgas and Hendrick, *William Crawford Gorgas*, 300.

31. Wickliffe Rose, "Yellow Fever: Feasibility of Its Eradication," October 27, 1914, Hench Collection; Wilbur A. Sawyer, "A History of the Activities of the Rockefeller Foundation in the Investigation and Control of Yellow Fever," *American Journal of Tropical Medicine and Hygiene* 17 no. 1 (1937): 35.

32. WCG to Wickliffe Rose, March 14, 1916, RF, IHB, RG 5 (FA115), Box 14.

33. Account Book, WCG, 1915–1916, WCGP.

34. "To Exterminate Germ: General Gorgas Stops Here before Sailing for South America Trip on Rockefeller Fund," *Baltimore Sun*, June 11, 1916.

35. WCG, "Suggestions as to Organization for Board to Investigate Yellow Fever," n.d., WCGP.

36. Journal, William Crawford Gorgas, partial typescript copy, 1919, WCGP (hereafter cited as WCG Journal, 1916 and 1919). Note: This typescript has almost two hundred pages, most of which are from 1916.

37. WCG Journal, 1916 and 1919, WCGP.

38. WCG to Wickliffe Rose, June 29, 1916, RF, IHB, RG 5 (FA115), Box 14.

39. Farley, *To Cast Out Disease*, 92. Farley argues that this balance shifted under subsequent leadership at the IHB in the 1920s and 1930s.

40. WCG to Wickliffe Rose, July 4, 1916, RF, IHB, RG 5 (FA115), Box 14.

41. WCG Journal, 1916 and 1919, WCGP.

42. WCG to Wickliffe Rose, July 18, 1916, RF, IHB, RG 5 (FA115), Box 14; WCG Journal, 1916 and 1919.

43. WCG Journal, 1916 and 1919, August 9, 1916, WCGP.

44. Anecdotes from the life of Gorgas, # 3579, WCGP.

45. WCG to Wickliffe Rose, August 23, 1916, RF, IHB, RG 5 (FA115), Box 14.

46. WCG to Thomas Suri Calcedo, August 19, 1916, RF, IHB, RG 5 (FA115), Box 14.

47. WCG Journal, 1916 and 1919, August 17, 1916, WCGP.

48. J. M. Montaye to WCG, December 6, 1916, WCGP.

49. WCG Journal, 1916 and 1919, August 26, 1916, WCGP.

50. WCG to Dick, September 5, 1916, WCGP.

51. WCG to Wickliffe Rose, July 4, 1916, RF, IHB, RG 5 (FA115), Box 14.

52. Christopher Abel, "External Philanthropy and Domestic Change in Colombian Health Care: The Role of the Rockefeller Foundation, ca. 1920–1950," *Hispanic American Historical Review* 75 (1995): 340.

53. Elizabeth Nix, "In 1916, German Terrorists Launched an Attack on American Soil," History.com website, August 31, 2018.

54. WCG Journal, 1916 and 1919, August 31, 1916 and September 3, 1916, WCGP.

55. "Report of the Surgeon General," *WDAR*, 1916, 475.

56. WCG Journal, 1916 and 1919, October 2, 1916, WCGP.

57. WCG Journal, 1916 and 1919, October 4, 1916, and September 27, 1916, WCGP.

58. WCG Journal, 1916 and 1919, October 16 and 23, 1916, WCGP.

59. Alan P. Marcus, *Confederate Exodus: Social and Environmental Forces in the Migration of U.S. Southerners to Brazil* (Lincoln: University of Nebraska Press, 2021).

60. WCG Journal, 1916 and 1919, November 7, 1916, WCGP.

61. "The Yellow Fever Expedition of the Rockefeller Foundation," *Science* 48 (December 1918): 595–96; T. C. Lyster, "Diplomatic Notes, September 9, 1916," on Maracaibo visit; Juan Guiteras, "City of Guayaquil, Republic of Ecuador: Report on Public Health Organization," July 4, 1916, unpublished reports for the Yellow Fever Commission of the Rockefeller Foundation, Gorgas Papers, Box 25, LoC; R. B. Fosdick, *Story of the Rockefeller Foundation* (New York: Harper, 1952), 60.

62. Gorgas and Hendrick, *William Crawford Gorgas*, 301.

63. WCG and Rockefeller correspondence, January and February 1917, WCGP; Sawyer, "A History of the Activities of the Rockefeller Foundation in the Investigation and Control of Yellow Fever," 35–50.

64. "The Yellow Fever Expedition of the Rockefeller Foundation," *Science* 48 (December 1918): 595–96; Kean, unpublished autobiography, 188.

## *Chapter 15*

1. Major W. N. Kenzie and Associates of the Medical Reserve, ed., *Year Book, Medical Officers' Training Camp, Fort Riley, Kansas, 1917–1918* (Kansas City, MO: Union Bank Note, 1918).

2. Mary C. Gillett, *The Army Medical Department, 1917–1941* (Washington, DC: Center for Military History, United States Army, 2009), 10, 16.

3. James M. Phalen, "Chiefs of the Medical Department, U.S. Army 1775–1940, Biographical Sketches," *Army Medical Bulletin* 52 (1940): 92.

4. Kean, unpublished autobiography, 247.

5. Merritte Ireland memoir, 2

6. WCG to Henry Carter, March 19, 1917, Hench Collection.

7. WCG to William Polk, March 20, 1917, WCGP.

8. WCG to Samuel Darling, March 22, 1917, WCGP.

9. WCG to Henry Carter, May 18, 1917, Hench Collection.

10. Edward Champe Carter, *The Lone Scout: A Tale of the United States Public Health Service* (Boston: Cornhill Com., 1920). Gorgas wrote a short foreword to the book.

11. Marian Moser Jones, *The American Red Cross from Clara Barton to the New Deal* (Baltimore: Johns Hopkins University Press, 2013).

12. Nancy K. Bristow, *Making Men Moral: Social Engineering During the Great War* (New York: New York University Press, 1997).

13. Samuel Gompers to WCG, April 27, 1917, and WCG to Gompers, May 1, 1917, WCGP.

14. WCG to Daniel Kiefer, April 11, 1917, and Daniel Kiefer to WCG, June 23, 1917, WCGP.

15. WCG to Daniel Kiefer, April 11, 1917, WCGP.

16. Leonard Porter Ayres, *The War with Germany: A Statistical Summary* (Washington, DC: GPO 1919), 13.

17. Leonard Porter Ayres, *The War with Germany: A Statistical Summary* (Washington, DC: GPO 1919), 13–19; Army War College (US), Historical Section, US Department of the Army, Office of Military History, *Order of Battle of the United States Land Forces in the World War* (Washington, DC: US GPO: 1931–1949), 3:374.

18. *WDAR, 1919*, vol. 1, pt. 1, 80–81, and pt. 2, 1431–32; Nancy Gentile Ford, *Americans All! Foreign-Born Soldiers in World War I* (College Station: Texas A&M University Press, 2001); Thomas A. Britten, *American Indians in World War I* (Albuquerque: University of New Mexico Press, 1997), 59–60, 198 n. 28.

19. Carol R. Byerly, *Good Tuberculosis Men: The Army Medical Department's Struggle with Tuberculosis* (Fort Sam Houston, TX: Borden Institute, 2013), chapter 4.

20. See correspondence in RG 112, Entry 29, Box 183, NARA.

21. War Department, Office of the Surgeon General, *The Medical Department in the World War*, vol. 6 (Washington, DC: GPO, 1921–1929) (hereafter cited as *MDWW*); War Department, Special Regulations No. 28, "Sanitary Regulations and Control of Communicable Diseases" (Washington, DC: GPO, 1917).

22. W. C. Gorgas, "Drug Addicts in the Military Service," June 22, 1918, RG 112, Entry 29, Box 130, NARA.

23. Łukaz Kamieński, "Drugs," in *1914–1918-Online. International Encyclopedia of the First World War*, ed. Ute Daniel, Peter Gatrell, Oliver Janz, Heather Jones, Jennifer Keene, Alan Kramer, and Bill Nasson (Berlin: Freie Universität Berlin, 2019).

24. *WDAR, 1917*, 346.

25. Victor C. Vaughan and George T. Palmer, "Communicable Diseases in the National Guard and National Army of the United States during the Six Months from September 29, 1917, to March 29, 1918," *Military Medicine* 41 (September 1918): 251.

26. *MDWW*, vol. 6, 137.

27. Victor C. Vaughan, "Measles and Pneumonia in Our Camps," *Journal of Laboratory and Clinical Medicine* 3 (January 1918): 248–57; Victor C. Vaughan, "The Responsibilities of the Medical Profession in This War," *Military Surgeon* 41 (December 1918): 651–58.

28. After the war, for example, the Medical Department noted that "no such detention camps were provided in the original plan of the cantonments." *MDWW*, vol. 1, 265.

29. Office of the Surgeon General, "Organization Charts Office of the Surgeon General," prepared June 22, 1918, RG 112, Entry 29, NARA; Franklin Martin, *Major General William Crawford Gorgas* (Chicago: Gorgas Memorial Institute, 1933), 56.

30. Martin, *Digest of the Proceedings of the Council of National Defense*.

31. *MDWW*, vol. 1, 789–90; See "An Imperative Appeal for Medical Officers," *Boston Medical and Surgical Journal* 178 (May 8, 1918): 646; *JAMA* 70 (April 13, 1918): 1100; *American Journal of Public Health* 8 (May 1918): 381–82, among other journals.

32. H.R. 5531, to Provide a Pharmaceutical Corps in the Army, Hearings before the House Committee on Military Affairs, March 19, 1918; H.R. 5407, Osteopathic Physicians for Military Service, Hearings before the House Committee on Military Affairs, March 15, 1918. Osteopathic physicians were not admitted to the Medical Corps until 1966.

33. "Medical Preparedness Movement Taking Shape," *Minneapolis Morning Tribune*, July 1, 1916.

34. Gillett, *Army Medical Department, 1865–1917*, 23–25, 111.

35. "Officers and Members of the Academy, November 20, 1918," *Proceedings of the National Academy of Sciences* 4 (1918): vii–viii; J. K. Gilman, "The Brief Military Career of Dr. William H. Welch," *Military Medicine* 182 (2017): 1831–34.

36. George Bushnell quoted in Franklin Martin, *Major General William Crawford Gorgas* (Chicago: Gorgas Memorial Institute, 1933), 39.

37. Memorandum for the Chief of Staff, "Medical Officers for Research and Special Laboratory Work," November 2, 1916, RG 165, Entry 296, Box 401, NARA.

38. WCG to Stanhope Bayne-Jones, June 17, 1915, Ms 155, Stanhope Baybe-Jones Papers, William C. Gorgas Papers, Hans Zinsser Papers, 1870–1969, Box 8, NLM.

39. War Department General Order No. 80, June 30, 1917, and quoted in Richard V. N. Ginn, *The History of the U. S. Army Medical Service Corps* (Washington, DC: Office of the Surgeon General and Center of Military History, 1997), 57. The Sanitary Corps was the precursor of the Medical Service Corps.

40. WCG to Charles Willcox, August 23, 1918, WCGP.

41. Bailey Ashford, *A Soldier in Science: The Autobiography of Bailey K. Ashford* (New York: William Morrow, 1934), 195; Gillett, *Army Medical Department, 1917–1941*, 16.

42. W. Douglas Fisher and Joann H. Buckley, *African American Doctors of World War I: The Lives of 104 Volunteers* (Jefferson, NC: McFarland, 2016); John M. Hyson Jr. "African-American Dentists in the U.S. Army: The Origins," *Military Medicine* 161 (July 1996): 375–81; Herbert M. Morais, *The History of the Negro in Medicine* (New York: Publishers Company, 1967), 111; Jane Lang Scheiber and Harry N. Scheiber, "The Wilson Administration and the Wartime Mobilization of Black Americans, 1917–18," *Labor History* 10 (June 1969): 433–58; *MDWW*, vol. 7, 262–76. Also, Adriane Lentz-Smith, *Freedom Struggles: African Americans and World War I* (Cambridge: Harvard University Press, 2009).

43. Emmett J. Scott, *Scott's Official History of the American Negro in the World War* (Chicago: Homewood Press, 1919), 108–9.

44. Hyson Jr., "African-American Dentists," 378.

45. Surgeon General, "Separation of White and Colored Patients," March 22, 1918, RG 112, Entry 91, Box 4610, NARA.

46. Mary Roth Walsh, *Doctors Wanted, No Women Need Apply: Sexual Barriers in the Medical Profession, 1835–1975* (New Haven: Yale University Press, 1977); Ellen S. More, *Restoring the Balance: Women Physicians and the Profession of Medicine, 1850–1995* (Cambridge: Harvard University Press, 1999).

47. WCG to Lucy Waite, March 16, 1907, Gorgas Papers, Box 22, LoC.

48. Kimberly Jensen, "Women, Citizenship and Civic Sacrifice: Engendering Patriotism in the First World War," in *Bonds of Affection*, ed. John Bodnar (Princeton: Princeton University Press, 1996), 139–59.

49. Kimberly Jensen, "'The Open Way of Opportunity': Colorado Women Physicians and World War I," *Western Historical Quarterly* 27 (Autumn 1996): 341–42.

50. Benjamin S. Warren and Charles F. Bolduan, "War Activities of the United States Public Health Service," *PHR* 34 (June 6, 1919): 1243–68; Henry Pomeroy Davison, *The*

*American Red Cross in the Great War* (New York: Macmillan, 1919); Sarnecky, *History of the Army Nurse Corps*, 101.

51. House Committee on Military Affairs, Army Appropriations Bill, 1919, 1166.

52. Proposed Legislation Affecting the Medical Corps of the United States Army, Hearings before the House Committee on Military Affairs April 16, 20 and June 7, 1918, 65th Cong., 2nd sess., 64.

53. House Committee on Military Affairs, Army Appropriations Bill, 1919, 1166. The Army Reorganization Act of 1920 did authorize relative rank for army nurses beginning in August of that year. Sarnecky, *History of the Army Nurse Corps*, 142–47.

54. On the Army School of Nursing, see "The Army Nurse Corps," *MDWW*, vol. 13, pt. 2; RG 112, Entry 283, Box 27, NARA.

55. Quoted in Scott, *Official History*, 448–49.

56. Beth Linker, *War's Waste: Rehabilitation in World War I America* (Chicago: University of Chicago Press, 2011), 61–78.

57. *MDWW*, vol. 8, 58.

58. Alfred Keogh to General Gorgas, April 9, 1917, WCGP.

59. WCG to Keogh, May 1, 1917, WCGP.

60. T. H. Goodwin to MG, November 20, 1920, WCGP.

61. Col. Goodwin of Royal Army Medical Corps, "Practical Hints to Medical Officers," *Military Surgeon* 40 (1917): 240–44; Col. T. H. Goodwin, "Sanitation in War," *Military Surgeon* 40 (October 1917): 377–87; Thomas Goodwin, *Notes for Army Medical Officers, War Department; Medical War Manual No. 2* (Philadelphia: Lea & Febiger, 1917).

62. WCG to Goodwin, January 1, 1918, WCGP.

63. *MDWW*, vol. 1, 126.

64. Martin, *Digest of the Proceedings of the Council of National Defense*, 306. Martin said that Gorgas attended practically every meeting of the council. Martin, *Major General William Crawford Gorgas*, 53.

65. Quoted by Congressman Francis M. Royal to Woodrow Wilson, October 9, 1917, RG 112, Entry 29, Box 414, NARA.

66. Correspondence regarding the antivaccination campaign can be found in RG 112, Entry 29, Boxes 413 and 414, NARA.

67. G. E. Bushnell, "Memorandum for the Secretary of War: Vaccination and Inoculation," n.d., RG 112, Entry 29, Box 414, NARA.

68. Surgeon General to S. Hubert Dent, Committee on Military Affairs, House, RG 112, Entry 29a, Box 19, NARA.

69. Allan M. Brandt, *No Magic Bullet: A Social History of Venereal Disease in the United States since 1880*, 2nd ed. (New York: Oxford University Press, 2020).

70. Woodrow Wilson, "God Keep and Guide You, Soldiers of the National Army," *Journal of Social Hygiene* 3 (1917): 454.

71. "Syllabus Accredited for the Use in Official Lectures on Sex Hygiene and Venereal Diseases," November 1917, RG 112, Entry 29, Box 129, NARA.

72. Published as W. C. Gorgas, "Venereal Diseases and the War," *American Journal of Public Health* 8 (February 1918): 107–11.

73. *WDAR, 1917*, 338.

74. William C. Gorgas, "The Credit Side of Our War Ledger," *Collier's* (June 8, 1918): 11; also, William C. Gorgas, "The Doctor and the War," *Journal of Social Hygiene* 3 (October 1917): 476; William C. Gorgas, "Because We Went to War," *Journal of Social Hygiene* 4 (1918): 218.

75. Ashburn, *History of the Medical Department of the U.S. Army*, 317.

76. *MDWW*, vol. 2, 39.

77. *MDWW*, vol. 2, 244–50.

78. *MDWW*, vol. 2, 350.

79. Martin, *Major General William Crawford Gorgas*, 52.

80. "Statement by Lieut. Col. Robert E. Noble, Medical Corps, October 26, 1917, on the Inspection of Various Camps," RG 112, Entry 29, Box 416, NARA.

81. Committee on Public Information, *Official Bulletin* (November 7, 1917): 5.

82. *Army Appropriation Bill, 1919, Hearings before the House Committee on Military Affairs*, December 1917, January and February 1918, 65th Cong., 2nd sess.; *Investigation of the War Department, Hearings before the Senate Committee on Military Affairs*, December 1917, January, February and March 1918, vols. 1–8, 65th Cong., 2nd sess.

## *Chapter 16*

1. Martin, *Digest of the Proceedings of the Council of National Defense*, 145.

2. H. C. Coe, "Obedience to Orders," *Military Surgeon* 43 (May 1918): 564.

3. W. C. Gorgas, essay, "Cooperation in our Departmental Personnel," n.d., RG 112, Entry 29, Box 13, NARA.

4. *WDAR, 1918*, 486.

5. Vaughan, "Measles and Pneumonia in Our Camps," 248–52; *WDAR, 1918*, 480.

6. *WDAR, 1918*, 480–88; *MDWW*, vol. 9, 409–50; Medical Department of the United States Army, Office of the Surgeon General, *Preventive Medicine in World War II: Volume IV. Communicable Diseases Transmitted Chiefly through Respiratory and Alimentary Tracts* (Washington, DC: Office of the Surgeon General, Department of the Army, 1958), 129–30.

7. *MDWW*, vol. 9, 414.

8. Vaughan, "Measles and Pneumonia in Our Camps," 257. For the Medical Department's rehearsal of their efforts to implement these policies, see *MDWW*, vol. 1, 991–92; *MDWW*, vol. 6, 68–69, 173–85; War Department, Special Regulations No. 28, "Sanitary Regulations and Control of Communicable Diseases," 28.

9. *MDWW*, vol. 1, 987–89; *MDWW*, vol. 6, 70.

10. "List of Sanitary Inspections Made by Officers of the Inspection Section during the Period of the World War," RG 112, Entry 29, Box 417, NARA; *MDWW*, vol. 1, 249–56.

11. *MDWW*, vol. 6, 151–52.

12. *MDWW*, vol 6, 66; "Personal Recollections of General Gorgas by Victor Vaughan," WCGP.

13. Memo, Vaughan to WCG, "Communicable Diseases in Camps," December 23, 1917, 68–69, and WCG to Chief of Staff, "Detention and Quarantine Camps," December 20, 1917, in *MDWW*, vol. 6, 175–76.

14. William Crawford Gorgas, *Sanitary Conditions at Army Camps: Communications*

*from the Surgeon General of the Army to the Chief of Staff upon the Sanitary Conditions of the Army Camps and Cantonments*, H. doc. No. 806, 65th Cong., 2nd sess. (Washington, DC: GPO, 1918). The original report can be found in RG 112, Entry 31, Box 75 (Camp Funston).

15. "Fear Is Shown by Gorgas," *Cincinnati Enquirer*, November 30, 1917; "Gorgas Reports Troops at Camps Crowded, Ill-Clad," *NYT*, December 19, 1917.

16. "Winter Clothing Is Now at Camps," *NYT*, December 20, 1917.

17. The records of the Office of the Surgeon General include several boxes of these inquiries. See RG 112, Entry 29, Boxes 391, 393, and 394, NARA.

18. H. Res. 205, A Resolution Proposing That an Inquiry Be Made into the Hospital and Health Records of Camp Mills, Hempstead, Long Island, December 18, 1917, 65th Cong., 2nd sess.

19. Gorgas, "Sanitary Conditions at Army Camps," *Congressional Record*, January 8, 1918, 1024–25.

20. "Maj. Gardner Dies at Camp Wheeler," January 15, 1918, *NYT*; Daniel R. Beaver, *Newton D. Baker and the American War Effort, 1917–1919* (Lincoln: University of Nebraska Press, 1966), 87–93.

21. Ernest Lester Jones to Newton Baker, January 31, 1918, Baker Papers, LoC, reel 5.

22. "Chamberlain Repeats His Charges," *NYT*, January 25, 1918.

23. Senator Chamberlain, speaking on a point of personal privilege concerning a war cabinet, 65th Cong., 2nd sess., *Congressional Record* (January 24, 1918): 1199–1200.

24. "Chamberlain Repeats His Charges," *NYT*, January 25, 1918.

25. "Editorial," *NYT*, January 23, 1918.

26. Senate, Committee on Military Affairs, *Investigation of the War Department*, 1989, 1994, and 2000.

27. "Gorgas Ascribes Deaths to Haste," *NYT*, January 26, 1918.

28. "Soldiers Dying in Camps from Lack of Clothing and Being Overcrowded," *Atlanta Constitution*, December 19, 1917; "Overcrowding and Poor Sanitary Conditions Blamed for Epidemics in Camps," *Hartford Courant*, December 19, 1917; "Camp Greene Is Unsanitary says Gorgas," *San Francisco Chronicle*, February 14, 1918.

29. Representatives Reavis and Campbell speaking on health conditions in the army training camps, *Congressional Record*, January 18, 1918, 65th Cong., 2nd sess., 1019.

30. Clarence Cramer, *Newton D. Baker: A Biography* (Cleveland: World, 1961), 143; Beaver, *Newton D. Baker*, 103.

31. Senate Committee on Military Affairs, *Investigation of the War Department*, 1732.

32. *Congressional Record*, January 31, 1918, 1426.

33. Senate Committee on Military Affairs, *Investigation of the War Department*, 1926, 1939.

34. Senate Committee on Military Affairs, *Investigation of the War Department*, 1931; Byerly, *Fever of War*, 59–61.

35. Surgeon General to Adjutant General, February 4, 1918, RG 112, Entry 29, Box 130, NARA; "Gen. Gorgas to Weed Out 'Medical Incompetents,'" *NYT*, December 22, 1917; *Army Appropriations, 1919, Hearings before the House Committee on Military Affairs*, January 28, 1918, 65th Cong., 2nd sess., 1154.

36. *Army Appropriations, 1919*, January 28, 1918, 1174–75.

37. *Army Appropriations, 1919*, January 28, 1918, 1163.

38. *Army Appropriations, 1919*, January 28, 1918, 1180.

39. *Army Appropriations, 1919*, letter from George W. Sparks, January 28, 1918, 1232–33.

40. Quoted in Gorgas and Hendrick, *William Crawford Gorgas*, 321.

41. WCG to Mamie, February 2, 1918, WCGP.

42. WCG to Keogh, January 28, 1918, WCGP.

43. Keogh to WCG, February 20, 1918, WCGP.

44. Rep. Edwin Webb of North Carolina, *Congressional Record*, February 22, 1918, 65th Cong., 2nd sess., 2546–50.

45. Surgeon General, "Request that next draft be delayed," n.d., and 2nd endorsement, March 2, 1918, RG 112, Entry 29, Box 181, NARA.

46. Paul A. C. Koistenen, *Mobilizing for Modern War: The Political Economy of American Warfare, 1865–1919* (Lawrence: University of Kansas Press, 1997), chapter 9; Frederic L. Paxson, "The American War Government, 1917–1918," *American Historical Review* (October 1920): 54–76; John Dickinson, *The Building of an Army: A Detailed Account of Legislation, Administration, and Opinion in the United States, 1915–1920* (New York: Century, 1922).

47. *WDAR, 1918*, 334.

48. *Order of Battle*, vol. 3, pt. 1, 248; Leonard Porter Ayres, *The War with Germany: A Statistical Summary* (Washington, DC: GPO 1919), 131–33.

49. *MDWW*, vol. 3, 34.

50. *MDWW*, vol. 3, 87–106.

51. *Order of Battle*, vol. 3, pt. 1, 248; Ayres, *War with Germany*, 131–33.

52. *MDWW*, vol. 3, 87–93.

53. *MDWW*, vol. 10, *Neuropsychiatry*, passim. Also, Ben Shephard, *A War of Nerves: Soldiers and Psychiatrists in the Twentieth Century* (Cambridge: Harvard University Press, 2001).

54. Beth Linker, *War's Waste: Rehabilitation in World War I America* (Chicago: University of Chicago Press, 2011); Jessica Adler, *Burdens of War: Creating the United States Veterans Health System* (Baltimore: Johns Hopkins University Press, 2017); Stephen R. Ortiz, ed., *Veterans' Policies, Veterans' Politics: New Perspectives on Veterans in the Modern United States* (Gainesville: University Press of Florida, 2012).

55. WCG to Secretary of War, November 7, 1917, "Plan for Physician Reconstruction and Training," *MDWW*, vol. 8, *Physical Reconstruction and Vocational Education*, 9–28; J. E. Goldthwait, *The Division of Orthopaedic Surgery in the A. E. F.* (Norwood, MA: Priv. print. at the Plimpton Press, 1941), 26.

56. *Legislative, Executive, and Judicial Appropriation Bill, 1919, Hearings before the House Committee on Appropriations*, January 22, 1918, 65th Cong., 2nd sess., 743.

57. Linker, *War's Waste*, 7.

58. Quoted in Linker, *War's Waste*, 155.

59. *MDWW*, vol. 13, 9–10, 38; Linker, *War's Waste*, 79.

60. WCG, "Administration of Great War Medical Service Which Keeps Up Fighting

Forces and Conserves the Stricken," *Chicago Commerce*, November 1, 1917; "Address by Gen. Gorgas," January 3, 1918, WCGP, audience unknown.

61. Harvey Cushing to MG, September 23, 1923, WCGP; Fulton, *Harvey Cushing*, 419.

62. W. C. Gorgas, "The Activities and Growth of the Medical Department," June 7, 1918, RG 112, Entry 29, Box 160, NARA.

63. See correspondence in RG 112, Entry 29, Box 183, NARA.

64. Furbush to B. R. Tillman, April 22, 1918, RG 112, Entry 29, Box 130.

65. "Surgeon General Gorgas and the Responsibility of the Medical Department of the Army," *JAMA* 70 (May 18, 1918): 1460.

66. "Men Who Are Winning the War," *Leslie's Weekly* (November 1917): 722.

67. "Your Man in Service," *Ladies' Home Journal* 35 (October 1918): 27.

68. Mary B. Mullett, "The Chances of Getting Killed or Hurt in This War: An Important Message to American Magazine Readers from Surgeon General Gorgas," *American Magazine* 85 (1918): 41–43.

69. Gorgas, "The Credit Side of Our War Ledger."

70. "Journal of William C. Gorgas, Chairman, Yellow Fever Commission Partial Typescript Copy, 1919," 47, WCGP.

71. "Memorandum of Sick Record of Major General William C. Gorgas," January 14,1919, Gorgas Papers, Box 6, LoC; Editorial, "Surgeon-General Gorgas Is Sixty-Three Years Young," *Southern Medical Journal* 11 (May 1918): 400–401.

72. Louis Post, to WCG, August 14, 1917, WCGP; WCG to W. H. Whiting, May 28, 1918, Gorgas Papers, Box 6, LoC.

73. WCG to George Denegre, November 15, 1917, WCGP. In the story it was actually a crocodile who had consumed a ticking alarm clock.

74. Victor C. Vaughan, "Major General Gorgas," *Journal of Laboratory and Clinical Medicine* 5 (August 1920): 749–52; "Personal Recollections of General Gorgas by Victor Vaughan," WCGP.

75. Kean, unpublished autobiography, 205, 214.

76. Gillett, *Army Medical Department, 1865–1917*, 46–50, 224–27; McGovern, *George W. Goethals*, 188–93.

77. "Memoir about W. C. Gorgas—by Colonel Ford" [probably Joseph H. Ford], 56–67, WCGP.

78. First lieutenants earned $2,000 per year ($166 per month, compared to the $30 for privates); majors, $3,000; colonels $4,000; and generals, such as Gorgas, earned $8,000 per year. US Department of War, *Register of the Army of the United States for 1918* (Washington, DC: GPO, 1918), 1156.

79. Martin, *Fifty Years of Medicine and Surgery*, 380; emphasis added. See also Martin to MG, January 22, 1923, WCGP.

80. *Advanced Rank for Army Medical Officers, Hearing before the Senate Committee on Military Affairs,* March 15, 1918, 65th Cong., 2nd sess., 13.

81. Newton Baker to Chairman, Senate Committee on Military Affairs, January 31, 1918, Record Group 165, Records of the Office of the Chief of Staff (hereafter cited as RG 165), Entry 296, Box 401, NARA.

82. *Advanced Rank for Army Medical Officers*, March 15, 1918, 65.

83. *Proposed Legislation Affecting the Medical Corps of the United States Army, Hearings before the House Committee on Military Affairs*, April 16, 20 and June 7, 1918, 65th Cong., 2nd sess., 41, 58.

84. See Office of the Chief of Staff, "Additional Personnel for the Medical Department," May 1918, RG 165, Entry 296, Box 401, NARA.

85. *Advanced Rank for Army Medical Officers*, March 15, 1918, 13–15.

86. *Army Appropriations, 1919*, House Committee on Military Affairs, 1214–15.

87. "The Owen-Dyer Bill for Increased Rank," *America Medical Association Special Bulletin* 23 (February 1918); "Legislation for Increased Rank for Medical Officers," *JAMA* 70 (March 30, 1918): 926.

88. "Appeal by Gorgas from Baker Ruling," *Washington Post*, March 16, 1918; Martin, *Major General William Crawford Gorgas*, 48.

89. "Gorgas Appeals Direct to Congress," and "Insubordinate, but with Good Reason," *NYT*, March 16, 1918.

90. Woodrow Wilson to Franklin Martin, March 5, 1918, RG 112, Entry 29, Box 19, NARA; Gillett, *Army Medical Department, 1917–1941*, 226.

91. Martin, *Major General William Crawford Gorgas*, 50.

92. Senator Robert Owen speaking on the grades of medical officers, *Congressional Record*, July 20, 1917, 65th Cong., 1st sess., 5330–34.

93. Quoted in Martin, *Major General William Crawford Gorgas*, 54.

94. Baker quoted in Franklin Martin's review of Gorgas and Hendrick, *William Crawford Gorgas*, in *Chicago Daily Tribune*, January 24, 1925.

## *Chapter 17*

1. Franklin H. Martin, *Fifty Years of Medicine and Surgery* (Chicago: Surgical Publishing Company of Chicago, 1934), 35.

2. Martin, *Digest of the Proceedings of the Council of National Defense*, 482.

3. Gibson, *Physician to the World*, 250–52; "William C. Gorgas," Wikipedia, October 29, 2022.

4. Byerly, *Fever of War*, 65–67.

5. WCG to Carter, February 13, 1918, Hench Collection.

6. "Surgeon-General Gorgas and the Responsibility of the Medical Department of the Army," *JAMA* 70 (May 18, 1918): 1461.

7. "Demand for Gorgas to Be Kept at Work," *Birmingham Age-Herald*, May 25, 1918; "Surgeon-General Gorgas Is Sixty-Three Years Young," *Southern Medical Journal* 11 (May 1918): 400–401.

8. Robert Owen to President Wilson, May 23, 1918, Baker Papers, LoC, Container 8, Reel 6.

9. President Wilson to Secretary Baker, May 25, 1918, Baker Papers, LoC, Container 8, Reel 6.

10. Martin, *Digest of the Proceedings of the Council of National Defense*, 476–77.

11. "Experientia Omnia Docet," editorial, *Military Surgeon* 43 (August 1918): 213; also, "Our Resources in Medical Personnel," editorial, *Military Surgeon* 43 (August 1918): 207–9.

12. WCG to John Ross, August 19, 1918, Gorgas Papers, Box 6, LoC.

13. "Your Man in Service," *Ladies' Home Journal* 35 (October 1918): 27. Also, on an August 9 inspection tour of the Mayo Clinic in Rochester, Minnesota, Gorgas told the medical personnel, "In actual accomplishment we have reasons to pat ourselves on the back on what has been done so far." See "Army Medical Corps Has Fine Record, Says Gorgas," *Minneapolis Morning Tribune*, August 10, 1918.

14. On the influenza pandemic, see Alfred W. Crosby, *Americas Forgotten Pandemic: The Influenza of 1918* (Westport, CT: Greenwood Press,1989); Nancy Bristow, *American Pandemic: The Lost Worlds of the 1918 Influenza Pandemic* (New York: Oxford University Press, 2012); John M. Barry, *The Great Influenza: The Epic Story of the Deadliest Plague in History* (New York: Viking, 2004); Susan Kingsley Kent, *The Influenza Pandemic of 1918–1919: A Brief History in Documents* (Boston: Bedford/St. Martin's, 2013); Byerly, *Fever of War*.

15. Jeffery K. Taubenberger, "The Origin and Virulence of the 1918 'Spanish' Influenza Virus," *Proceedings of the American Philosophical Society* 150 (2006): 86–112.

16. Victor C. Vaughan, "An Explosive Epidemic of Influenzal Disease at Fort Oglethorpe," *Journal of Laboratory and Clinical Medicine* 3 (June 1918): 560–68.

17. "Spanish Influenza Is Raging in the German Army," *NYT*, June 27, 1918; "Topics of the Times," *NYT*, June 28, 1918; "The War Situation," *NYT*, July 15, 1918.

18. *MDWW*, vol. 4, 49; "Grip Now Epidemic throughout the Country," *NYT*, October 16, 1918; Edgar Sydenstricker, "Preliminary Statistics of the Influenza Epidemic," *PHR* 33 (December 27, 1918): 2305–21; W. H. Frost, "Statistics of Influenza Morbidity," *PHR* 35 (March 12, 1920): 584–97.

19. *MDWW*, vol. 6, 353.

20. Victor C. Vaughan et al., *Epidemiology and Public Health* (St. Louis: C. V. Mosby, 1926), vol. 1, 8.

21. *MDWW*, vol. 4, 49–50; George A. Soper, "The Pandemic in the Army Camps," *JAMA* 71 (December 7, 1918): 1899–1909.

22. *MDWW*, vol. 1, 1000–1003; *MDWW*, vol. 6, 352–71.

23. Robert G. Torrey and Lawrence C. Grosh, "Acute Pulmonary Emphysema Observed during the Epidemic of Influenza Pneumonia at Camp Hancock, Georgia," *American Journal of Medical Science* 157 (1919): 172.

24. Charles L. Mix, "Spanish Influenza in the Army," *New York Medical Journal* 108 (October 26, 1918): 712.

25. On dispersion of influenza, see K. David Patterson and Gerald F. Pyle, "The Geography and Mortality of the 1918 Influenza Pandemic," *Bulletin of the History of Medicine* 65 (June 1991): 4–21; Edgar Sydenstricker, "Preliminary Statistics of the Influenza Epidemic," *PHR* 33 (December 27, 1918): 2305–21.

26. Military Service Cards, Camp Wadsworth, RG 112, Entry 91, Box 2633, NARA.

27. Memorandum, C-362, September 24, 1918, RG 120, Entry 2109, Box 5493, NARA; *MDWW*, vol. 1, 998.

28. "Surgeon General Asks for More Home Care," *NYT*, October 13, 1918.

29. Andrew Noymer and Michel Garenne, "Long-Term Effects of the 1918 'Spanish' Influenza Epidemic on Sex Differentials of Mortality in the USA," in *The Spanish Influenza*

*Pandemic of 1918–1919: New Perspectives*, ed. Howard Phillips and David Killingray (New York: Routledge, 2003), 202–18.

30. Jefferson R. Kean war diary, Ms C14, Jefferson R. Kean Papers, NLM.

31. W. C. Gorgas, "Diary, William Crawford Gorgas, September–October 1918." 1918, WCGP, (hereafter cited as Gorgas Diary, 1918).

32. Gorgas Diary, 1918, WCGP. See also "Notes on trip to France with Secretary of War Baker, typescript copy, 1918," WCGP.

33. Gorgas Diary, 1918, September 3, 1918, WCGP.

34. Gorgas Diary, 1918, September 6, 1918, WCGP.

35. Merritte Ireland memoir, 38–39.

36. Gorgas Diary, 1918, September 3, 1918, WCGP.

37. Gorgas Diary, 1918, September 10, 1918, WCGP.

38. On American medical services, see Gillett, *Army Medical Department, 1865–1917*, 327–47.

39. Itinerary from the William Crawford Gorgas, U.S. Army, retired, *Inspection of Medical Services with American Expeditionary Forces: Confidential Report to Secretary of War* (Washington, DC: GPO, 1919).

40. Gorgas Diary, 1918, September 16, 1918, WCGP.

41. Harry W. Goodhall, "Report on Gas Hospital, Justice Hospital Group," *MDWW*, vol. 14, 840–46.

42. Goldthwait, *Division of Orthopaedic Surgery in the A. E. F.*, 80.

43. Harvey Cushing, *From a Surgeon's Journal, 1915–1918* (Boston: Little, Brown, 1936), 145. Cushing mistakenly places this incident in 1917, but Gorgas was not in France then.

44. Ward J. MacNeal, "The Influenza Epidemic of 1918 in the American Expeditionary Forces in France and England," *Archives of Internal Medicine* 23 (June 1919): 681.

45. Kean, unpublished autobiography, 226–27.

46. WCG to MG, September 23, 1918, WCGP.

47. Gorgas Diary, 1918, WCGP.

48. Letter from Stan to Uncle George, October 15, 1918, Ms 155, Stanhope Bayne-Jones Papers, William C. Gorgas Papers, Hans Zinsser Papers, 1870–1969, NLM.

49. "Notes on trip to France with Secretary of War Baker, typescript copy, 1918," WCGP.

50. "Notes on trip to France with Secretary of War Baker, typescript copy, 1918," WCGP.

51. Gorgas Diary, 1918, October 3, 1918, WCGP.

52. Newton Baker to MG, July 4, 1920, WCGP.

53. WCG to MG, October 10, 1918, WCGP.

54. Editorial, *New York Medical Journal* 108 (October 12, 1918): 643.

55. WCG to MG, October 10, 1918, WCGP.

56. Gorgas Diary, 1918, 28, WCGP.

57. Gorgas Diary, 1918, October 15, 1918, WCGP.

58. William C. Gorgas, *Inspection of Medical Services with the AEF: Confidential Report to the Secretary of War* (Washington, DC: Government Printing Office, 1919), 20–21.

59. Gorgas, *Inspection of Medical Services with the AEF*, 47.

60. Gorgas, *Inspection of Medical Services with the AEF*, 28.

61. Jefferson Kean WWI diary, Ms C14, Jefferson R. Kean Papers, NLM.

62. *WDAR, 1919*, vol. 1, pt. 2, 2755.

63. Col. A. N. Stark, "Medical Activities of the American Expeditionary Forces in the Zone of the Armies," *Military Surgeon* 46 (August 1920): 172.

64. *WDAR, 1919*, vol. 1, pt. 2, 1469.

65. Margaret Humphreys, "The Influenza of 1918: Evolutionary Perspectives in a Historical Context," *Evolution, Medicine, and Public Health* (2018): 220.

66. *MDWW*, vol. 9, 66–67.

67. William C. Gorgas, "Thrift in Health—Application of Lessons of Military Sanitation to Peace Times," paper presented at the Twelfth Annual Meeting of the Association of Life Insurance Presidents, New York, December 6, 1918, Gorgas Papers, LoC.

68. See Byerly, *Fever of War*, chapter 6.

69. Victor Vaughan, *A Doctor's Memories* (Indianapolis: Bobbs Merrill, 1926), 432.

70. "Report of Gen. Pershing," *Congressional Record*, 65th Cong., 3rd sess. (December 30, 1918), 914–17; Baker, *WDAR 1919*, vol. 1, pt. 1, 623.

71. H. J. Res. 333, A Resolution to Aid in Combating the Disease Known as Influenza, *Congressional Record* (September 28, 1918), 10895–97, 10900–17, 65th Cong., 2nd sess; Senate Committee on Appropriations, *Suppression of Spanish Influenza*, 65th Cong., 2nd sess.; S. J. Res. 63, A Resolution to Establish a Reserve for the Public Health Service, *Congressional Record* (October 15, 1918), 11267–88, 65th Cong., 2nd sess.

72. Baker to Gorgas, October 26, 1918, Gorgas Papers, Box 6, LoC.

73. Welch to WCG, November 27, 1918, WCGP.

74. Special Orders 269–0, November 16, 1918, Gorgas Papers, Box 6, LoC; Army General Order, signed by Peyton C. March, War Department, Washington, DC, December 27, 1918, Distinguished Service Medal, WCGP.

75. WCG to A. W. Hedrich, June 26, 1918, WCGP. No Nobel prizes were awarded from 1915 to 1918, due to the war.

76. Martin, *Major General William Crawford Gorgas*, 5; Martin to MG, September 2, 1924, WCGP.

77. Ashburn, *A History of the Medical Department of the U.S. Army*, 359.

78. "Address of Hon. Newton D. Baker," 1920, WCGP.

79. War Department, Office of the Surgeon General, *The Medical Department in the World War* (Washington, DC: GPO, 1921–29), vols. 1–15.

80. United States Army, *Medical and Surgical History of the War of the Rebellion*, 6 vols. (Washington, DC: GPO, 1870–88); Fielding H. Garrison, "Medical and Surgical History of the War," *Military Surgeon* 43 (September 1918): 347–50.

81. William C. Gorgas, "Clinical Research in United States Army Base Hospital." *Medical Clinics of North America* 2 (1918): 313–19.

82. Kean reported on the first editorial board meeting in his "Autobiographical Sketch," 248–49.

## *Chapter 18*

1. "Memorandum of Sick Record of Major General William C. Gorgas," January 14, 1919, Gorgas Papers, Box 6, LoC.

2. WCG to Jessie, December 19, 1918, WCGP.

3. The bust was executed by Sgt. P. Bryant Baker, a sculptor for the Medical Department who made plaster casts of wound victims to help prepare prosthetics. "Bust of Gorgas in the Surgeon General's Library," *Southern Medical Journal* 12 (March 1919): 167–69; "Secretary of War Pays Glowing Tribute to Former Head of Medical Department," *The Come-Back*, Washington, DC, March 1919; *Bust of William C. Gorgas*, NLM Digital Collections, Image ID B013211.

4. "Housing Under Way for 4,675 Families," *NYT*, June 30, 1919. There is no record that Gorgas and Catt ever met.

5. Anecdotes from the life of Gorgas, # 3579, WCGP.

6. Randall M. Packard, *A History of Global Health: Interventions into the Lives of Other Peoples* (Baltimore: Johns Hopkins University Press, 2016).

7. William C. Gorgas, "Journal of William C. Gorgas, Chairman, Yellow Fever Commission, Partial Typescript Copy, 1919," April 14, 1919, WCGP (hereafter cited as "WCG Journal, Yellow Fever Commission, 1919").

8. W. W. Rasor, "The New Guayaquil," *Pan-American Magazine* 31 (1920): 281–89.

9. "Rockefeller Foundation Annual Report, 1919" (New York, 1919), Rockefeller Foundation website; W. W. Rasor, "Who's Who on the Equator Today," *Pan-American Magazine* 31 (1920): 303–4.

10. W. C. Gorgas, "Memorandum of Yellow Fever Work in Guayaquil, Ecuador," and W. C. Gorgas to Victor Heiser, January 22, 1920, RF, IHB, RG 5 (FA115), Box 47.

11. "WCG Journal, Yellow Fever Commission, 1919," 28–31.

12. "WCG Journal, Yellow Fever Commission, 1919," 33, 35, 38.

13. "WCG Journal, Yellow Fever Commission, 1919," 28–31.

14. Photograph of William and Marie Gorgas with some fifty women, *El Guante*, Guayaquil, Ecuador, May 23, 1919, WCGP.

15. "WCG Journal, Yellow Fever Commission, 1919," 66.

16. Lois F. Parks and Gustave A. Nuremberger, "The Sanitation of Guayaquil," *Hispanic American Historical Review* 23 (1943): 197.

17. Gorgas, "Report on the Sanitation of Guayaquil," 71.

18. "WCG Journal, Yellow Fever Commission, 1919," 50–53.

19. "Diary, WCG, June–November 1919," WCGP.

20. "Diary, WCG, June–November 1919," 34, WCGP.

21. "Diary, WCG, June–November 1919," 55–56, WCGP.

22. "Anecdotes," August 1919, WCGP.

23. Anecdotes on life of W. C. Gorgas, taken from correspondence with the International Health Board and from his personal diary, 1916–1920, June 1919, WCGP; WCG, "Journal, Yellow Fever Commission, 1919," 58.

24. WCG to Jessie, August 6, 1919, and September 3, 1919, WCGP.

25. Anecdotes, August 1919; WCG, "Journal, Yellow Fever Commission, 1919," 62–63.

26. WCG to Henry Carter, September 15, 1919, Hench Collection.

27. Anecdotes, Guayaquil, August 1919, WCGP.

28. WCG to Ria, October 3, 1919, WCGP.

29. WCG to Dick, November 4, 1919, WCGP.

30. Anecdotes, October 1919, WCGP.

31. W. C. Gorgas to Victor Heiser, January 22, 1920, RF, IHB, RG 5 (FA115), Box 47.

32. Henry Hanson, "Three Years Study of Sanitary Conditions in Peru," circa 1922, Hench Collection.

33. "Journal, WCG, February 28, 1920, Partial Typescript, 1920" (and 1916), 2, WCGP.

34. WCG to RG, February 27, 1920, WCGP.

35. "Anecdotes on life of W. C. Gorgas, taken from correspondence with the International Health Board and from his personal diary, 1916–1920," March 1920, WCGP.

36. H. R. Carter, "Carter's Tribute to Gorgas," *Southern Medical Journal* (September 1920): 688; Henry Carter to Laura Amistad Carter, June 16, 1920, Hench Collection.

37. Henry Carter to J. Gil Cardenas, July 23, 1920, Hench Collection.

38. R. B. Fosdick, *Story of the Rockefeller Foundation* (New York: Harper, 1952), 61; "Rockefeller Foundation Annual Report, 1919," 17.

39. "Henry Carter to the Rockefeller Foundation." n.d., c. 1920, Hench Collection; Rupert Boyce, "The History of Yellow Fever in West Africa," *British Medical Journal* (February 1911): 301–6; Raymond E. Dumett, "The Campaign against Malaria and the Expansion of Scientific Medical and Sanitary Services in British West Africa, 1898–1910," *African Historical Studies* 1 (1968): 153–97; Curtin, "The End of the 'White Man's Grave'?," 63–88.

40. Mark Sullivan to WCG, May 4 and 19, 1920, WCGP.

41. Typescript, at sea *S. S. Victorian*, May 11, 1920, WCGP.

42. Typescript, at sea *S. S. Victorian*, May 11, 1920, WCGP.

43. WCG to Jessie, May 26, 1920, WCGP.

44. Gorgas and Hendrick, *William Crawford Gorgas*, 334; Thomas E. Bowen, "William Crawford Gorgas, Physician to the World," *Military Medicine* 148 (December 1983): 917–20.

45. The Tate Museum now occupies the hospital site.

46. Gorgas and Hendrick, *William Crawford Gorgas*, 335.

47. "Note concerning health of Gorgas and the thoughts of King George V, June 8, 1920," WCGP; "The Most Distinguished Order of Saint Michael and Saint George," *Encyclopedia Britannica*, online, January 17, 2011.

48. MG to Dick, June 9, 1920, WCGP.

49. "Gorgas Very Ill," *Tallahassee Daily Democrat*, June 17, 1920.

50. Forwarded by Letter from Williamson S. Howell, Second Secretary of Embassy, London, to MG, July 6, 1920, WCGP.

51. Theo to MG, July 1, 1920, WCGP.

52. Gorgas and Hendrick, *William Crawford Gorgas*, 335.

53. E. Langahan Buzzard (actually, E. Farquhar Buzzard) to Lady Gorgas, July 9, 1920, WCGP.

54. C. H. Mayo to L. B. Schmidt, January 30, 1931, WCGP.

55. T. H. Goodwin to Mr. MacAlister, March 7, 1920 [misdated, actually July 3, 1920], WCGP.

56. Robert Ernest Noble, "William Crawford Gorgas," *American Journal of Public Health* 11 (March 1921): 250–56.

57. "General Gorgas Dies in London at 66," *Washington Post*, July 4, 1920, WCGP.

58. Newton D. Baker to MG, July 4, 1920, WCGP.

59. Henry (not Carter, as it says in the archives—no last name, a younger man; Birmingham, AL) to MG, July 4, 1920, WCGP.

60. Julia Le Prince to MG, July 10, 1920, WCGP.

61. Pershing to MG, August 19, 1920, John J. Pershing Papers, LoC.

62. WCG to Minnie, December 18, 1914, WCGP.

63. My thanks to Alice Goodman, who traveled with me to London to retrace William and Marie's last days in that city.

64. "General Gorgas's Funeral Is Held in St. Paul's," *Atlanta Constitution*, July 11, 1920, WCGP.

65. "Funeral Service for General Gorgas at St. Paul's," *British Medical Journal* (July 17, 1920): 88; "Order of Service for the Funeral of Major-General William Crawford Gorgas," July 9, 1920, WCGP.

66. Newspaper clipping, Harvey Cushing, letter to the editor, "The Funerals of General Gorgas and of Lord Fisher," n.p., July 15, 1920, WCGP.

67. May Thomas to MG, July 12, 1920, and poem "To Mrs. Gorgas," July 12, 1920, WCGP.

68. Goodwin to MG, July 13, 1920, WCGP.

69. Daisy S. Phillips (likely John L. Phillips's widow) to MG, August 18, 1920, WCGP.

70. Edith B. Denegre to MG, August 23, 1920, WCGP.

71. J. D. Rockefeller to George Vincent, August 17, 1920, RF, IHB, RG 5 (FA115), Box 47.

72. "Body of Gen. Gorgas Saluted from Fort," *NYT*, August 13, 1920; Cablegram from acting military attaché, London, England, to Adjutant General, Washington, D.C., July 22, 1920, WCGP.

73. "Order of Service for the Funeral of William Crawford Gorgas," August 16, 1920, WCGP.

74. Gibson, *Physician to the World*, 280.

75. RHG to Jessie, August 16, 1920, WCGP.

76. "Site for Interment of Gorgas Unknown," *Tuscaloosa News and Times-Gazette*, July 12, 1920, WCGP.

77. Operations Orders, Number 1, Military Funeral of the Late Major General William C. Gorgas, Camp Meade, Maryland, August 12, 1920, WCGP; and newspaper clipping photo, "Funeral Procession of the Late Major General William C. Gorgas," *NYT*, n.d., probably August 22, 1920, WCGP.

78. Arlington National Cemetery was established in 1861 on the lawn of the Curtis-Lee mansion in northern Virginia, where Robert E. Lee lived before he left to lead the Army of the Confederacy.

79. "Address of Hon. Newton D. Baker," 1920, WCGP.

80. Arlington National Cemetery website, "William Crawford Gorgas."

## *Epilogue*

1. "Surgeon General Gorgas," *London Times*, July 5, 1920.

2. Gandy et al., "The Statesmanship of William Crawford Gorgas," provides a summary of many of these honors.

3. "Gorgas in St. Paul's Today," *New York City Telegram,* July 9, 1920; "Maj. Gen. William C. Gorgas," *Confederate Veteran* 28 (August 1920): 283; "General Gorgas," *Nashville Banner*, July 5, 1920; "William C. Gorgas," *Peoria Illinois Transcript,* July 6, 1920; "Major General Gorgas," *Dayton Ohio News*, July 6, 1920; "Major General Gorgas," *Stockton California Evening Record*, July 9, 1920. These are collected in "Typed copies of newspaper articles on death of W. C. Gorgas, July–September 1920," WCGP.

4. "General William C. Gorgas, Wholesale Saver of Human Lives," *Literary Digest* 66 (1920): 50–52; John Bassett Moore, "Gorgas, Redeemer of the Tropics," *Review of Reviews* 65 (1922): 188–94.

5. "Career of Gorgas Lauded by Nations," *Washington Post,* January 17, 1921; "Maj. Gen. William C. Gorgas," *Confederate Veteran* 28 (August 1920): n.p.

6. Southern Society of Washington, *Memorial Services Held in Honor of Major General William Crawford Gorgas*, S. doc. No. 390, 66th Cong., 3rd sess. (Washington, DC: GPO, 1921), 64.

7. "Program on the Life and Work of William Crawford Gorgas for Gorgas Day, 1921," WCGP; Leah Rawls Atkins, *Developed for the Service of Alabama: The Centennial History of the Alabama Power Company, 1906–2006* (Birmingham: Alabama Power, 2006), 53, 73.

8. My thanks to Rev. Peter Gray, Buck Butler, and others at the University of the South for help in providing a photograph of the window.

9. A. W. Schwartz, "William C. Gorgas and the Gorgas Hospital," *Scalpel and Tongs* 43 (July–October 1999): 54, 65; translated Western Union telegram from Mayor Juan Frage, Marcelina de Villegas, to War Department, March 28, 1921; John W. Weeks to MG, April 5, 1921; L. R., Havana, to MG, December 30, 1926, WCGP.

10. American College of Surgeons website, "Murphy Doors Present Six Important Contributors to Medical Science," originally published in an ACS newsletter, *Erie News*, March 1986. The other two were Lister and Ephraim McDowell.

11. E. R. Squibb & Son, "The Cleansing of the Tropics," *Ladies' Home Journal* (December 1928).

12. London School of Hygiene and Tropical Medicine website, "History," November 2022. The other vectors are the flea, tsetse fly, housefly, bedbug, body louse, tick, rat, and snake.

13. "Gorgas and the *Stegomyia*," *Philadelphia Evening Ledger,* September 6, 1920, in WCGP; "The Gorgas Memorial," *Science* 56 (1922): 245–46; W. C. Braisted, "The Gorgas Memorial," *Pan American Union* 52 (1921): 48–53; Public Law No. 350, 1923.

14. "Memorial Bust of General Gorgas for Panama," *Pan American Union* 52 (1921): 581–82; Willard Hull Wright, *40 Years of Tropical Medicine Research: A History of the Gorgas Memorial Institute of Tropical and Preventive Medicine, Inc., and the Gorgas Memorial Laboratory* (Baltimore: Reese Press, 1970).

15. "Hoover Gives Prize for Gorgas Essay," *Washington Post,* May 24, 1929; President Presents Award to Winner of Gorgas Essay Contest, Washington, DC, May 16, 1938, LoC online catalog, #LC-H21- C-861 [P&P].

16. "The Gorgas Memorial," *Southern Medical Journal* (June 1922): 517–18; "The Gorgas Courses in Tropical Medicine," Heersink School of Medicine website, University of Alabama at Birmingham, 2022.

17. See Gorgas: Instituto Conmemorativo Gorgas de Estudios de la Salud website, Panama, Republica de Panama, 2022.

18. *Monument to Maj. Gen. William C. Gorgas*, Sen. Rpt. 906, April 27, 1928, 70th Cong., 1st sess.

19. "Extract from letter from Marie Gorgas, 1929," WCGP.

20. See Gorgas House Museum, University of Alabama Museums website for a virtual tour.

21. NavSource Online, *USAT General W. C. Gorgas*, ID 1365.

22. Today the Gorgas Science Foundation is located on the Sabal Palm Sanctuary, Brownsville, Texas.

23. D. Wayne Johnson, "Hall of Fame for Great Americans at NYU," Medal Collectors of America website, 2004; "Dr. Gorgas Named to Hall of Fame," *American Journal of Public Health* 41 (1951): 146.

24. Gorgas Memorial Library, Walter Reed Army Institute of Research, located in Silver Spring, MD.

25. US Bureau of Labor Statistics, CPI Inflation Calculator website.

26. Newspaper clipping, "Gorgas Might Have Become Millionaire," n.d., circa 1925, WCGP; "Which of These Two Men Is Greatest," *Denver Labor Bulletin*, November 16, 1920. I am grateful to Todd Laugen for bringing this to my attention.

27. "Marie Doughty Gorgas," House Committee on Pensions, 67th Cong., 2nd sess., House Report 930, April 25, 1922; "Pension to Marie Doughty Gorgas, Widow of Maj. Gen. William Crawford Gorgas, United States Army," Committee on Pensions, S. Rpt. 566, March 16, 1922; "Mrs. Gorgas's Pension," *NYT*, September 25, 1922.

28. Sue McNamara, "Washington Woman Collected Old Spanish Silver," *Detroit Free Press*, November 7, 1928. The silver is now housed in the Gorgas Family Museum, University of Alabama, Tuscaloosa.

29. "Burton J. Hendrick, 1870–1949," LibraryThing.com website.

30. Gorgas and Hendrick, *William Crawford Gorgas*, "Yellow Fever Meets Its Master," *World's Work* (April 1924): 637.

31. Hendrick to Kean, May 5, 1924, Hench Collection; Jefferson Randolph Kean, "Reed, Gorgas, and Yellow Fever," April 27, 1924, *NYT*, Hench Collection, italics in the original.

32. Pointed out in *Panama Times*, August 29, 1925, in Hench Collection.

33. Gorgas and Hendrick, *William Crawford Gorgas*, 132.

34. "*William Crawford Gorgas: His Life and Work*," *Southern Medical Journal* (April 1925): 312; "*William Crawford Gorgas: His Life and Work* (book review)," *Boston Transcript* (1924): 5; "*William Crawford Gorgas: His Life and Work* (book review)," *American Review of Reviews* 71 (1925): 221; John K. Baxter, "Book Reviews for *William Crawford Gorgas: His Life and Work*," *Panama Times* (August 29,1925); E. C. Beckwith, "*William Crawford Gorgas: His Life and Work* (book review)," *Saturday Review of Literature* 2 (1925): 106; C. H. Gaines, "*William Crawford Gorgas: His Life and Work* (book review)," *North American Review* 221 (1925): 575.

35. Franklin Martin, "Hendrick's Life of Gorgas Well Worth Reading," *Chicago Daily Tribune*, January 24, 1925.

36. Jefferson Randolph Kean, "William Crawford Gorgas," *Military Surgeon* (March 1925): 1–5.

37. Kean to Cushing, June 30, 1925; Cushing to Kean, July 1,1925; Richard A. Strong, Harvard University Medical School, March 24, 1925, Hench Collection.

38. MG to Kean, March 19, 1925, Hench Collection.

39. "Mrs. W.C. Gorgas Dies at Her Home in Washington," *New York Herald Tribune*, November 10, 1929.

40. Kean to Albert E. Truby, April 25, 1936, Hench Collection.

41. Robin Lampson, author of *Death Loses a Pair of Wings*, thought that Gorgas, a "truly great American[,] deserves to be more 'in the hearts of his countrymen'—in their textbook and on their tongues—than he now is." See "Memorandum from Robin Lampson," 1937, Hench Collection.

42. Clara Judson, *Soldier Doctor: The Story of William Gorgas* (New York: Scribner's, 1942); Beryl Williams and Samuel Epstein, *William Crawford Gorgas: Tropic Fever Fighter* (New York: J. Messner, 1953); Edward F. Dolan and H. T. Silver, *William Crawford Gorgas: Warrior in White* (New York: Dodd, 1968).

43. Gaylord W. Anderson, "Review of *Physician to the World: The Life of General William C. Gorgas*, John M. Gibson," *American Historical Review* 56 (1951): 921–22; John E. Baur, "Review of *Physician to the World: The Life of General William C. Gorgas*, John M. Gibson," *Pacific Historical Review* 20 (1951): 174–75; David Lowenthal, "Review of *Physician to the World: The Life of General William C. Gorgas*," *Hispanic American Historical Review* 31 (1951): 708–9.

44. H. C. Coe to MG, January 31, 1923, WCGP.

45. Kean, "Text of Speech Jefferson Randolph Kean Gave upon the Receipt of the Gorgas Medal," Hench Collection. The Medal was awarded until 2009, when it was replaced by the annual William Gorgas Preventive Medicine Award. See AMSUS, Society of Federal Health Professionals website, "AMSUS Annual Awards Program."

46. "Jefferson Randolph Kean's Answers for a Questionnaire from Philip Showalter Hench," May 25, 1946.

47. For example, he interviewed Reed's children Lawrence and Emily Reed, but even though Kean gave him Aileen's name and address, Hench did not contact her or Gorgas's surviving sisters. Philip S. Hench, "Interview with Lawrence Reed and Blossom Reed," November 21, 1946; and "Remarks to Be Given at the Unveiling of Dean Cornwell's Painting *Conquerors of Yellow Fever*," 1941, Hench Collection. The Hench Collection has an extensive collection of correspondence and preliminary sketches for the Cornwell painting.

48. Hench shared the medal with Edward C. Kendall and Tadeus Reichstein. Biographical information for Philip Showalter Hench, Hench Collection.

49. "Outline for the Conquest of Yellow Fever, by Philip Showalter Hench," 1947, Hench Collection.

50. R. B. Fosdick, *Rockefeller Foundation* (New York: Harper, 1952), 58. Farley calculates that 37 percent of the foundation's disease budget was devoted to yellow fever from 1914 to 1950. See *To Cast Out Disease*, 20.

51. W. C. Gorgas et al., "Report on Yellow Fever," 1916, Gorgas Papers, Box 25, LoC.

52. Farley, *To Cast Out Disease*, 88–106.

53. Crosby, *American Plague*, 223–28.

54. "Locally Acquired Cases of Malaria in Florida and Texas," Centers for Disease Control and Prevention, Health Alert Network Health Advisory, July 7, 2023.

55. "Malaria Fighters' Latest Chemical Weapon May Not Last Long," *Science* 369 (September 4, 2020): 1153.

56. "Mosquitoes," Centers for Disease Control website; "Vector-Borne Diseases," World Health Organization website.

# Select Bibliography


## PRIMARY SOURCES

### Archives and Special Collections

University of Alabama Libraries Special Collections, Tuscaloosa

*William Crawford Gorgas Papers*
*Josiah Gorgas Family Papers*

John Hay Library, Brown University, Providence, Rhode Island

*William W. Keen Papers*

Library of Congress, Washington, DC

*William Crawford Gorgas Papers*
*George W. Goethals Papers*
*Canal Zone Library-Museum Papers*

National Library of Medicine, Bethesda, Maryland

*Walter Reed Memorial Association Records, 1904–1909*
*Merritte Ireland Papers*
*Stanhope Bayne-Jones Papers, William C. Gorgas Papers, Hans Zinsser Papers, 1870–1969*
*Jefferson R. Kean Papers*

National Archives and Records Administration

*RG 94, Records of the Adjutant General's Office*
*RG 112, Records of the Army Surgeon General*
*RG 165, Records of the Office of the Chief of Staff*
*RG 185, Records of the Panama Canal*
*RG 383, Records of the US Continental Army*

Rockefeller Archive Center, New York, New York

*Rockefeller Foundation Records, International Health Board/Division Records*

Tennessee State Library and Archives

*John Walton Ross Papers*

University of Florida, George A. Smathers Libraries

*Panama Canal Museum Collection*

## GOVERNMENT DOCUMENTS

Congressional Hearings and Senate and House Proceedings on the Construction of the Panama Canal, 1904–1920

Congressional Hearings and Senate and House Proceedings on the Conduct of the War, 1917–1918

Congressional Hearings and Senate and House Proceedings on Memorializing William C. Gorgas

Martin, Franklin H. *Digest of the Proceedings of the Council of National Defense during the World War*. Washington, DC: Government Printing Office, 1934.

US Congress. *Report of the Commission Appointed by the President to Investigate the Conduct of the War Department in the War with Spain*. Vols. 1–9. US 56th Cong., 1st sess. Sen. Doc. 221. Washington, DC: Government Printing Office, 1900.

US Congress. Committee on Public Health and National Quarantine. *Yellow Fever: A Compilation of Various Publications: Results of the Work of Maj. Walter Reed, Medical Corps, United States Army and the Yellow Fever Commission*. Edited by 61st Congress, U.S. Senate, 3rd sess. Washington, DC: Government Printing Office, 1911.

War Department. Office of the Surgeon General. *The Medical Department in the World War*. Vols. 1–15. Washington, DC: GPO, 1921–1929.

War Department Annual Reports, 1880–1921

## SELECT PERIODICALS

*American Journal of Public Health*
*British Medical Journal*
*Canal Record*
*Journal of Laboratory and Clinical Medicine*
*Journal of the American Medical Association*
*The Lancet*
*Medical Record*
*Military Surgeon*
*New York Times*
*North American Review*
*Outlook*
*Public Health Reports*
*Science*
*Scientific American*
*Scribner's*

*Southern Medical Journal*
*Washington Post*
*World's Work*

## PRIMARY SOURCES, PUBLISHED

Bishop, Joseph Bucklin. *The Panama Gateway*. New York: Scribner's Sons, 1913.

———. *Goethals—The Genius of the Panama Canal*. New York: Harper's and Brothers, 1930.

Cushing, Harvey. *From a Surgeon's Journal, 1915–1918*. Boston: Little, Brown, 1936.

Finlay, C. E. "Carlos Finlay and Yellow Fever." *Journal of Parasitology* 28 (1942): 172–74.

Forbes-Lindsay, Charles. *The Panama Canal Today*. Boston: L. C. Page, 1910.

Gorgas, Marie D., and Burton J. Hendrick. *William Crawford Gorgas, His Life and Works*. Garden City, NY: Doubleday, Page, 1924.

Gorgas, W. C. *Sanitation in Panama*. New York: Appleton, 1915.

Guiteras, John. "Experimental Yellow Fever at the Inoculation Station of the Sanitary Department of Havana with a View to Producing Immunization." *American Medicine* (November 23, 1901).

Hibbard, M. Eugenie. "Cuba: A Sketch." *American Journal of Nursing* 4 (1904): 840–46.

Kelly, Howard A. *Walter Reed and Yellow Fever*. Classic Reprints rev. ed. New York: McClure, Phillips, 2012. Originally published 1907.

Le Prince, Joseph A., A. J. Orenstein, and L. O. Howard. *Mosquito Control in Panama: The Eradication of Malaria and Yellow Fever in Cuba and Panama*. New York: G. P. Putnam's Sons, 1916.

Martin, Franklin. *Major General William Crawford Gorgas*. Chicago: Gorgas Memorial Institute, 1933.

Martin, Thomas W. *Doctor William Crawford Gorgas of Alabama and the Panama Canal*. New York: Newcomen Society of England, American Branch, 1947.

Owen, William O. *A Chronological Arrangement of Congressional Legislation Relating to the Medical Corps of the United States Army, 1785–1917*. Chicago: American Medical Association, 1918.

Wiggins, Sarah Wolfolk, ed. *The Journals of Josiah Gorgas, 1857–1878*. Tuscaloosa: University of Alabama Press, 1995.

## SECONDARY SOURCES

### Books, Dissertations, and Articles

Aboul-Enein, Faisal H. "Dr. William Gorgas and His Style of Management against Yellow Fever during the Construction of the Panama Canal: A Historical Case Study." University of Texas Health Science Center, ProQuest, 2009.

Adams, Kevin. *Class and Race in the Frontier Army: Military Life in the West, 1870–1890*. Norman: University of Oklahoma Press, 2009.

Anderson, Warwick. "Immunities of Empire: Race, Disease, and the New Tropical Medicine, 1900–1920." *Bulletin of the History of Medicine* 70 (1996): 94–118.

Barrios, J., and J. P. O'Leary. "Brigadier General Theodore C Lyster [Correction of

Lister], MD: Father of American Aviation Medicine." *American Surgeon* 66 (July 2000): 706–7.

Bayne-Jones, Stanhope. *The Evolution of Preventive Medicine in the United States Army, 1607–1939.* Washington, DC: Office of the Surgeon General, 1968.

Bell, Andrew McIlwaine. *Mosquito Soldiers: Malaria, Yellow Fever, and the Course of the American Civil War.* Baton Rouge: Louisiana State University Press, 2010.

Bruce-Chwatt, L. J. "Ronald Ross, William Gorgas, and Malaria Eradication." *American Journal of Tropical Medicine and Hygiene* 26, no. 5, Pt 2 Suppl (September 1977): 1071–79.

Byerly, Carol R. *Fever of War: The Influenza Epidemic in the United States Army during World War I.* New York: New York University Press, 2005.

Cashman, T. M. "William Crawford Gorgas: He Set the Standard of Military Preventive Medicine." *Hawaii Medical Journal* 57, no. 1 (January 1998): 377–80.

Chaves-Carballo, Enrique. *American Medicine and the Panama Canal: Proceedings of the Medical Association of the Isthmian Canal Zone.* Morgan Hill, CA: Bookstand, 2014.

———. "Ancón Hospital: An American Hospital during the Construction of the Panama Canal, 1904–1914." *Military Medicine* 164, no. 10 (October 1999): 725–30.

———. "Carlos Finlay and Yellow Fever: Triumph over Adversity." *Military Medicine* 170 (October 2005).

———. "The Cost of Running American City Hospitals: The Gorgas 1910 Survey." *Southern Medical Journal* 93 (February 2000): 191–94.

———. *The Tropical World of Samuel Taylor Darling: Parasites, Pathology and Philanthropy.* Sussex Academic Press, 2007.

Cirillo, Vincent J. *Bullets and Bacilli: The Spanish-American War and Military Medicine.* New Brunswick, NJ: Rutgers University Press, 2004.

Conniff, Michael L. *Black Labor on a White Canal: Panama, 1904–1981.* Pittsburgh: University of Pittsburgh Press, 1985.

Cosmas, Graham. *An Army for Empire: The United States Army in the Spanish American War.* Columbia: University of Missouri Press, 1971.

Cowdrey, Albert E. *War and Healing: Stanhope Bayne-Jones and the Maturing of American Medicine.* Baton Rouge: Louisiana State University Press, 1992.

Craddock, W. L. "The Achievements of William Crawford Gorgas." *Military Medicine* 162 (May 1997): 325–27.

Crosby, Molly Caldwell. *The American Plague: The Untold Story of Yellow Fever, the Epidemic That Shaped Our History.* New York: Berkley Books, 2006.

Cueto, Marcos. "Sanitation from Above: Yellow Fever and Foreign Intervention in Peru, 1919–1922." *Hispanic American Historical Review* 72 (1992): 1–22.

Espinosa, Mariola. *Epidemic Invasions: Yellow Fever and the Limits of Cuban Independence, 1878–1930.* Chicago: University of Chicago Press, 2009.

———. "The Question of Racial Immunity to Yellow Fever in History and Historiography." *Social Science History* 38 (2014): 437–53.

Farley, John. *To Cast Out Disease: A History of the International Health Division of the Rockefeller Foundation, 1913–1951.* Oxford: Oxford University Press, 2004.

Gandy, Roy E., Raven M. Christopher, and Charles B. Rodning. "The Statesmanship of William Crawford Gorgas, M.D., Surgeon General, Medical Corps, United States Army." *American Surgeon* 83 (March 2017): 221–32.

Gibson, John M. *Physician to the World: The Life of General William C. Gorgas*. Durham, NC: Duke University Press, 1950.

Gillett, Mary C. *The Army Medical Department, 1865–1917*. Washington, DC: Center for Military History, United States Army, 1994.

———. *The Army Medical Department, 1917–1941*. Washington, DC: Center for Military History, United States Army, 2009.

Greene, Julie. *The Canal Builders: Making America's Empire at the Panama Canal*. New York: Penguin Press, 2009.

Hoffman, Jon T., et al. *The Panama Canal: An Army's Enterprise*. Washington, DC: United States Army Center for Military History, 2009, 2019.

Humphreys, Margaret. *Yellow Fever and the South*. New Brunswick, NJ: Rutgers University Press, 1992.

Ives, Stephen, dir. *American Experience: Panama Canal: Gateway to the American Century*. Video documentary. 2011. 1:30.

Johnston, Mary Tabb, with Elizabeth Johnston Lipscomb. *Amelia Gayle Gorgas*. Tuscaloosa: University of Alabama Press, 2003.

Lampson, Robin. *Death Loses a Pair of Wings: The Epic of William Gorgas and the Conquest of Yellow Fever: A Novel in Cadence*. New York: Charles Scribner's Sons, 1939.

Litsios, Socrates. "William Crawford Gorgas (1854–1920)." *Perspectives in Biology and Medicine* 44 (Summer 2001): 368–78.

Lopez Sanchez, Jose. *Carlos J. Finlay: His Life and His Work*. La Habana, Cuba: Editorial Jose Marti, 1999.

McCallum, Jack. *Leonard Wood: Rough Rider, Surgeon, Architect of American Imperialism*. New York: New York University Press, 2006

McCullough, David. *The Path between the Seas: The Creation of the Panama Canal, 1870–1914*. New York: Touchstone, 1977.

McGuinness, Aims. *Path of the Empire: Panama and the California Gold Rush*. Ithaca: Cornell University Press, 2008.

McNeill, J. R. *Mosquito Empires: Ecology and War in the Greater Caribbean, 1620–1914*. New Approaches to the Americas. Edited by Stuart Schwartz. Cambridge: Cambridge University Press, 2010.

Mehra, Akhil. "Politics of Participation: Walter Reed's Yellow-Fever Experiments." *American Medical Association Journal of Ethics* 2, no. 4 (April 2009): 326–30.

Nuwer, Deanne Stephens. *Plague among the Magnolias: The 1878 Yellow Fever Epidemic in Mississippi*. Tuscaloosa: University of Alabama Press, 2009.

Parker, Matthew. *Panama Fever: The Epic Story of One of the Greatest Human Achievements of All Time—the Building of the Panama Canal*. 1st US ed. New York: Doubleday, 2007.

Patterson, Gordon. *The Mosquito Crusades: A History of the American Anti-Mosquito Movement from the Reed Commission to the First Earth Day*. New Brunswick, NJ: Rutgers University Press, 2009.

Patterson, K. David. "Yellow Fever Epidemics and Mortality in the United States, 1693–1905." *Social Science Medicine* 34 (1992): 855–65.

Pierce, John R., and James V. Writer. *Yellow Jack: How Yellow Fever Ravaged America and Walter Reed Discovered Its Deadly Secrets*. Hoboken, NJ: Wiley, 2005.

Rogers, J. David. "The American Engineers That Built the Panama Canal." *ASCE Global Engineering Conference: A Centennial Retrospective* (Reston, VA: American Society of Civil Engineers, 2014), 112–349.

Sarnecky, Mary. *A History of the Army Nurse Corps*. Philadelphia: University of Pennsylvania Press, 1999.

Standlee, Mary W. *Borden's Dream: The Walter Reed Army Medical Center in Washington, D.C.* Washington, DC: Borden Institute, 2009. Originally published 1952.

Stepan, Nancy. "The Interplay between Socio-Economic Factors and Medical Science: Yellow Fever Research, Cuba and the United States." *Social Studies of Science* 8 (November 1978): 397–423.

Stern, Alexandra Minna. "The Public Health Service in the Panama Canal: A Forgotten Chapter of U.S. Public Health." *Public Health Reports* 120 (2005): 675–79.

———. "Yellow Fever Crusades: US Colonialism, Tropical Medicine, and the International Politics of Mosquito Control, 1900–1920." In *Medicine at the Border: Disease, Globalization, and Security, 1850 to the Present*, edited by Alison Bashford, 41–59. UK: Palgrave Macmillan, 2007.

Sutter, Paul S. "'The First Mountain to Be Removed': Yellow Fever Control and the Construction of the Panama Canal." *Environmental History* 21 (2016): 250–59.

———. "Nature's Agents or Agents of Empire? Entomological Workers and Environmental Change during the Construction of the Panama Canal." *Isis* 98 (2007): 724–54.

Tone, John Lawrence. "How the Mosquito (Man) Liberated Cuba." *History and Technology* 18 (2002): 277–308.

———. *War and Genocide in Cuba, 1895–1898.* Chapel Hill: University of North Carolina Press, 2008.

Wiggins, Sarah Woolfolk. "Josiah Gorgas, a Victorian Father." *Civil War History* 32 (1986): 229–46.

———. *Love and Duty: Amelia and Josiah Gorgas and Their Family*. Tuscaloosa: University of Alabama Press, 2005.

# Index

*Page numbers in italics refer to illustrations.*


Adams, Charles Francis, 186

*Aedes aegypti* mosquito: and chikungunya and Zika viruses, 315; eradication of, in Panama, 147–54; Finlay's theory of, as agent infecting people with yellow fever, 4, 7, 98, 333n11; life cycle of, *9*; Reed's experiments confirming theory of, as transmitter of yellow fever, 4–5, 94; transmission of yellow fever, 2, 8, 98; transmittal of deadly diseases beyond yellow fever, 315

African American physicians in Medical Corps, segregated training camp at Fort Des Moines, Iowa, 247–48

African American soldiers: assigned to segregated units and lower salaries at frontier posts, 45; Buffalo Soldiers, Twenty-Fourth and Twenty-Fifth African American infantries, charge of San Juan heights, 69; Ninth Volunteer Infantry "immune" regiment sent to Cuba, and loss of life, 75–76

African American women: barred by Army Medical Department from service as nurses, 72, 75, 249–50; hired as nurses to care for African American soldiers in Cuban hospitals, 75; small number of nurses admitted at end of World War I to care for Black soldiers only, 250

Afro-Cubans, press for economic and political power, 66

Agramonte, Aristides: adviser on yellow fever to Army Medical Department, 69, 96; and Reed Commission experiments on human volunteers, 100–102; and US Army Yellow Fever Commission, *97*

Aiken, Hugh Kerr, 19, 22

Aiken, Mary (nèe Gayle), 21

Alabama, secession from Union, 21

Albertini, Antonio Diaz, Havana yellow fever board, 86, 102, 103

Alger, Russell, secretary of war under McKinley, 68

Amador Guerrero, Manuel, first President of Panama, 132, 151

Ambulance Americaine, 220

American Expeditionary Forces in France (AEF): creation of Chief Surgeon's Office to support, 254; establishment of rest camps to care for men near the battlefields and specialized hospitals for shell shock victims, 265; Gorgas's inspection tour, 279–85; influenza within, 277–79, 285–87; need for medical officers to support, 246–47; tension between OTSG and AEF medical services, 254–55; tuberculosis cases among the US troops, 244

American Medical Association (AMA): award of Gold Medal to Gorgas, 213; election of Gorgas as president, 1909,

183; Gorgas speech at 1916 annual meeting, "Yellow Fever," 229, 361n19, 362n27; public relations campaign for doctors to sign up for Medical Corp, 246; support for Gorgas on Isthmian Canal Commission, 119; support for promotions for medical officers, 271
American Red Cross: mobilization of, for World War I, 220–21, 243; nursing program, 250
American Single Tax Committee, 191
Ancón Hospital, Panama: became largest hospital in Latin America, 154–55; medical staff, 1906, *156*; mowed lawn and screened buildings of, *172*; new facility, 202; renamed as Gorgas Hospital, 306; renovation of, 148
*Anopheles* mosquito: Darling's groundbreaking work on, 170, 175; Gorgas's battle with, in Panama, 168–75, 184; Le Prince's experiments with, 171–73; Ross's proof of transmittal of malaria, 85, 98
Anthony, Carolina M., 77
antiseptic surgery, advent of, 267
Appleton, William W., 309; and three-volume series on Panama, 218, 358n41
Arlington National Cemetery, 377n78; burial of Marie Gorgas next to William, 310; burial of William Crawford Gorgas with high military honors, 2, 303–4; Confederate Memorial, 319n16; exclusion of Gorgas from roster of "Medical Figures" in, 7
Army Corps of Engineers, lobbying for representative on Panama Canal project, 119
Army Medical Corps: Civil War, and increase in experience and knowledge, 45; development of medical transport system, 45; establishment of Army Medical Museum, 45; Gorgas's recruitment of physicians to serve in World War I, 228, 246, 247; high standards for medical education and skill, 44; increase in officers, nurses, hospital workers, and hospital beds during war, 264; permission for medical officers to pursue private practice, 44, 56; resentment of Gorgas within, 211–12, 313; segregation by race and sex through World War I, 247–49; white, male, and allopathic, 3, 246, 364n32. *See also* Army Medical Department; frontier medicine
Army Medical Department: barring of African American women from service as nurses, 72, 75; construction and supply of hospitals in occupied Philippines, Puerto Rico, and Cuba, 85; conversion of passenger ships into hospitals in Cuba, 69–70, 328n20; and eradication of *Stegomyia* in Panama, 147–54; failure to fully embrace female nursing until World War I, 157; *Medical and Surgical History of the War of the Rebellion*, 45, 288. *See also* Army Medical Department, and World War I
Army Medical Department, and World War I, 245–50; establishment of reconstructive medicine, 265–66; establishment of tuberculosis hospitals, 244; and Hospital Corps and Army Nurse Corps, 227; implementation of sanitation and preventive measures in camps, 244; lack of resources and authority to protect health of men in training camps, 245, 364n28; *The Medical Department in the World War*, 288; new responsibilities for gas masks and military psychiatry, 264–65; preparedness for, 220–21, 226, 227; screening of war recruits for health, 244; urgent need for doctors, 246
Army Medical Museum, 45
Army Nurse Corps, 249–50, 329n33
Army Reorganization Act of 1920, authorization of rank for army nurses, 366n53

Army School of Nursing, 249, 288
Arthur, Maj. William H., 77
Ashford, Bailey: at Army Medical School at Langres, 247; discovery of hookworm, 227
Association of Military Surgeons of the United States, 55
Atwater, Nicholas, 38, 41
Aviation Board of the Army Signal Corps, 228

Baker, Newton, Secretary of War, 216, 231–32, 237, 245, 256; and compulsory vaccination in army, 252; condolences to Marie upon death of William, 300; and defense of war mobilization at expense of Medical Corp, 260, 261–62; and Gorgas's "retired for age" trip, 276, 279–84; and Gorgas's successor as SG, 276; graveside eulogy for Gorgas, 303; laudatory letter to Gorgas, 287
Baldwin, Benjamin J., 38
Barquerizo, Alfredo, president-elect of Ecuador, 234–35
Barton, Clara, 71
Bayne, Ria (née Gayle), 22, 23
Bayne, Thomas L., 22, 24, 25, 29, 33, 39
Bayne-Jones, Stanhope, 190, 283
Beeks, Gertrude, 160
Bellevue Hospital Medical College, New York, 36–38; employment of women nurses, 71; Gorgas's acceptance at, 35; leader in medical science education, 36, 37; obstetrical service and requirement of sanitation practices, 38; one of first hospitals to have ambulance service, 37
beriberi, research on, 227
Beverly, Edward P., 130
Bingham, Hiram, 192
Birmingham, H. P., 237, 251
Bishop, Joseph Bucklin: Isthmian Canal Commission (ICC), 1909–1914, *183*; *The Panama Gateway*, 218; promotion of Goethals as master of the Panama Canal, 217–18, 358n37
Black, Col. William, 85, 122
Black workers, Panama Canal. *See* Panama Canal, US occupation, and Black workers
Bliss, Maj. Gen. Tasker, pallbearer for Gorgas, 303
Blue, Rupert: General Medical Board, Council of National Defense, *251*; and influenza pandemic of 1918, 279
Bogotá, Colombia, 235
Borden, Maj. William C., 114
Bovay, Harry, 142–43
Bowen, John, 38, 41
Bradley, H. C., AEF chief surgeon, 254
Braisted, William, General Medical Board, Council of National Defense, 251
breast cancer, early twentieth century: "Halsted Method" of breast cancer surgery, 134; little understanding of cause or treatment, 134, 341n28; Plates X and XI from Halsted's 1894 paper, *135*; question of removal of ovaries, 134, 136; radical and dangerous procedures, 136, 139, 342n38, 342n56; X-ray treatment, 136, 139
Bridgman, V. H., 46, 60–61
British Royal Medical Corps, liaison with Gorgas, 250–51, 283
British Royal Medical Society, 2, 298
Brooke, Maj. Gen. John R., 84
Bryan, William Jennings: *The Commoner*, 191, 202; *The Commonwealth*, 191; populism, 3; as secretary of state, 202, 205, 212, 213, 225; visit to Panama, 192
Bryce, James, 192
bubonic plague, spread by flea bites, 99
Buffalo Soldiers, Twenty-Fourth and Twenty-Fifth African American infantries, charge of San Juan heights, 69
Bunau-Varilla, Philippe, 118, 120–21, 191
Bushnell, George, 244, 247, 365n36

Calhoun, John C., 16
Camp Beauregard, Louisiana, 258
Camp Columbia, Havana, 85, 92, 93
Camp Devens, Massachusetts, 278
Camp Funston, Kansas, 258, 277
Camp Greene, North Carolina, 262
Camp Lazear, Havana, 102, 103
Camp Mills, Long Island, 259
Camp Sever, South Carolina, 258
Camp Thomas, Chickamauga, Georgia, and typhoid fever, 77
Camp Wheeler, Georgia, 258
Caracas, Venezuela, 237
Cárdenas, President Alejandro, 198
Caribbean: "conquest" of, by Spanish explorers largely through disease, 65, 66; first recorded cases of yellow fever from Spanish slave ships, 66; smallpox epidemic from 1518 to 1520, 65–66
Carr, Carrie Chapman, 291
Carroll, James: depiction in Cornwell's *Conquerors of Yellow Fever*, 1939, 6–7, *7*; and "filterable virus" as infecting agent, 103, 110; first experimental case of yellow fever observed to be caused by mosquito bite, 100–101, 117, 334n25; paper on yellow fever work at 1901 American Public Health Association annual conference, 109; and Reed Commission experiments on human volunteers, 4–5, 100–101; and US Army Yellow Fever Commission, *97*
Cartagena, Colombia, 235, 236
Carter, Henry Rose, 205; belief that yellow fever could be eradicated, 314; and conditions in Panama, 129, 150, 185; inspection of army grounds for malaria, 222; marine sanitation and quarantine operations in Panama, 125, 132, 137; Rockefeller Foundation Yellow Fever Commission members, c. 1916, *233*; theory of "extrinsic incubation," 99, 334n20; and theory of "key centers" or "seed-beds" of yellow fever, 231; trip to Ecuador with yellow fever commission, 1919, 291, 297; trip to South America with yellow fever commission, 232, 236
Carter, Laura, 150
Central America, yellow fever commission trip to, 1919, 295–96, 297
Chagas disease, 238
Chagres River, Panama, 164, 191
Chamberlain, George E., 260
chikungunya virus, and *Aedes aegypti* mosquito, 315
Chinese Exclusion Act, 161
City Insane Asylum, Blackwell's Island (now Roosevelt Island), 44
Civil War: as defining childhood experience for Gorgas, 15, 21–24; and increase in experience and knowledge of Army Medical Department, 45
Cole, Rufus, investigation of influenza of 1918, 277, 278
Coley fluid treatment, 136, 342n38
Colombia, Republic of: Gorgas's visit with Rockefeller Yellow Fever Commission, 235–36; Muzo mines, 235–36; Panamanian revolution against, 120, 197; Panama's merger with, 117; US military intervention in province of Panama between 1856 and 1903, 118
Colón, Panama, 120–21, 123, 130
Compromise of 1877, 35
Confederate Memorial in Arlington National Cemetery, 319n16
Connor, Dr. Michael E., 292, 293
Cornwell, Dean, *Conquerors of Yellow Fever*, 1939, 6–7, *7*, 313, 380n47
Council of National Defense, General Medical Board, 229, *251*, 251–52, 270
Crawford, Sarah (née Gayle), 17
Crawford, William Bones, 17, 18
Crile, Dr. George, 220; and Base Hospital #4, 242, 246
Crowder, Enoch, 49, 52, 325n8
Cuba, history: Afro-Cubans, 66; collapse of Amerindian population from disease

in early 1500s, 66; Creole (Cuban-born) landowners, and ten-year war, 66, 68; 1895 rebellion against Spain, 66; history of yellow fever, 66, 68, 69; world's largest sugar producer by mid-nineteenth century, 66
Cuba, US occupation government: army command removed from Havana, 85; cleanup of Havana, 1899, 84–86; and disbanding of Cuban insurgent military, 84; entrance into Spanish-American–Cuban War, 65–67; and Foraker Amendment, 83–84; and Platt Amendment, 110, 111; and Teller Amendment, 83. *See also* Havana, Cuba; yellow fever, Cuba
Cuban Republic, 110–11
Culebra Cut, Panama, 165, 167, 176, 191, 202
Cushing, Dr. Harvey, 220, 266, 270, 282, 301, 373n43; and Base Hospital #5, 242, 246

Daniels, Josephus, General Medical Board, Council of National Defense, *251*
Darling, Samuel, 192; Ancón Hospital medical staff, 1906, *156*; groundbreaking work on *Anopheles* mosquito, 170, 175; research on broad array of diseases, 174–75; trip to South Africa with Gorgas, 203, 207
Davis, Gen. George, governor of canal zone through ICC, 121, 131, 132, 151, 158, 159
Davis, Jefferson, 23, 27
Dean, William H., 101
Deeks, Dr. W. E., 156, 184
Delano, Jane, head of Red Cross nursing program, 250
De Lesseps, Ferdinand, 118
Denegre, Edith, 302
Denegre, George, 267, 370n73
Devol, C. L., 179
Dodge Commission, 79–80, 330n79
Donnelly, Florence O'Brien, 252
Doughty, Marie. *See* Gorgas, Marie (nèe Doughty) (wife of William)
Doughty, Martha "Mattie." *See* Lyster, Martha "Mattie" (née Doughty)
Doughty, Martha (mother of Marie), 49
Doughty, William (father of Marie), 49
Dyer, Leonidas, 270

Ecuador: offer to Gorgas to oversee sanitation work, 293; Rockefeller Foundation Yellow Fever Commission trips to, in 1919, 291–93, 294–95; Rockefeller Foundation Yellow Fever Commission trip to, in 1916, 234–35; sanitation visit and recommendations by Gorgas and team, 1912, 197–99
Ehrlich, Paul, 220

Farquhar Buzzard, Sir Edward, 299, 300
Federation of Women's Clubs, Panama, 160
Finlay, Dr. Carlos Juan: adviser on yellow fever to Army Medical Department, 69; death of, in 1915, 224, 360n76; education, 96, 98; gala and bronze statue to honor discovery, 103; Havana yellow fever board, 86, 102, 103; met with skepticism and ridicule as "mosquito man," 98; mosquito mitigation methods, 104; theory of *Aedes aegypti* mosquito as agent infecting people with yellow fever, 4, 7, 98, 333n11
Finsen, Niels, development of ultraviolet light treatment and receipt of Nobel Prize in Medicine, 342n38
Flexner, Simon: director of Rockefeller Institute for Medical Research, 230; wartime work for OTSG, 247
fomite theory: discredited by Reed Commission experiments, 103; and yellow fever transmission, 72
Foraker Amendment, 83–84
Fort Adams, Rhode Island, 54

Fort Barrancas, Pensacola Bay, Florida, 54
Fort Brown, Texas, and yellow fever, 45, 48, 49–50
Fort Clark, Texas, 45
Fort Duncan, Texas, 45
Fort Jay, Governors Island, 302
Fort Leavenworth, Kansas, 54
Fort McIntosh, Texas, 45
Fort Randall, Dakota Territory, 54–55
Fort Reno, Oklahoma Territory, 54
Fort Riley, Kansas, Medical Officers Training Camp 1917–1918 yearbook, dedication to Gorgas, 240
Forts, Gorgas assigned to from 1885 to 1894, 54
Fort Sill, Oklahoma Territory, 54, 326n43
Fort Snelling, Minnesota, 54
Fort Sumter, Battle of, 21–22
frontier medicine, 55–57
Furbush, C. L. (Charles Lincoln): as health officer of Panama City, 156–57; as office manager of OTSG under Gorgas, 213, 251, 266, 275; veteran of Spanish-American–Cuban War, 226; wartime trip to France with Gorgas, 280–85

Gaillard, David Dubose, 218; death from brain tumor, 203; engineer for Panama Canal, 167, 202; Isthmian Canal Commission (ICC), 1909–1914, *183*
Gaillard, Katherine, 202, 203, 309, 311
Garrison, Lindley, first secretary of war under Wilson, 203, 221, 225
Gayle, Clarissa (stepmother of Amelia), 16
Gayle, John (father of Amelia), 16, 319n2
Gayle, Mary. *See* Aiken, Mary (nèe Gayle)
Gayle, Matthew, 17, 22
Gayle, Ria. *See* Bayne, Ria (née Gayle)
Gayle, Richard, 22
Gayle, Sarah. *See* Crawford, Sarah (née Gayle)
Gayle, Sarah (mother of Amelia), 16
General Medical Board, Council of National Defense, 229, *251*, 251–52; proposed legislation to increase rank, pay, and benefits for medical officers, 270
George, Henry: *Progress and Poverty*, 215; and single-tax movement, 3, 51, 215
germ theory of medicine, 2, 34, 37, 40
Gibson, John M., *Physician to the World*, 4, 313, 341n16
Goethals, Effie Rodman, 178
Goethals, George Washington: books on Panama, 358n41; depiction of, by Marie Gorgas, 167–68; disparagement of Gorgas's work in Panama, 202; interference in mosquito control and increase in malaria cases in Panama, 179–80; Isthmian Canal Commission (ICC), 1909–1914, *183*; military discipline and strict chain of command, 165–67, 182; and Sanitation Department budget, 187–90; struggle with Gorgas over cutting grass, 178–80; versus Gorgas, 167, 176–78, 182, 187–90; writings by Bishop and others celebrating his role in the canal, 217–18
Gómez, Gen. Máximo, 69
Gompers, Samuel, 216, 243
Goodwin, Sir John: British Army Medical Services, 299; as British liaison to OTSG during war, 250–51, 283; and funeral party for Gorgas, 301; oversight of Gorgas's care in last weeks of life, 299
Gorgas, Aileen Lyster. *See* Wrightson, Aileen Lyster Gorgas
Gorgas, Amelia (née Gayle) (mother of William): allegiance to South and Confederacy, 16, 21, 26, 29, 90–91; baptism in St. Paul's Episcopal Church, Richmond, 23; daughter of former Alabama governor, 15, 16; death in 1913, 16, 199–201; and death of husband, 52; and education of William, 34; encouragement of William to marry,

53; and Marie (wife of William), 147; marriage to Josiah Gorgas, 1853, 18; nursing care in Confederate hospitals, 15, 22; portrait of, 1890, *200*, 354n26; post–Civil War flight to Maryland, 1865–1866, 26–27; post–Civil War support of family, 25; University of Alabama hospital matron, 15, 16; University of Alabama library named for, 201; University of Alabama library work, 191

Gorgas, Christine Amelia "Minnie" (sister of William), 18, 23, 31, 199–200, 300–301

Gorgas, Jessie (sister of William): William's correspondence with, 18, 22, 23, 31, 35, 42, 52, 53, 181, 190, 192, 201, 211, 222, 290; William's last letter to, 298

Gorgas, Josiah (father of William): allegiance to South, 21; appointment to West Point, 16; attempt to obtain nomination for William to West Point, 34; born to Pennsylvania farm family, 15, 19, 319n9; command of Mount Vernon Arsenal in 1853, 17; as department headmaster at University of the South, 30, 41; escape south after fall of Richmond, 24, 25; journal as instruction for children, 19, 20, 23; marriage to Amelia Gayle, 1853, 18; objections to army and medical career for William, 33, 34, 42, 44; ordnance officer for Confederate Army in Richmond and promotion to brigadier general, 16, 22, 23; portrait of, c. 1863, *17*; post at Frankford Arsenal in 1860, 20–21; post–Civil War business failures in South, 28–30; post–Civil War loss of health and family fortune, 25; as president of University of Alabama at Tuscaloosa, 41–42; stroke and death in 1883, 51–52, 323n36; stroke and paralysis in 1879, 42; survived yellow fever, 16; view of slavery, 19–20

Gorgas, Marie Bayne "Ria" (sister of William), 18, 22, 53, 141

Gorgas, Marie C., and Burton J. Hendrick, *William Crawford Gorgas, His Life and Works*, 4, 309–10, 336n59

Gorgas, Marie (nèe Doughty) (wife of William), 16, 19; admiration of Gorgas's skill and demeanor as doctor, 57; with Aileen, c. 1891, *58*; assistance to Gorgas in writing *Sanitation in Panama*, 218; birth of daughter in 1889, 57; courted by and marriage to William Gorgas, 51–54; death in 1929 and burial in Arlington National Cemetery, 310; depiction of Goethals, 167–68; description of Havana and study of Spanish, 82–83, 84, 85; development of yellow fever at Fort Brown, 49–50; on Gorgas's work in Panama, 131, 132; health issues and treatment for breast cancer, 57, 60, 124, 134, 136–39, 141; on husband's mosquito mitigation campaign, 105; life in Panama with William after surgeries, 90, 130, 147, 158, 159–61, 166, 178, 192; public profile, 224; receipt of government pension, 309; Red Cross work in wartime Washington, 267; return to New York with William's casket, 302; Rockefeller Foundation Yellow Fever Commission members, c. 1916, *233*; Spanish silver collection, 309, 379n28; trip to Ecuador with yellow fever commission, 1919, 291, 292, 293; trip to Egypt with Gorgas, 114–15; trip to South America with yellow fever commission, 232, 234–35, 236, 239; unhappiness with life on frontier army forts, 54–55; and William's last illness, 298–300; and William's return from Cuba with typhoid fever, 79. *See also* Gorgas, Marie C., and Burton J. Hendrick, *William Crawford Gorgas, His Life and Works*

Gorgas, Mary Gayle "Mamie" (sister of William), 16, 18, 19, 180, 191, 201, 203
Gorgas, Richard Haynesworth "Ritchie" or "Dick" (brother of William): correspondence with William, 18–19, 23, 45, 46–47, 114, 137, 141, 203, 295, 296; and William's funeral, 302, 303
Gorgas, William Crawford, early life and education: attendance at Munford Academy, Richmond, 22; birth in 1854, 2; boarding school in Alabama and Marshall School in New Orleans, 28–29; Civil War as defining childhood experience, 15, 21–24; color blindness, and inability to pursue laboratory science, 42, 44; efforts to obtain nomination to West Point, 34; enslaved boy as playmate, 19; law study in New Orleans with uncle, 33–34; medical education and internship at Bellevue Hospital Medical College, 33–34, 37–38, 39–41; medical education and internship at City Insane Asylum, Blackwell's Island, 44; moves with family to army posts in various states, 15, 20; post–Civil War life, 24–26; preparatory school and graduation from the University of the South, Sewanee, Tennessee, 30–32, 33; records of income and expenditures during medical education, 38–39
Gorgas, William Crawford, and Frontier Army Medical Corps: advice for brother Richard, 46–47; care for Marie's medical needs, 57; cities and towns lived in, and army installations assigned to, *43*, 44–45; commission as first lieutenant and assistant surgeon, 44; commitment to preventive medicine and sanitation, 3, 4; first physician at Fort Barrancas to conduct antiseptic surgery, 60; at Fort Barrancas, 60–62; at Fort Randall, Dakota Territory, 54; forts assigned to from 1885 to 1894, 54; and horse named Traveler, 54, 326n45; ledgers of medical work, 56; lifelong practice of sending money to parents, 44; noted for compassion, 46, 60–61; promotion to full colonel, and ensuing resentment of colleagues, 5; publication of first medical article and contributions of medical specimens to Army Medical Museum, 60; and qualifying examinations, 44; stricken with yellow fever at Fort Brown, and subsequent immunity, 3, 11, 48, 49; study with leaders in medicine and adoption of new surgical and treatment techniques, 55. *See also* frontier medicine; Gorgas, William Crawford, yellow fever work; Gorgas, William Crawford, yellow fever work, Havana
Gorgas, William Crawford, last illness, death, and funeral: burial with high military honors in Arlington Cemetery, 2, 303–4; death on July 3, 1920, 1, 2; decorated with Most Distinguished Order of St Michael and St George by King George V, 299; funeral, 302–4; gravestone inscription, 304; honored with funeral ceremony at St. Paul's Cathedral, 1, 301; repose in Church of the Epiphany, Washington, DC, 302; stroke on May 29, 1920, 298–99
Gorgas, William Crawford, overseas travels, 1898–1920: Brazil, 1916, 237–39, 297; Central America, 1919, 295–96; Colombia, 1919, 293–94; Colombia and Venezuela, 1916, 235–37; decision to accept position of Peru's director of sanitation, 296–97; Ecuador, 1912, 197–99, 354n18, 354n20; Ecuador, 1919, 291–93, 294–95; Ecuador and Peru, 1916, 234–35; Guatemala, 1918, 290; last trip, 297–301; map of, *196*; Peru, 1919, 291–93, 294–95, 296–97; Rhodesia, 206–7; Royal Society of Medicine and Royal College of

Physicians, London, 207–8, 356n71; South Africa, 1913–14, 203–7
Gorgas, William Crawford, personal life and interests: concern for Marie's health, 57, 60, 141; courtship of and marriage with Marie Doughty, 50–54; deep-sea fishing, 60; editing of father's multivolume diary, 191; health issues in 1915, 224; health issues in 1918, 267; horseback riding, walking and hiking, and canoeing, 190–92; library and reading interests, 191; marriage of Aileen, 201; monthly payments to sisters and granddaughter, 222–23; mother's death, 199–201, 354n25; net worth increase for 1910–1914, 222–23; plans to resign army commission to be with Marie, 134, 136, 137; political groups, 191; purchase of residential lots in Washington, DC, 203
Gorgas, William Crawford, and race, class, and nation, 91; admiration for Bryan's sympathy for "common people," 212; advancement of white American imperialism and dominance, 3, 183–84, 194, 219; anti-imperialism, 91; comparison of "industrial slavery" to chattel slavery, 217; "The Conquest of the Tropics for the White Race," 3, 183–84, 217; declined to work with Black officers, 75–76; display of Southern Cross of Honor on uniform, 91; linking of good sanitation with expansion of white civilization, 189; mourning for Lost Cause of the Confederacy, 3, 91; on poverty as single greatest cause of poor sanitation and health, 216–17; support for Henry George's single tax, 216, 243, 291; support for populism, 3; views softened by innate empathy over time, 212; white supremist views, 3, 76, 84, 161, 193–94
Gorgas, William Crawford, as surgeon general: appointment in 1914, 2, 206; articles between 1915 and 1916 on yellow fever and tropical sanitation, 229; assessment of his leadership of Medical Department, 288; as chair of Rockefeller Yellow Fever Commission, 1, 231; dispatch of ambulance units to Texas during Mexican insurgency, 226; division between war preparation and war against mosquitoes and yellow fever, 225, 229, 255; increase in support for pharmacy, dentistry, nursing, anesthesiology, and X-ray medicine, 213; promotion from brigadier to major general, 213; promotion from colonel to brigadier general, 206; trips to investigate suspected cases and conditions for diseases, 222; and typhus commission to Serbia, 221–22
Gorgas, William Crawford, and World War I: and advances in treatments of the wounded, 267; African American women nurses and Army Nurse Corps, 249–50; award of Distinguished Service Medal, 287; budget requests to Congress for Medical Department, 264–65; commission of African American physicians, 248; concern over surgical challenges caused by new war weapons, 227; dispatch of medico-military observers to Europe, 226; establishment of Army School of Nursing, 249, 288; and General Medical Board of the Council of National Defense, 251–52, 366n64; inspection tour to France, 279–85; management of chemical warfare and treatment of shell shock, 288; measles in training camps, and army rejection of medical recommendations, 257–59; medical preparedness for war in Europe, 213, 220–22; recommendations for housing of trainees, 245, 258, 364n28; and reconstructive medicine and rehabilitation, 265–66, 288; resegregation of

Medical Department hospital wards, 248; "retired for age," 275–85; "Sanitary Conditions at Army Camps" ("Gorgas Report"), 259–60; sexually transmitted disease among troops, speech on, 253; tensions between Medical Department and War Department during congressional investigations, 256–57, 260–64; tensions with AEF medical services, 254–55; tensions with General Staff over rank and promotion of medical officers, 268, 270–72, 276, 370n78; testimony to Congress, 227–29, 251, 361n9; use of national media to assure public of commitment to soldiers' health, 266–67; welcomed by troops in France, 284

Gorgas, William Crawford, yellow fever work: army expert on yellow fever in 1880s and 1890s, 2; belief that disease could be eradicated, 314; contracting of yellow fever at Fort Brown, and subsequent immunity, 3, 11, 49; management of outbreak at Fort Barrancas, 61–62; Paris public health conference adoption of his recommendations on yellow fever, 120; tracking of epidemic of 1878, 3, 11. *See also* yellow fever, story of

Gorgas, William Crawford, yellow fever and sanitation work, Panama, 2; approach to sanitation work through education, incentives, and penalties, 151, 153; battle with malaria and *Anopheles* mosquito, 168–75, 184; blame of Goethals for failure of ICC to rid zone of malaria, 179–80, 218; bureaucratic challenges, 129–33, 139–46, 176–80, 187–90; campaign for physician and sanitarian to be named to Panama Canal commission, 112, 113, 121; compassionate management of patients and staff, 157–58; distribution of monthly reports to health officials, scientists, and Congress, 189; employment of women nurses, 157; eradication of *Stegomyia* and control of yellow fever, 147–54; first case of yellow fever, 133; first trip to Panama, April 1904, 121–24; hiring of African American physicians to care for Black patients in segregated hospitals and clinics, 162; modernization of Panama medical system, 154–57; only senior official to *see* the Panama Canal from beginning to end, 182; open door policy for staff, 131; plans for Medical Department role in Panama Canal project, 118, 119–20, 123; president of clubs in Canal Zone and popularity as speaker, 160–61; recruitment of best medical professionals in US, 155–56; speaker at Pan-American Scientific Congress, Santiago, Chile, December 1908, 178, 349n50; struggle with Goethals over cutting grass, 178–80; struggle with Goethals over Sanitation Department budget, 187–90; success determined by choice of men and attitudes of staff toward his leadership, 130–31; survey of hospital expenses in major US cities in comparison with ICC costs, 188–89; trip to medical congress in Cairo, Egypt, and tour of Suez Canal, 114–15; visits from leading medical scientists and public health officials, 192

Gorgas, William Crawford, yellow fever work, Havana, 74, 89; appointment as chief sanitary officer of Havana, 89; appointment as chief surgeon of Havana, 86; care for persons infected by Reed Commission experiments, 101; in charge of yellow fever hospital at Siboney, 74–75; clearing of Havana of mosquitos and yellow fever in ninety days, 2, 5, 103–6; close relationship with Cuban physicians, 84; education of community about mosquito control,

104–5; establishment of first nurses' training school in Cuba, 77; experiments with Guiteras on yellow fever vaccine, 95, 108–9, 252; four steps for control of yellow fever, 11, 113, 340n7; on Havana yellow fever board, 86, 102, 103; hesitancy in accepting mosquitoes as only source of transmission, 106–8; lower death-rate of patients than army-wide rate, 74; monthly reports on falling rates of disease in Havana, 108; mosquito mitigation as scientific and public health endeavor, 104; paper on yellow fever work at 1901 American Public Health Association annual conference, 109; patient histories, 81, 87–88; promotion to full colonel for yellow fever work, 116–17; revision of yellow fever treatment protocols, 72–73; skepticism toward Finlay's mosquito theory, 98; statistical studies of Havana public health, 90; treatment of yellow fever patients from 1899 to 1901 at Las Animas hospital, 81, 86

Gorgas Medal, Medical Reserve Corp Association, 313, 380n45

Gorgas Science Foundation, 309, 379n22

Grant, Ulysses S., 24, 25, 29

Grayson, Rear Adm. Cary, 252, 273, 303

Grunsky, Carl E., 140

Guayaquil: high mortality rates for yellow fever and plague, 197; mosquito mitigation, 292; Rockefeller Yellow Fever Commission visits, 1916 and 1919, 234, 238, 291–92, 297; sanitation visit and recommendations by Gorgas and team, 1912, 197–99

Guiteras, Juan: adviser on yellow fever, Army Medical Department, 69; excluded from "Roll of Honor" of Reed Commission work, 5; experiments with Gorgas for yellow fever vaccine, 108–9, 252, 336n77; at Gorgas funeral, 301; Havana yellow fever board, 86, 102, 103; plan for trip to West Africa with Gorgas, 297; Rockefeller Foundation Yellow Fever Commission members, c. 1916, *233*; trip to South America with yellow fever commission, 232, 236

Gustamante, Tranquilina, 160, 208, 294

*Haemogogus* mosquito, transmittal of yellow fever, 314, 318n17

Haiti, Napoleonic troops devastated by yellow fever and other diseases, 66

Halsted, William, 38; "Halsted Method" of breast cancer surgery, 134, *135*

Harris, Seale, 212, 276

Hasson, Ester V., 70, 71

Havana, Cuba: Army Medical Department construction of Camp Columbia, 85; cleanup of, by American sanitary engineers, 1899, 1900, 84–86, 89–91; eradication of mosquitoes, 103–6; first Cuban nurses' training school, 88; immigrants from Spain and US in 1899 and 1900, 90; mosquito mitigation methods used in, 95, 103–6; yellow fever board, 86, 102, 103; yellow fever deaths, fall in numbers to zero in 1901, 105–6; yellow fever deaths between 1871 and 1900, 90; yellow fever in 1899 and 1900, 86–92, 101. *See also* yellow fever, Cuba

Havard, Valery, 78, 116

Hench, Philip: influenced by Kean's minimization of Gorgas's role in yellow fever work, 7, 313–14, 380n47; 1950 Nobel Prize for Physiology and Medicine, 313, 380n48. *See also* Philip Hench Walter Reed Collection, University of Virginia

Hendrick, Burton J., 4, 309

Henry George Lecture Association, 191, 216

Hibbard, Mary Eugenie, chief nurse for Panama hospital system, 125, 157

Hispaniola, collapse of Amerindian population from disease, 66
hookworm: discovery of, 227; and IHB drive to fight in American South, 230
humoral medical treatment: based upon Aristotelian and Galenic theory, 36; transformation of, to scientific method, 2, 37

immunization, US Army, opposition to, 252, 360n5. *See also* vaccine
Indian Wars, 35, 55
infant mortality: for Black babies in 1859, 319n8; high rates at turn of century, 36; for white babies in mid-nineteenth century, 319n8
influenza pandemic of 1918, 277–79, 372n13; alarming symptoms and high morbidity, 278–79; arrival in US, 278; cyanosis, 279; failure of modern science to contain, 286–87; Kean's record of cases in US and Europe, 285–86; reduction in life expectancy by twelve years in 1918, 279
Ireland, Merritte W.: criticism of Gorgas as Surgeon General, 241; pallbearer for Gorgas, 303; second-in-charge to AEF chief surgeon, 254–55; successor to Gorgas as surgeon general, 276, 279, 280, 281; veteran of Spanish-American–Cuban War, 226
Isthmian Canal Commission (ICC), 117; 1909–1914, *183*; abolishment of, and formation of Panama Canal agency, 213; Department of Sanitation public health policy as progressive, 162–63; employment of more than 50,000 people from more than one hundred countries, 161; failure to perceive importance of sanitary work and mosquito mitigation in Panama, 125, 132, 133, 341n16; hiring of American women workers, 160; memorial dedicated to those who died in construction of the canal, 187; new commission's approval of Department of Sanitation budget and salary increases, 146; payment system reinforcing racial stratification, 161–62; provision of accessible and affordable public medical care in Panama, 155; recruitment of foreign workers from Jamaica and Barbados, 161; Roosevelt's appointment of first members, 121

Jackson, Thomas "Stonewall," 23
*JAMA*: announcement of medical opportunities in Panama, 156; Gorgas's use of, to assure public of soldier's health, 266; and Panama as tourist destination, 192; praise for Gorgas's recruitment of physicians to medical service, 276; publication of Gorgas's monthly reports on yellow fever, 108; publication of Gorgas's reports and articles on sanitation in the tropics, 188, 189; public relations campaign for doctors to sign up for Medical Corp, 246; report on Gorgas's "Conquest of the Tropics" speech, 184; review of Gorgas's *Sanitation in Panama*, 219; support for Gorgas's proposals for military medical readiness, 228; support for modern sanitation measures in canal zone, 119
Jenner, Edward, 94, 108
Jim Crow laws: Panama Canal Zone, 161; US, and lynching of sixty-nine African Americans in 1909, 184
Johnson, Andrew, 25, 26–27, 29
Jones, Dr. Willis W., 184

Kavanaugh, Anne, 19
Kean, Cornelia, 317n11
Kean, Jefferson Randolph, 142; announcement that malaria, yellow fever, and filarial infection were transmitted by mosquitoes, 103; and care for Reed's widow and legacy, 114; contracting of

yellow fever in Havana, 96; criticism of Gorgas for promotions of medical staff, 268; criticism of Gorgas's lateness in embracing mosquito theory, 106; critique of Marie Gorgas biography of Gorgas, 310, 311–12; desire to succeed Gorgas as chief of sanitation in Panama, 163; first person to be awarded the Gorgas Medal, 313, 380n45; against Gorgas as surgeon general, 212; and Gorgas's struggle with ICC and Goethals, 142, 144, 146, 189; historical effacement of Gorgas's memory, 4–7, 289, 305, 311–12, 374n82; omission of Gorgas and Cuban scientists from Reed Commission "Roll of Honor," 5–6; orders to army camps for mosquito mitigation, 101–2, 103, 107; record of emergence of influenza among troops, 279, 285; resentment over publicity and favors received by Gorgas, 317n11; responsibility for historical inaccuracy of commissioned painting, *Conquerors of Yellow Fever*, *6*, 6–7; veteran of Spanish-American–Cuban War, 226

Keen, Dr. William: recruited by Gorgas for Medical Corps, 228, 247; surgeon for Marie, 136–37, 138–39, 180

Keogh, Alfred, 250, 251

Kiefer, Daniel, 240, 243

Kissinger, John, 102

Kligler, Israel, 291

Knopf, S. A., 313

Knox, Philander C., Secretary of State, 199

Koch, Robert, 37, 38, 220; germ theory of medicine, 37, 94; identification of tuberculosis "germ," 68

Ku Klux Klan, 29, 35

La Garde, Maj. Louis: in charge of Panama City hospital, 125, 137; in charge of Siboney Hospital and dedicated yellow fever hospital, 71, 72; development of yellow fever, 74; plans with Gorgas for Panama Canal work, 119–20; replaced as head of Ancón Hospital, 143; trip to Panama, April 1904, 122

Lambert, Alexander, 122, 140–41, 144, 192, 219, 247

Lampson, Robin: *Death Loses a Pair of Wings*, 312; "Memorandum from Robin Lampson," Hench Collection, 380n41

Lane, Franklin, 216

Las Animas hospital, Havana: Gorgas's treatment of yellow fever patients from 1899 to 1901, 81, 86–91; Las Animas ambulance, 87; low rate of patient loss to yellow fever, 89

Laveran, Alphonse: award of Nobel Prize in Medicine in 1907, 334n15; discovery of parasite in blood of malaria patients, 98

Lazear, Jesse: contract surgeon at hospital laboratory at Camp Columbia, 96; death of yellow fever, 94, 101, 334n28; depiction in Cornwell's *Conquerors of Yellow Fever*, 1939, 6–7, *7*; and Reed Commission experiments on human volunteers, 4–5, 100–101; study of malaria and mosquitos in Italy, 96; and US Army Yellow Fever Commission, *97*

Lazear, Mabel, 101

Lee, Robert E., 23, 25, 30, 377n78

Le Prince, Joseph, 119; with Ancón Hospital medical staff, *156*; chief sanitary inspector in charge of mosquito mitigation in Panama, 125, 133, 143, 148, 150–51; condolences upon death of Gorgas, 300; experiments on *Anopheles* mosquitoes, 171–73, 219, 348n30, 359n44; exploration of Panamanian jungle, 190; in Guayaquil, 198–99; inspection of US army grounds for malaria, 222; *Mosquito Control in Panama*, *149*; as expert on mosquito control, 170, 171

Le Prince, Julia, condolences upon death of Gorgas, 300
Lincoln, Abraham: assassination of, 25; election of, in 1860, 21; reelection in 1864, 23
Lister, Joseph, 37
Longstreet, Gen. James, 23
Longstreet, Helen, 23
Lost Cause of the Confederacy, 3, 30, 91, 191
Ludlow, General, military governor of Cuba, 87, 89
lynching, Reconstruction and Jim Crow era, 31, 184
Lyster, Aileen (niece of Marie), 48
Lyster, Lua (wife of Theodore), 48, 291, 292
Lyster, Martha "Mattie" (née Doughty), 49, 51, 53, 299
Lyster, Theodore, 116, 119; assigned by Gorgas to Aviation Board of the Army Signal Corps, 228–29; in charge of Siboney yellow fever hospital, 77; concerns about Gorgas's health, 180; contracting of typhoid fever and evacuation from Cuba on hospital ship *Missouri*, 78; joined Gorgas on *Relief* hospital ship to Cuba, 70; last letter to Marie and William, 299–300; leading ear, nose, and throat physician and pioneer in aviation medicine, 50; as medical officer in Panama, 125, 155; promotion to brigadier general by end of World War I, 247; sent by Gorgas to investigate health conditions in Vera Cruz, 215; surgery on patients in need of nose and throat work, Guayaquil, 292; treated by Gorgas for yellow fever at Fort Brown, 50, 70; trip to Ecuador and Peru with yellow fever commission, 1919, 291, 294; trip to South America with yellow fever commission, 232, 236
Lyster, William, 49, 50, 51, 53–54, 325n10
Maass, Clara, 109
MacMurray, Capt. Junius W., 61–62
Magoon, Charles E., 143, 146
malaria: battle in Panama Canal Zone, 168–75; chart showing reduction in number of ICC employees admitted to hospital for malaria by month as percentage of workforce, *175*; decrease in Havana after mosquito mitigation, 107; life cycle of malaria parasite *plasmodium*, *169*; in Muzo mines, Colombia, 236; research showing transmission of, through *Anopheles* mosquitos, 85; swamp draining against, 85
Manson, Patrick: discovery of cause of filariasis (elephantiasis), 98; "Father of Tropical Medicine," 192
March, Gen. Peyton C., 263, 268, 270, 271, 284, 303
Marine Hospital Service, lobbying for representative on Panama Canal project, 119
Marti, José, 216
Martin, Dr. Franklin: chair of General Medical Board, Council of National Defense, 229, *251*, 252; examination of housing plans for trainee camps, 245; on Gorgas's enthusiasm for epidemics in tropics, 255; on Gorgas's open-door policy as SG, 275; on Gorgas's retention as SG, 276–77; on Gorgas's style of command, 288; and Owen-Dyer Bill, 270, 271; review of Marie Gorgas's biography of William Gorgas, 310; survey of medical profession, 246
Mayo, Charles: and Gorgas's funeral, 301; visit to Gorgas on day before death, 300; wartime work for OTSG, 247
Mayo, William, wartime work for OTSG, 247
McCreery, Dr. George, 74–75, 78
McCulloch, Champ, 61
McKinley, William: appointment of John Brooke as military governor of Cuba,

84; and Dodge Commission, 79–80; investigation of sanitary conditions in Havana, 86
measles, in army training camps, 257–59
*Medical and Surgical History of the War of the Rebellion*, Army Medical Department, 45, 288
*Medical Department in the World War, The*, Army Medical Department, 288–89
medical practice and education: frontier medicine, 55–57; and high infant and child mortality rates and low life expectancy, 36–37; introduction of new technologies and epidemiological tracking of diseases, 37; reputation of, during nineteenth century and Civil War, 34, 36; transformation from practice based on humoral theory to practice grounded in scientific germ theory, 2, 36–37. *See also* Army Medical Corps; Army Medical Department, and World War I
Mercedes Hospital, Havana first nurses' training school in Cuba, 88
Meuse-Argonne, battle of, 281, 283
Mexican Civil War of 1914, 213; occupation of Vera Cruz by US Marines, 213–14
Mexico, as endemic center for yellow fever, 296
Miles, Gen. Nelson, 68
military psychiatry, new field of, 265
*Military Surgeon* (later *Military Medicine*), 55, 88, 256, 277, 310, 312, 326n50
Miraflores Hospital, Panama, 132–33
Moran, John, 103
mosquitoes: evolving resistance to pesticides, 315; more than one species able to transmit yellow fever, 314; ubiquity of, in Cuba during rainy season, 96. *See also Aedes aegypti* mosquito; *Anopheles* mosquito
mosquito mitigation: effectiveness of oil to destroy larvae, 104; Finlay's methods, adopted by Gorgas, 104; Gorgas's recommendations for, in Rhodesia, 206–7; ICC's failure to perceive importance of, 125, 132, 133, 341n16; Le Prince's mosquito mitigation in Panama, 125, 133, 143, 148, 150–51; methods used in Havana, 95, 103–6; as model for disease control in twentieth century, 11, 104, 318n25

National Board of Health (1879–1883), 40, 68
National Defense Act of 1916, 228–29, 268, 361n11
National Single Tax League, 243
Native American "Indian scouts," 45
Navy Bureau of Medicine, lobbying for representative on Panama Canal project, 119
New York Single Tax League, 216
*New York Times*: on the "Gorgas Report," 259, 260, 261; on Gorgas's "Conquest of Tropics" speech, 184; on Gorgas's popularity in Cuba, 113–14; inaccurate report of Gorgas's position in Serbia, 222; on the Owen-Dyer Bill," 271; on Panama as tourist destination, 192; publication of Kean's critique of Marie Gorgas's biography of William Gorgas, 3103; report of dysentery and malaria among troops in Cuba, 76; report of typhoid in army training camps in 1898, 77; report on yellow fever in Havana, 93; tracking of influenza deaths in military camps, 278
Nightingale, Florence, 37, 71
Noble, Ella, 297, 302
Noble, Robert: consideration as Gorgas's successor, 276; continuation to West Africa after service for Gorgas, 302; and death of Gorgas, 300; entrance to St. Paul's Cathedral with Marie, 301; and Gorgas's last trip, 297, 298;

investigation of health of soldiers in training camps, 255; South African trip with Gorgas, 203, 207; South American trip with Gorgas, 198; veteran of Spanish-American–Cuban War, 226
Noguchi, Hideyo, 296
Noland, Lloyd, 130, 131
Nott, Dr. Josiah Clark: "scientific" defense of slavery, 319n7; theory of mosquito transmission of yellow fever and malaria, 18
nurses, women: African American women barred by Army Medical Department from service as nurses, 72, 75; Army Nurse Corps as single-sex, white organization, 249; Army School of Nursing established in 1918, 249; Dodge Commission criticism of War Department for failure to recognize value of nurses, 80; enlisted in Army Medical Department during and after Spanish-American–Cuban War, 71–72; and establishment of first nurses' training school in Cuba, 77

Office of Surgeon General (OTSG): dossiers on Reed and Gorgas after promotions for work on yellow fever, 112; establishment of Research Division in Army Medical School, 247; support for Gorgas on Isthmian Canal Commission, 119; twenty-four divisions reporting to surgeon general as of June 1918, 246; and vaccination policy and sexually transmitted diseases among troops, 252; in wartime, 250–53. *See also* Gorgas, William Crawford, as surgeon general; Gorgas, William Crawford, and World War I
O'Reilly, Robert M., Surgeon General: appointment surgeon general, 113; dispatch of Gorgas to Egypt and Suez Canal, 114; objection to low salary for Gorgas in Panama, 124–25; recommendation that Gorgas be promoted to full Colonel, 116; and replacement of Gorgas's staff in Panama, 142; support for Gorgas as successor as Surgeon General, 163; support for Gorgas on Isthmian Canal Commission, 118; support for Gorgas struggle with ICC, 143, 144, 146
Osler, Dr. William, 2, 189, 204, 208, 226; *Principles and Practice of Medicine*, 4e, 113
Owen, Robert L., 270, 271, 276
Owen, William O., 270
Owen-Dyer Bill, 270, 271–72

Palma, Tomás Estrada, 113
Panama and canal, history of: American interest in, and Isthmian Canal Commission, 117, 118; De Lesseps' attempt to build canal, 118; French effort to build canal thwarted by yellow fever, 112, 130; Panamanian declaration of independence from Spain in 1821, 117; Panama Railroad Company construction of railroad across Isthmus, 117–18; Spanish transport of silver from Inca Empire across Isthmus, 117; US military intervention in Colombian province of Panama between 1856 and 1903, 118; US purchase of French holdings in Panama and lease for canal zone, 118; US treaty with Republic of Panama for canal, 120–21, 153
Panama Canal, US occupation: accidents and injuries, 186–87; Afro-Caribbean residents from Barbados and Jamaica, 130, 161; American Zone, 130; Culebra Cut, 165, 167, 176; Department of Sanitation medical staff, 155–56, *156*; domestic and social activities for white American families, 159–61; government medical aid and support for indigent and disabled workers, 187; new mosquito breeding grounds as result of

construction, 179; Panama medicine, 185–87; racial disparities in illnesses, 185–86; as tourist destination, 192; white supremacy and Jim Crow segregation, 161–63, 184. *See also* Gorgas, William Crawford, yellow fever and sanitation work, Panama; Isthmian Canal Commission (ICC); yellow fever, Panama
Panama Canal, US occupation, and Black Workers: Black physicians hired to care for Black patients in segregated hospitals, 162, 185; prevalence of pneumonia and malaria among West Indian workers due to poor living conditions, 180, 185–86; and racial stratification in payment system, 161–62, 184; subject to Jim Crow practices, 161–63
Panama Canal Act of 1912, 193, 213
Panama City, 123, 130
Panama Railroad Company, 117, 165, 213; *SS Allianca*, 122
Panama Women's Club, 178
Pardo y Barreda, José, President of Peru, 235
Pasteur, Louis, 37, 94, 108
pellagra, 244
Pershing, Gen. John: appointment of Ireland as chief medical officer for AEF, 276; condolences upon Gorgas's death, 300; pallbearer for Gorgas, 303; "punitive expedition" to Mexico against paramilitary action, 226; repeated requests for more soldiers, supplies, and weapons for AEF, 243, 246, 254–55, 259
Peterson, Maj. Matt R., 92
Peterson, Mrs. (wife of Matt R.), suicide, 92–93
Philip Hench Walter Reed Collection, University of Virginia, 313–14, 380n47
Phillips, Daisy, 302
Phillips, John L., 192, 208, 213, 224
*plasmodium*, malaria parasite, life cycle of, *169*
Platt Amendment, 110, 337n86
*Plessy v. Ferguson*, 161
pneumonia vaccine, 205
Polk, Frank, 33
Polk, William Mecklenburg: Gorgas's boyhood memory of, as his "ideal," 33; Gorgas's correspondence with, 242; Marie Gorgas's surgeon, 122, 134, 322n1
Porras, President of Panama, 294, 306
Post, Louis F., 358n26
Progressive movement, 212, 243
Prohibition, 244
Public Health Service (PHS): and influenza of 1918, 279, 287; quarantine protocol, Cuba, 90; quarantine protocol, Panama, 132; responsibility for health conditions around army training camps, 132; and yellow fever vaccine, 314
Puerto Rico, collapse of Amerindian population from disease, 66
Purnell, Dr. John, 107, 156

Queen Alexandra Military Hospital, London, 1, 299, 301, 376n45
quinine, therapeutic and preventive drug for malaria, 123, 171, 348n24
Quito, Ecuador, 198

radiation therapy, 1904, 136
Radical Republicans, 27, 29
railroads, lack of coordination during World War I, 254
Rand Mines of South Africa, 203
Rankin, Jeanette, 259
Reavis, Charles, 261
Reconstruction Era: and Compromise of 1877, 35; Gorgas's coming of age in, 26–32
Red Cross. *See* American Red Cross
Reed, Charles A. L., indictment of ICC management in Panama, 139–40, 141

Reed, Dr. Walter, 183, 333n1; appointment to typhoid board of 1898, 79, 96; colleague of Gorgas, 2; death in 1902, 5, 114; disparagement of Cuban doctors and Finlay, 106; experiments confirming theory of *Aedes aegypti* mosquito as transmitter of yellow fever, 4–5, 94; experiments discrediting fomite theory, 103; investigation of yellow fever in army laboratory in Washington DC, 96; and naming of new army hospital in Washington after, 5, 117; one of first instructors at Army Medical School, 96; paper on yellow fever work at 1901 American Public Health Association annual conference, 109; research effort to find yellow fever germ, 113; study of bacteriology at Johns Hopkins Hospital, 95–96; and US Army Yellow Fever Commission, *97*. *See also* Reed Commission

Reed Commission: consideration of all methods of yellow fever infection, including mosquitoes, 99; disproof of Sanarelli and Reed theories of yellow fever cause, 98; "The Etiology of Yellow Fever," 103; review of Finlay's experiments and testing of mosquito theory on human volunteers, 99–103, 333n1; simplified story of, 94. *See also* yellow fever, story of

Reed Commission "Roll of Honor," erasure of Gorgas and Cuban scientists from history of yellow fever eradication, 5–6

Reed Emilie (wife of Walter Reed), 114, 117

Rhodesia: affliction with malaria and "Blackwater Fever," 206; Gorgas's recommendations for mosquito mitigation and worker conditions, 206–7

Richard, Brig. Gen. Charles, 251, 278

RMS *Lusitania*, sinking of, 220, 225, 227

Robertson, Jim, 76, 78

Rockefeller, John D., 230, 239

Rockefeller Foundation: distinction between charity and philanthropy, 230, 234, 362n39; International Health Board (IHB), 230, 231, 239; 37 percent of disease budget devoted to yellow fever from 1914 to 1950, 380n50; and power of public health to connect nations, 239; pursuit of vaccine for yellow fever, 314; typhus commission to Serbia, 221–22, 360n69

Rockefeller Foundation Yellow Fever Commission: born in meeting between Rose and Gorgas, 230–31; investigative trip to South America, 1916, 232–39; members, c. 1916, *233*; trip to Central America, 1919, 295–96; trips to Ecuador, Colombia, and Peru, 1919, 291–95; trip to West Africa, 297, 302

Rockefeller Institute for Medical Research, 230

Röntgen, Wilhelm, 136, 220

Roosevelt, Edith, 158

Roosevelt, Theodore, 2; appointment of Isthmian Canal Commission (ICC), 121; appointment of new ICC in 1907 under Goethals' leadership, 165; call for preparedness for war, 225; directed support and resources for Gorgas in Panama, 144; dismissal of ICC and appointment of three-man body, 143; efforts to compete with world powers in Europe and Asia, 182–83; law authorizing canal with locks, 164; and segregation in Panama, 161; and Spanish-American–Cuban War, 76, 77; support for canal across Central America, 118, 120; support for Gorgas, 178; support for Panamanian revolution against Colombia, 120, 197; visit to Canal Zone in 1906, 158–59

Root, Elihu, Secretary of War, 2, 89, 110, 189; appointment of Gorgas to Pan-American Scientific Congress of 1908,

178; naming of O'Reilly as surgeon general, 113; recommendation for promotions of Reed and Gorgas, 112, 116; request of Gorgas to advise on cleaning up Guayaquil, 197
Rose, Wickliffe, 221, 230–31, 234, 237; "Yellow Fever: Feasibility of Its Eradication," 231
Ross, John R., 89, 121, 146, 206, 212; in charge of hospitals along Panama Canal route, 125; forced to leave Panama because of malaria, 136; interest in Panama Canal work, 119; trip to Panama, April 1904, 122; US Navy Surgeon and lifelong friend of Gorgas, 60
Ross, Ronald, 183, 189, 204; awarded Nobel Prize in Medicine in 1902, 192, 334n15; proof that *Anopheles* mosquitoes transmit malaria, 85, 98, 208; and quinine, 171
Rough Riders: charge of San Juan heights, 68; illness from dysentery and malaria in Cuba, 76; and Maj. Gen. Leonard Wood, 84
Rousseau, Harry H.: Isthmian Canal Commission (ICC), 1909–1914, *183*; military engineer on Panama Canal, 167

Salvarsan, 253
Sanarelli, Giuseppe: announcement of bacterium *Bacillus icteroides* as yellow fever germ, 95; Reed Commission disproof of theory, 98
Scott, Winfield, expedition to Vera Cruz during Mexican War, 16
*Scribner's Magazine*, articles by Bishop lionizing Goethals' role in the Canal, 217–18, 358n37
Selective Service, heath screening, and multiple health problems, 244
Semmelweis, Ignaz, 38
Serbia, typhus outbreak, 221, 360n69
sexually transmitted diseases, in military, 252–53
Shakespeare, E. O., 79
shell shock (Post-traumatic Stress Disorder), 251, 265, 288
Sherman, Gen. William Tecumseh, 46
Shonts, Theodore, 141, 143, 144
Sibert, William L.: *The Construction of the Panama Canal* (with John F. Stevens), 218, 358n41; engineer for locks and dams of canal, 167; on Gorgas's "polished pertinacity," 179; Isthmian Canal Commission (ICC), 1909–1914, 182, *183*
single tax movement, 215–16, 357n19, 358n26
*Single Tax Review*, 216
Sisters of Charity nurses, 157
smallpox: Caribbean epidemic from 1518 to 1520, 65–66; introduction of vaccine, 37, 94; vaccination against in Cuba, 84, 85, 86; vaccination against in Panama, 155; Washington's inoculation of Continental Army against, 252
South Africa: Gorgas's recommendations for miners' condition, 205; miners afflicted by pneumonia, meningitis, typhoid, and tuberculosis, 203, 205
South America, Rockefeller Foundation Yellow Fever Commission investigative trips, 232–39, 291–95, 296–97
Spanish-American–Cuban War: American occupation and governance of Cuba in 1899, 83; demonstration of value of hospital ships and women's nursing, 71, 80; and Dodge Commission, 79–80; and enlistment of women nurses in Army Medical Department, 71–72; entrance of United States, 65–67; and Theodore Roosevelt, 76, 77; Treaty of Paris, 80, 83; typhoid fever, 79. *See also* Gorgas, William Crawford, yellow fever work, Havana; yellow fever, Cuba
St. Dominique, Napoleonic troops decimated by yellow fever and other diseases, 66

St. Luke's Episcopal Church, Panama, 161
St. Mihiel, battle of, 281–82
*Stegomyia fasciata (Culex fasciatus). See Aedes aegypti* mosquito
Sternberg, George Miller, Surgeon General, 183; addition of Cuban scientists to Medical Department, 69; appointment of typhoid board to investigate propagation in training camps, 79; first bacteriology textbook published in the US, 68; focus in Cuba on typhoid, 85; modernization of Army Medical Department and Corps, 68; naming of *Bacillus X* as yellow fever germ, 95; promotion of Gorgas to major and second in command in Cuba, 70; and Reed Commission, 96; report to Dodge Commission on camp conditions during Spanish-American–Cuban War, 80; support for Reed Commission experiments on volunteers, 100; survival of yellow fever, 68; three unsuccessful commissions seeking yellow fever germ, 95; warnings of deadly disease in Cuba, 67, 68, 176
Sternberg, Martha, 68
Stevens, John, second chief engineer of Panama Canal, 143, 144, 162, 164–65, 218
Stimson, Harry L., 193
sylvan yellow fever, 314
syphilis: and Salvarsan, 253; and Wasserman blood test, 253

Taft, William Howard, as president, 189, 192, 198
Taft, William Howard, as secretary of war, 2; appointment of Gorgas as acting governor in Panama during ICC transition, 143; and investigation of Panama situation, 139, 140, 153; of Isthmian Canal Commission (ICC), 121; proposed salary for Gorgas in Panama, 124; and segregation in Panama, 161; support for Gorgas on Isthmian Canal Commission, 118; visit to Panama, 192
Teller Amendment, 83
Texas cattle fever, transmittal by ticks, 99
Thatcher, Maurice, Isthmian Canal Commission (ICC), 1909–1914, *183*, 218
Theiler, Max, 314
Thomas, May: attended funeral service for Gorgas and wrote poem for the occasion, 1, 301–2; loss of son to yellow fever and comfort from Gorgas, 1, 294, 301
Tillman, Benjamin, 266
Tivoli Hotel, Panama, 158, 167, 171, 192, 294
Torney, George H., Surgeon General, 70, 177, 179, 205
training camps, World War I: measles in training camps, and army rejection of medical recommendations, 257–59; OTSG implementation of sanitation and preventive measures in training camps, 244–45; Public Health Service (PHS) responsibility for health conditions around army training camps, 132; "Sanitary Conditions at Army Camps" (Gorgas Report), 259–60
Transvaal Chamber of Mines, South Africa, 203
Treaty of Paris, 80, 83
trench fever and trench foot, 227, 250
tuberculosis: among AEF troops, 244; among South African miners, 203, 205; Koch's identification of tuberculosis "germ," 68; single greatest cause of death in nineteenth-century US, 36
typhoid fever: appointment of typhoid board in 1898 to investigate causes of propagation in training camps, 79, 330n78; caused by *Salmonella typhi* bacteria, 77; outbreak in Serbia, 221, 360n69; transfer from US army training camps to Cuba, 77–79, 106

typhoid vaccine, 77–78, 226

ultraviolet light treatment, 136, 342n38
United Fruit Company, 165, 232
University of the South, Sewanee, Tennessee, 30, 193
US Army: capture of Guantánamo Bay, 68; compulsory typhoid vaccination in 1909, 226; congressional reforms to improve conditions, 55; Hospital Corps of male attendants, 71; and immunizations, 252; intervention in Colombian province of Panama between 1856 and 1903, 118; "non-effective rate" of units or camps, 154; racially segregated units, 75; troops sent to Cuba in June of 1898, 68; Yellow Fever Commission, 40, *97*. *See also* Army Medical Corps; Army Medical Department; Spanish-American–Cuban War
US Navy: defeat of Spanish fleet in Santiago harbor, 69; destruction of Spanish fleet in Philippines, 67; movement of ships into Havana harbor, 66–67
USS *Maine*, sinking of, in Havana harbor, 62, 65, 67, 81
USS *Relief*, hospital ship sent to Cuba, 69–72, *70*

vaccine: Gorgas's experiments with Guiteras on yellow fever vaccine, 95, 108–9, 252; smallpox, 37, 84, 85, 86, 94, 155; yellow fever, 9, 314. *See also* immunization, US Army, opposition to
Vaughan, Victor C., 228, 268; appointed to typhoid board to investigate disease in training camps, 79; blame for disease on poor trainee living conditions, 257–58; examination of housing plans for trainee camps, 245; General Medical Board, Council of National Defense, *251*; investigation of influenza of 1918, 277, 278; on measles-associated-pneumonia in training camps, 257; Medical Reserve Corps officer during World War I, 270; sanitary inspections of trainee camps, 258; stricken with yellow fever in Siboney, 73–74; wartime work for OTSG, 247

Walker, Adm. John G.: and first Isthmian Canal Commission (ICC), 118, 119, 121, 124; hostility to mosquito theory of disease transmission, 131, 133
Wallace, John, chief engineer of Panama Canal, 131, 143, 218, 343n82
Wallace, William L., 87–88
War Department: assignment of Gorgas to ICC, Panama, 124; creation of alleged "immune regiments" of Black and white soldiers from southern states, 75; creation of Chief Surgeon's Office to support AEF in France, 254; failure to fulfill Gorgas's recommendations for training camps for World War I recruits, 245, 364n28; failure to grant military rank or privileges to women nurses, 249, 366n53; inadequacy to manage modern army, 254, 255, 259–60; isolation camp for troops evacuated from Cuba on Montauk Point, Long Island, 76; resentment of Gorgas by senior officials, 288; tensions with Medical Department during congressional investigations, 256–57, 260–64; training camps to prepare recruits to join Allied forces, 244
War Risk Insurance Act, 265
Washington, Gen. George, inoculation of Continental Army against smallpox, 252
*Washington Post*, 108, 117, 271; report of Gorgas's death, 300
Wasserman blood test, 253
Welch, Dr. William Henry, 2, 156, 174, 189, 287; and besieged OTSG during war, 266; examination of housing plans for trainee camps, 245; and General

Medical Board, Council of National Defense, *251*, 252; instruction of Gorgas at Bellevue Hospital, 38, 42; investigation of influenza of 1918, 277, 278; medical advice to Roosevelt about transmission of yellow fever, 144; Medical Reserve Corps Officer during war, 270; president of Rockefeller Institute for Medical Research, 230; sanitary inspections of trainee camps, 258; visit to Panama to *see* Gorgas's sanitation program, 192; wartime work for OTSG, 247
Wellcome, Henry, 189, 192
West African workers, Panama Canal construction, and high rates of malaria, 180
Weyler, Valeriano ("Butcher Weyler"), 66–67
White, Maj. James R., petitions to Gorgas to appoint Black physicians to Medical Corp, 248
white supremacy, and medicine: African American women barred by Army Medical Department from service as nurses, 72, 75, 249–50; and American imperialists' desire to make tropics hospitable to white race, 182–85; segregation of African American physicians in Medical Corps, 247–48; War Department creation of alleged "immune regiments" of Black and white soldiers from southern states, 75. *See also* Gorgas, William Crawford, and race, class, and nation; Panama Canal, US occupation, and Black workers
Whitmore, Eugene, 232, 234, 235, 236
*William Crawford Gorgas, His Life and Works* (Marie Gorgas and Burton J. Hendrick), 4, 309–10, 336n59
Wilson, Woodrow: appointment of Goethals as first governor of Panama Canal Zone, 2; appointment of Gorgas as army surgeon general in 1914, 2, 206; appointment of single taxers to cabinet, 216, 358n26; election to presidency, 202; endorsement and signing of Owen-Dyer Bill, 271, 272; exhortation of soldiers to be "Fit to Fight," 253; and Gorgas's successor as SG, 276; imposition of national economic planning to gain control of war effort, 263; and inadequacy of War Department to manage modern army, 254, 255, 259–60; neutrality stance in war, 220, 222, 225; "punitive expedition" to Mexico, 226; reelection to presidency, 241; request for declaration of war against Germany, 242; signing of National Defense Act of 1916, 228–29
women, in Medical Department: "women war workers" to support hospitals as dieticians and therapists, 250 (*See also* African American women; nurses, women; women physicians)
women physicians: barred from serving in Medical Reserve Corps until 1918, 249; could not formally serve in army until World War II, 249; desire of almost one-third to serve in war, 248–49; women physicians admitted to Sanitary Corps and as civilian "contract surgeons" during World War I, 249
Wood, Maj. Gen. Leonard, military governor of Cuba, 189, 225; economic, social, and political reforms in Havana, 89; orders to begin yellow fever eradication, 103; orders to Gorgas to continue investigations of yellow fever and mosquitos, 111; pallbearer for Gorgas, 303; public health measures, 84, 85; and special commission on yellow fever, 92, 96; support for Cuban independence, 110; support for Gorgas on Isthmian Canal Commission, 118
World War I: American military mobilization slowed by weak central government, 242–43, 259–60; armistice, 287; breakout in Europe, 215; congressional

hearings on inadequacies of Wilson's war mobilization, 259–60; Meuse-Argonne, battle of, 281, 283; shell shock (now Post-traumatic Stress Disorder), 251, 265, 288; St. Mihiel, battle of, 281–82; surgical challenges from new weaponry, 227; trench fever and trench foot, 227, 250; US declaration of war, April 1917, 221; Verdun and the Somme, 241; Zimmerman Telegram, 242. *See also* Gorgas, William Crawford, and World War I
World War I, US Mobilization: congressional granting of new executive powers to Wilson, 263; congressional hearings on inadequacies of Wilson's war mobilization, 259–60; and "Gorgas Report" on sanitary conditions at army camps, 259–60; hindered by weak central government and patchwork of institutions, 242–43, 259–60; military draft, 243; 4.8 million men in American armed services, 243; and Public Health Service, 243; Red Cross, 243; training camps, 243–45; voluntary organizations, 243; War Risk Insurance Act, 265. *See also* American Expeditionary Forces in France (AEF); Wilson, Woodrow
Wrightson, Aileen Lyster Gorgas (daughter of William and Marie), 296; birth of, 57; boarding school in New York, 80, 90, 136; donation of parents' papers to University of Alabama, 159; enroute to Peru at time of father's funeral, 302; marriage to William Daugherty Wrightson, 201; in Washington, DC, 267
Wrightson, Marie (daughter of William and Aileen), 211, 224
Wrightson, Pricilla (daughter of William and Aileen), 224
Wrightson, William Daugherty, 201; promotion to lieutenant colonel by end of World War I, 247; sent by Gorgas to investigate health conditions in Vera Cruz, 215; trips to Ecuador and Peru with yellow fever commission, 1919, 291, 292, 294; trip to South America with yellow fever commission, 232, 234, 235, 236
Wyeth Laboratories, and Gorgas Medal, 313

yellow fever: absence of, in Asia, 10; also known as "Yellow Jack," 54, 144, 318n18; caused by RNA *Flavivirus*, 8; discovery that more than one mosquito species could transmit yellow fever, 314; 1878 epidemic, 39–41, 68; epidemics in American history, 10–11, 17; first confirmed outbreak in North America, 10; first recorded outbreak in Western Hemisphere in Yucatán of Mexico, 10; at Fort Barrancas, Pensacola, Bay, Florida, 61–62; at Fort Brown, Texas, 48, 49–50; high mortality rate and frightening symptoms, 8–9, 40; historically confined to Africa and South America, 10; history of, in Cuba, 66, 68, 69; origin of, 9–10; prevailing theory in 1898 of spread by filth and fomites, 72, 95; prevention by vaccine but no effective treatments, 9, 314–15; sylvan yellow fever, 314; and theory of "key centers" or "seed-beds" of, 231; transmitted by bites of female *Aedes aegypti* mosquitos, 2, 8, 98, 169; transmitted by *Haemogogus* mosquito, 314, 318n17. *See also* yellow fever, story of
yellow fever, Cuba: cases in Havana, 1899 and 1900, 86–92, 101; deaths from in Havana between 1871 and 1900, 90; epidemic rates in ten years of rebellion against Spanish, 39; history of beginning with epidemic of 1648, 68; leading cause of death during

Spanish-American–Cuban War, 72; prevailing theory in 1898 of spread by filth and fomites, 72, 95; Sternberg's warnings of deadly disease in Cuba, 67, 68; yellow fever patients in hospital at Siboney, Cuba, July 1898, 72, *73*. *See also* Gorgas, William Crawford, yellow fever work, Havana; Havana, Cuba; Reed Commission; yellow fever, story of

yellow fever, Panama: eradication of *Stegomyia*, 147–54; fumigation brigades against yellow fever mosquitoes in Panama, *150*; Gorgas's battle with malaria and *Anopheles* mosquito, 168–75; Le Prince's experiments on *Anopheles* mosquitoes, 171–73; Le Prince's mosquito mitigation in, 125, 133, 143, 148, 150–51; plates of water to prevent leaf-cutter ant infestations in gardens, as habitat for mosquito breeding, *149*; yellow fever carried on ship to Colón, 137–38, 141, 143–44

yellow fever, story of: believed to be transmitted by fomites, 72, 95; and deaths of volunteers from experiments, 94, 333n1; Gorgas's effort to develop a yellow fever vaccine, 95, 108–9, 252; Gorgas's 1901 mitigation efforts in Havana, 95, 103–6; international search for causative agent or "germ," 95–96; Reed Commission demonstration that fever was caused by "filterable virus" rather than by bacteria, 95, 98, 110; Reed Commission experiments proving mosquito theory and disproving fomite theory, 95, 99–103

Zika virus, and *Aedes aegypti* mosquito, 315